MILK
OF
PARADISE

Also by Lucy Inglis

Georgian London

MILK
OF
PARADISE

A History of Opium

LUCY INGLIS

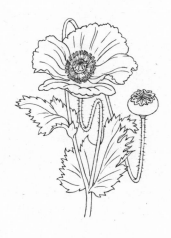

MACMILLAN

First published 2018 by Macmillan
an imprint of Pan Macmillan
20 New Wharf Road, London N1 9RR
Associated companies throughout the world
www.panmacmillan.com

ISBN 978-1-4472-8576-2 HB
ISBN 978-1-4472-8577-9 TPB

1 3 5 7 9 8 6 4 2

A CIP catalogue record for this book is available from the British Library.

Illustrations by Hemesh Alles
Map artwork by ML Design
Typeset by Palimpsest Book Production Ltd, Falkirk, Stirlingshire
Printed and bound by CPI Group (UK) Ltd, Croydon, CR0 4YY

To the memory of my father,
and his indefatigable curiosity.

And his delight in reading the closest thing to hand,
whether that was his trigonometry, cereal boxes,
the telephone book or the old newspapers when he should
have been lighting the fire. But never this book.

CONTENTS

LIST OF ILLUSTRATIONS

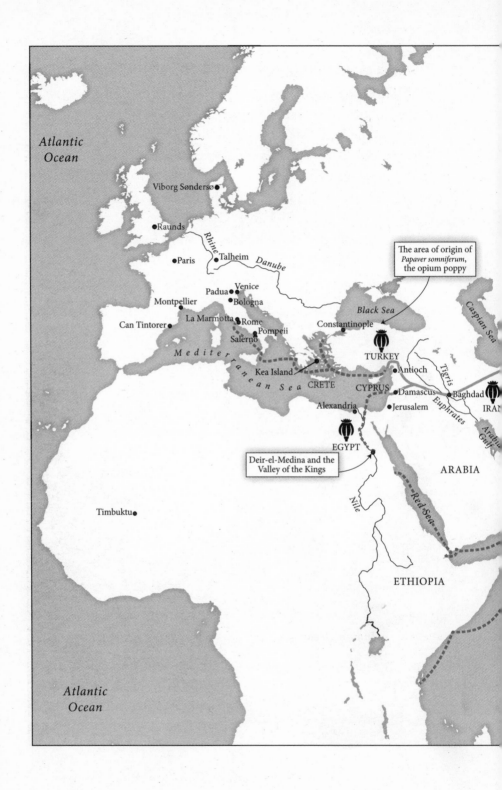

Atlantic
Ocean

Viborg Søndersø●

●Raunds

Rhine

●Talheim   *Danube*

●Paris

Venice
Padua●●
Montpellier●   ●Bologna
Can Tintorer●   La Marmotta●●Rome
●Salerno   ●Pompeii

Black Sea

Caspian Sea

Constantinople●

The area of origin of
Papaver somniferum,
the opium poppy

TURKEY

M e d i t e r r a n e a n   S e a
Kea Island●
CRETE
CYPRUS

●Antioch

Tigris

Damascus●   ●Baghdad
Alexandria●   ●Jerusalem   *Euphrates*

IRAN

EGYPT

Arabian Gulf

Deir-el-Medina and the
Valley of the Kings

ARABIA

Nile

Red Sea

Timbuktu●

ETHIOPIA

Atlantic
Ocean

Opium and the Ancient World

- Opium-growing regions
- Silk Roads
- Maritime Silk Roads

Aral
Sea

BADAKHSHAN   Kashgar   Taklamakan
                                   Desert

Yellow
River

AFGHANISTAN   Indus

CHINA   Xian

PAKISTAN

Ganges

Yangtze

Arabian
Sea

INDIA

Guangzhou

Bay of
Bengal

South
China
Sea

Mekong

Muziris

Indian Ocean

0	500	1000	1500	2000 miles
0	1000	2000		3000 kilometres

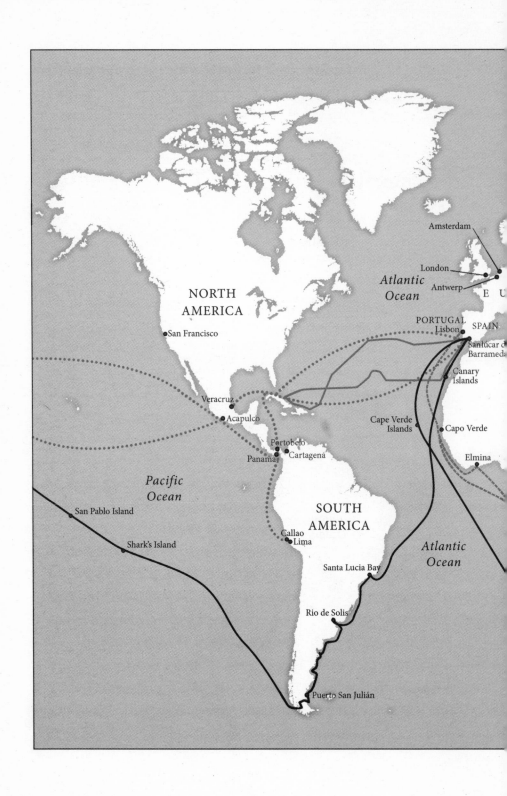

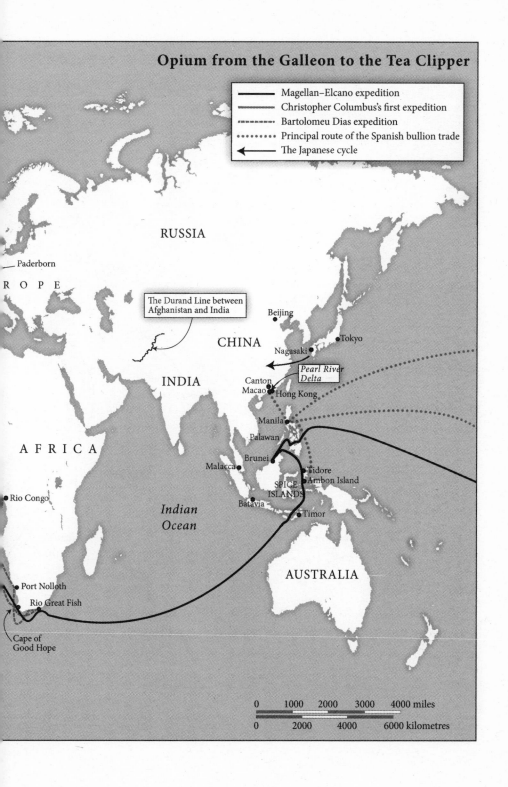

Opium from the Galleon to the Tea Clipper

Legend:
— Magellan–Elcano expedition
— Christopher Columbus's first expedition
---- Bartolomeu Dias expedition
···· Principal route of the Spanish bullion trade
← The Japanese cycle

RUSSIA

— Paderborn

ROPE

The Durand Line between Afghanistan and India

Beijing

CHINA

Tokyo

Nagasaki

INDIA

Canton
Macao
Hong Kong

Pearl River Delta

Manila

Palawan

AFRICA

Brunei

Malacca

Tidore
Ambon Island

SPICE ISLANDS

Batavia

Rio Congo

Indian Ocean

Timor

Port Nolloth

Rio Great Fish

AUSTRALIA

Cape of Good Hope

0	1000	2000	3000	4000 miles
0	2000	4000		6000 kilometres

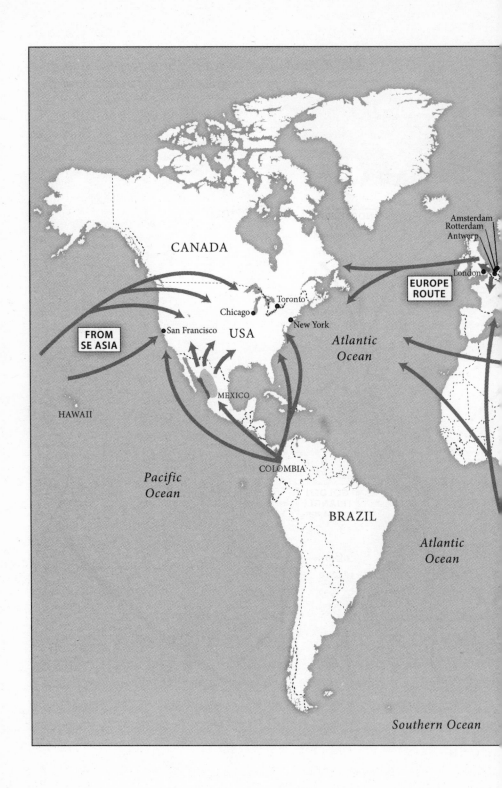

CANADA

Amsterdam
Rotterdam
Antwerp

London

EUROPE
ROUTE

Toronto

Chicago

New York

FROM
SE ASIA

San Francisco

USA

Atlantic
Ocean

MEXICO

HAWAII

COLOMBIA

Pacific
Ocean

BRAZIL

Atlantic
Ocean

Southern Ocean

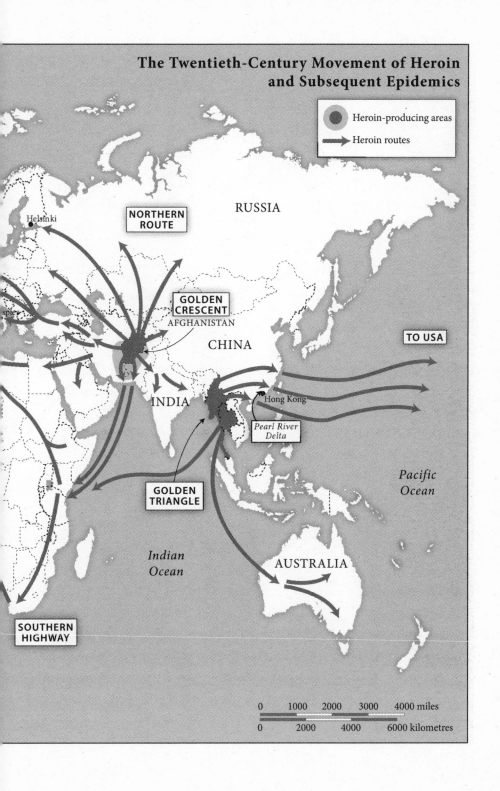

The Twentieth-Century Movement of Heroin and Subsequent Epidemics

Legend:
- Heroin-producing areas
- Heroin routes

RUSSIA

Helsinki

NORTHERN ROUTE

GOLDEN CRESCENT
AFGHANISTAN

CHINA

TO USA

INDIA

Hong Kong

Pearl River Delta

GOLDEN TRIANGLE

Pacific Ocean

Indian Ocean

AUSTRALIA

SOUTHERN HIGHWAY

0	1000	2000	3000	4000 miles

0	2000	4000	6000 kilometres

INTRODUCTION

'The only thing that is good is poppies. They are gold.'[1]

In mankind's search for temporary oblivion, opiates possess a special allure. For a short time, there is neither pain, nor fear of pain. Since Neolithic times, opium has made life seem if not perfect, then tolerable, for millions. However unlikely it seems at this moment, many of us will end our lives dependent upon it.

Indefensible but as yet indispensable, the opium poppy, and now its chemical mimics, endure and multiply. They cross continents, religions, cultures, languages and time. *Milk of Paradise* attempts to address this long history and the current, often galling compromises to be made as the world moves towards a model that is based increasingly upon the control of natural resources and expanding alternative economies. It is a journey from the ancient world to present-day America, along routes of legal and illegal commerce that belt the globe.

This book charts the evolution of one drug, although others feature in cameo roles. It seeks to provide a non-partisan view of this remarkable substance, and to dispel at least some of the myths surrounding opiates and the uses we put them to, and why. It began, in part, in London's Farringdon Station, in 2002, when I was forced by necessity to avail myself of the desperately squalid public convenience there at the time. As a child of the Reagans' 'Just Say No' campaign, the filthy, fluorescent-lit and heavily graffitied single cubicle was the stuff of bad dreams, only to be used in a dire emergency. By the sink, staring into the mirror, was a grubby young woman in baggy clothing who, startled by my urgent entrance, dropped what she was holding into the sink with a clatter. The obligatory tiny wrapped parcel, the spoon and syringe were there, and also a rubber band. 'I'm sorry,' she said immediately, flustered, and began to gather up her precious stuff. Pushing past me, out into what was not the gleaming commuter hub visible today, but at the time a grim focus for central London's flotsam of homeless and addicts, she apologized again. It wasn't me she was apologizing to.

Since that encounter, I have witnessed and experienced diamorphine used in medical surroundings, where everything is clean and warm, and I trusted those administering the drug. As a carer for dying family members, I have juggled my charges' morphine doses, wondering whether five milligrams more will mean we can just make it home, or through the night without incident, and drunk liquid morphine to prove that 'Come on, it's really not that bitter.' It really is that bitter. I have also watched as diamorphine induced respiratory failure in those people, over a period of hours and days, as their lives came to an end as peacefully as possible. And I have been impossibly grateful for a drug that allowed them to continue to live well, even as they were in the process of dying.

The research this book has entailed, although set in motion by personal experience and a cursed curiosity, has been both desk- and field-based. The former attempts, in the main, to reduce opiates, and now opioids, to a numbers game: kilograms seized, hectares burned, numbers arrested. The latter contains the human stories of addiction and recovery, of war, and treatment from both ends of the doctor–patient spectrum, but above all, the existential needs that drive humanity to seek the temporary relief opiates provide. It has been a transformative experience: exposing me to the reality of a global economy I had only a vague notion of before, and a redrawing of the world map not only in terms of borders, but a lack of them. Organized crime, in its purest form, is simply another economy, borderless and amoral. The importance of personal relationships and credit lines are not only mechanisms in the legal economy, they are equally if not much more powerful in illegal economies. These networks operate increasingly on efficient corporate models of collaboration and middle management. Notions of what is transgressive, illicit and ultimately illegal have changed dramatically over time, and continue to change as the world's governments and drug-enforcement agencies fight turf battles in an international war.

Milk of Paradise is divided into three parts: the stories of opium, morphine and heroin. Part One is a history of the opium poppy, its earliest relationships with mankind, and its transformation into one of the first commodities traded between the West and the East. Part Two concerns the isolation of morphine from opium, and the revolutionary scientific and political changes, as well as chemical discoveries that transformed the West in the nineteenth century, and set us on a course that, as it accelerated, changed the face of the world, from Tombstone, Arizona to the Durand Line dividing Afghanistan and Pakistan. The third and final part covers the twentieth and early twenty-first centuries, from the first years of commercially available heroin, the associated growth of Big Pharma and the present-day US opioid crisis, and charts the successive global wars on and involving drugs, as well as treatment, prohibition and attempts at the suppression of the trade in heroin and its derivatives. Because of the major roles they have played in the establishment and continuation of the opiate trade, the book focusses mainly on Britain, Europe and America.

Ultimately, *Milk of Paradise* is a tale of the many interwoven human stories that make up the history of our relationship with this fascinating compound. Taken together, they show us how opium has developed and how it will go forward. Historically, it is central to the advances in modern medicine, and the Eastern Triangular Trade, along with tea and bullion. The Opium Wars in the middle of the nineteenth century helped lay the foundations of Hong Kong, and of modern China. The drug has played a key role in conflicts from the American Civil War, to Vietnam and to Afghanistan, where Camp Bastion was a pioneering field hospital in the middle of the world's largest illicit poppy plantations. Scientifically, opium and its many derivatives lie at the heart of the surgical and pharmaceutical industries. Socially, the drug is both a tremendous force for good and an indescribable evil. It gives comfort to millions daily as part of a lucrative healthcare system, yet it creates addictions that fuel the worst kinds of degradation and exploitation, and plays a major role in all layers of worldwide crime. Our relationship with opium is a deep-seated part of our human history, and a critical part of our future.

Therefore, perhaps it is fitting that I write this introduction in Fort Cochin, an old colonial outpost on the Malabar Coast of southern India, which was once a great trading port with ties as far away as Mexico. An even greater one, Muziris, dominated by Jewish, Arab and Chinese traders and lost since 1346, has just been rediscovered by archaeologists some twenty miles up the coast. Once one of the world's greatest hubs for exotic goods and spices, the only map of Muziris – if it can be called a map at all – is a copy of one that may be as early as the fourth century AD, which resides in a museum in Vienna and which is itself a copy of a first-century BC map by Agrippa.

European and Middle Eastern travellers have been borne to this coast for millennia, albeit now by Boeing rather than across the ocean by the monsoon winds. Fort Cochin is a romantic place, at once familiar and exotic. Every few minutes the precarious passenger ferry spears up to the wharf and tips out a hundred or so commuters and a dozen auto-rickshaws from the mainland. People rush to go about their business against the backdrop of the huge, cantilevered fishing nets, introduced to this spot by Chinese traders in the fourteenth century. On a new, half-built rubble quay, day-labourers sit and drink whisky. Others sleep nearby, despite or perhaps because of the early hour. Cochin is like any large port: an amalgam of those it trades with, and Cochin has been trading for centuries. European influences, namely Portuguese, Dutch and British, are everywhere, from the tomb of legendary navigator Vasco da Gama and the church that houses it, just visible from my vantage point, to the quasi-British lanes of houses behind. A mosque and a synagogue – where a gravestone dating from 1268 bears the inscription 'Here Lies Sarah' – sit only a short walk apart. One Dutch writer of the 1660s recorded how the inhabitants of the coast lived well, eating from coconut cups, drinking coconut toddy, the soldiers eating opium for strength, which the Dutch, of course, attempted to ban. Later, from a dusty pavement, I will stop and stand outside the wall of a school and hear the girls singing 'Auld Lang Syne' over the noise as they clear their steel thali plates away from lunch. A few minutes after that, I ask at the government, female-run pharmacy for a legally contentious cough medicine I know contains morphine, and some codeine pills. The neat, stern pharmacist will tut at me, and then point to another pharmacy across the road, where men sit outside, and what I ask for is readily available, for the equivalent of around £1.80. The elderly man next to me has enough coins for a strip of generic beta-blockers and two blue low-dose morphine pills, which he dry-swallows immediately. Just down the road, the government beer and wine shop is doing a roaring trade, even as this part of India edges towards alcohol prohibition.

But for now, I look out towards the vast new port under construction on the other side of the river: Vallarpadam. Financed from over 1,700 miles away by the royal family of Dubai, it will be the largest-capacity container port in the world when the third phase of construction is complete. Unable to resist, I begin to scribble down rough, outrageous estimates of the amount of heroin that will pass through the port annually, based on comparable and laughably inadequate figures from Rotterdam. Thousands and thousands of kilos, billions of dollars, figures so large that zeros become redundant. In illegal opiates alone, Vallarpadam will be a city state to rival fifteenth-century Venice. As I write, the labourers continue to drink and sleep, and the passenger ferry arrives again with its cargo of office workers, housewives and hawkers. Behind it, colossal vessels come and go, fore and aft declaring their various origins across the world; but as Thomas Jefferson observed, 'Merchants know no country'.

Fort Cochin, February 2017

PART ONE

Ópion, afyūn, opium

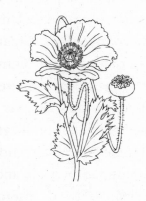

Chapter One

THE ANCIENT WORLD

Origins

There is no such thing as a wild opium poppy.[1] Its ancestor originated on the Anatolian coast of the Black Sea and no longer exists.[2] *Papaver somniferum* is a domesticated species and, along with coca, tobacco and the earliest wheat and barley cultivars, represents one of mankind's earliest attempts at genetic engineering, over 5,000 years ago.[3]

The origins of *Papaver somniferum* are elusive, and opinion remains divided on whether cultivation of the opium poppy began in the western Mediterranean, or in the Near East. Botanists and biogeographers believe the closest existing relative to the opium poppy is the wild, dwarf variety *Papaver setigerum*, widespread in the western Mediterranean for millennia.[4] The wild poppy, however, although it does contain small amounts of alkaloids in the latex (the milky liquid contained inside the head), does not contain them in sufficient levels to be of any medicinal or recreational use. Taxonomists around the world even vary on how many poppy species exist, identifying between 250 and 470.[5] In lieu of concrete evidence, all that remains is to trace botanical and archaeological clues to the use of the opium poppy through the ancient world.

3

Somewhere between 10,000 and 12,000 years ago, prehistoric man started to move away from the nomadic hunter-gatherer lifestyle of the past, towards a more settled culture. People began living in villages, domesticating plants and animals, and building social structures and religious models that are the foundations of the societies we live in today. The earliest known of these Neo-lithic sites lie between Greece and Iran, and stretch to the Black Sea in the north and the Sinai peninsula in the south.[6] A crescent of fortuitous agricultural conditions existed in Egypt, spreading east through modern Israel, Jordan, Lebanon and Syria, then down through southern Iraq to the Persian Gulf. On ancient maps these were Egypt, the Levant and Mesopotamia. This area had long been the meeting point of two different societies: the mountain people of the north, and the nomadic tribes who wandered the grasslands in shifting patterns of cultivation. Within both societies were many different tribes, making war and unrest a constant cycle.

This Fertile Crescent is often also called the Cradle of Civilization, referring to the development of the first cities, writing, and the study of history, trade, science and organized religion. It is an area of tremendous importance to the history of the modern human race.

The Natufians of the Levant were among the first settled people. Tell Abu Hureyra, their earliest known village, lies in Syria, where an abundant crop of wild cereals was turned into a farmed one perhaps as far back as 13,000 years ago. The site was excavated extensively, if rapidly, in 1972–3, before it was flooded to create Lake Assad. The Natufian community grew from a few hundred people hunting gazelle and foraging for food, into a large village of perhaps 2,000 individuals who kept sheep as well as cultivating the land.[7] They were not only coalescing into structured communities, but they were also forming relationships with the world around them: one of the earliest discoveries relating to human domestication of dogs was found at Ain Mallaha in Israel, sixteen miles north of the Sea of Galilee, where around 12,000 years ago an elderly human was buried with a puppy.[8] Modern man was becoming someone we could recognize today.

Although the Natufians are key to global agricultural history, there is no evidence that they were poppy farmers. They grew primarily first-wave Fertile Crescent crops, such as emmer and einkorn wheats, peas, lentils, chickpeas, bitter vetch and flax. The first evidence of human settlement coinciding with the poppy is that found at the early Neolithic site of Netiv Hagdud in the Jordan Valley, where plant remains have been carbon-dated to between 8,000 and 10,000 years ago, and include those of *Glacium flavum*, the horned poppy.[9] This variety of the *papaver* family is now widely regarded as highly poisonous, but it does contain glaucine, which like the opium poppy will relieve pain and suppress the respiratory system, and so help to alleviate persistent coughing. It also has the distinctive opiate side effect of causing agonizing stomach cramps in those unaccustomed to it, effectively preventing early humans overdosing as they conducted experiments on the flora around them. Glaucine is still used in some cough medications, and occasionally for doping canine competitors on the United Kingdom greyhound-racing circuit.[10]

Outside the Fertile Crescent, Neolithic settlements began to spring up around the world at broadly the same time, and they were first seen in Europe along the basin of the Danube River around 7,500 years ago. Villages were also appearing in Spain and south-western France. It is from Spain that the earliest evidence of the consumption of the opium poppy for narcotic or analgesic purposes is recorded, in a burial in the Can Tintorer mining complex of Gavà, near Barcelona. Can Tintorer was mined by these early people for callainite, a green mineral they used to make jewellery, and when the deposits played out, the mines were used for burials. A man was interred in Mine 28 with a poppy capsule stuck in his bad teeth, and his bones contained evidence of long-term opium consumption.[11]

The Neolithic people spread rapidly into what are now northern France and Belgium, and the Ukraine. The Ice Age had ended, the retreating ice leaving navigable rivers full of fish, a steady source of protein, and cross-continental overland routes were also becoming established. These river- and lake-dwelling Europeans, dating from 5,700 to 4,900 years ago, are known by historians and archaeologists as the *Linearbandkeramik*, or the LBK, for their distinctive pottery.

The relatively recent discovery, in 1989, of the Neolithic La Marmotta settlement under the waters of Lake Bracciano, during the building of a new aqueduct to supply Rome, twenty-five miles away, has been a revelation for historians of this early period. The La Marmotta site was only occupied for a short time, around 5700–5230 BC.[12] La Marmotta is remarkable, because it appears to be a fully formed community who arrived in boats from the Mediterranean. One of their seagoing canoes, thirty-five feet long, remains almost fully intact in the National Museum of Prehistory and Ethnography in Rome, and indicates that the Marmotta people may have come from Greece, or even the Near East.[13] With them, they brought women and children, pigs, sheep, goats, two different breeds of dog, and an array of their plants and seeds to grow in the fertile local soil, including opium poppies.[14]

The level of sophistication in the Marmotta village – such as super-sharp obsidian and stone tools, beads, plates, cups, artwork and other items, as well as their plentiful diet including cherries, figs and hazelnuts, as well as wild boar and venison – suggests they were better off than many contemporary early people. Their boats, of which they made small ceramic models for either decoration or demonstration, also suggest trade, or at the very least, exposure to other Mediterranean cultures. People such as 'La Marmottas' may also have been instrumental in introducing the second wave of Fertile Crescent crops, of olives, grapes, pomegranates and the opium poppy. At the same time, brewing of barley beer began in Assyria. Intoxicants had arrived in the Bronze Age world.[15]

The LBK lived mainly in timber, and wattle-and-daub longhouses at the edge of lakes or rivers, and their villages included buildings to shelter livestock and for specific work purposes, such as making their pottery. We know that these Neolithic European peoples grew and harvested opium poppies; what we don't know is if they used them medicinally or recreationally. The seed of *Papaver somniferum* is not poisonous, and the seed capsule is large, yielding a considerable harvest that can be pressed for a nutritious oil, or made into solid but nutritious cakes, and poppy stalks are a useful animal fodder.

What remains of these LBK villages suggests a peaceful agrarian lifestyle surrounded by livestock, dogs and children, where the poppy was perhaps used to treat severe toothaches, chronic joint pain or ease childbirth. Yet the reality of life on the shores of these European lakes and rivers was markedly different, and many were fortified with complex arrangements of fences and ditches. Evidence of three large – given average village size – massacres remain in the German Neolithic settlements of Talheim and Herxheim in the Rhine Valley, and Schletz-Asparn near Vienna. Dozens of individuals, mostly young men, were killed with the LBK-style farming adze, indicating they were not battling outsiders, but fighting amongst themselves, possibly within the same villages. A wider look at LBK societies, particularly those in western Germany, shows they suffered an almost unthinkable rate of violence during their lives: more than 32 per cent of the bodies show evidence of traumatic injury (2 per cent is indicative of a society engaged in war). Skull drinking cups and evidence of cannibalism have also been found at LBK sites, suggesting violence was not only sporadic, but endemic and, in some locations, ritualized.[16] In such settlements, a plant that could not only kill pain, but also induce oblivion, may well have been highly valued. Furthermore, later accounts of war in the ancient world indicate that soldiers drugged themselves before battle, which may also help to account for the horrifying injuries sustained in the LBK population.

Regardless, the level of opium poppy cultivation in various LBK settlements indicates an evolving system of trade and communication, and other finds indicate that the way *Papaver somniferum* was regarded changed quickly. The clearest evidence of Western opium trading at this early stage is found at Raunds in the Nene Valley of Northamptonshire. In the Long Barrow ditches at Raunds, amongst other detritus of Neolithic life, eight opium poppy seeds were discovered, dating from 3800 to 3600 BC. They are the earliest evidence of the opium poppy in Britain, and as a non-native species, must have been imported.[17] Another British Bronze Age find, although later, is that at Wilsford Shaft near Stonehenge in Wiltshire. The shaft itself is a ditch thirty metres deep, used for rubbish by a nearby Bronze Age settlement, and reveals a mixture of detritus from the daily lives of such villages, including discarded plant matter. *Papaver somniferum* seeds were discovered there when the trench was excavated, as well as poppy capsules from assorted species, but also present was *Hyoscyamus niger*, or henbane, often taken with opium to counteract the nausea and stomach cramps. With neither plant native to Britain, it is significant to find them both in the rubbish dump of a single village.[18]

The Raunds and Wilsford Shaft finds, while important, give little context as to how and why opium appears in Britain for the first time, but they do indicate that early civilizations valued it highly enough to travel with it. Some of the most significant evidence for how these early settlements regarded the opium poppy comes from a prehistoric site near Granada, in Spain. Cueva de los Murciélagos, often called the Bat Cave, had been used by early humans for many thousands of years, but a set of burial chambers dating from around 4000 BC revealed bodies buried with *Papaver somniferum* capsules in small woven bags, along with wheat and locks of hair. The bodies were decorated with *esparto* grass caps and gold jewellery, indicating high status and careful burial with some ceremony.[19] The veneration of the opium poppy by western European society was underway.

Then, just as rapidly as the Neolithic people settled in Europe, their cultivation of opium poppies slowed. The poppy retreats quietly but quickly from the West. Yet its story continues. Still without written language, the Bronze Age people of eastern Europe begin their relationship with opium, and back in the Fertile Crescent, other cultures begin to revere it in art and, later, in words.

The Bronze Age

By the time poppy cultivation declined among the Neolithic lake-dwellers, their trade routes had carried the opium poppy over the Alps and into the eastern Mediterranean. This area, where the West meets the East, was, in the time of the early metal ages, a place of trading, seagoing peoples and cults that worshipped strange gods. The general movement of the opium poppy at this time seems to have been, broadly, north-west to south-east, reflecting the influence of the lake-dwellers and the movement of trade.[20] The metal ages created a new era of commercialism. Previously, settlements had traded amongst themselves at gatherings and festivals. Stone tools were often objects of exquisite skill, but reliant upon the stone from which they were knapped. Metal, though still a skilled enterprise, could be forged, and had thousands of uses on both small and large scales, everything from pinning cloaks to pinning cartwheels. The Bronze Age, dependent as it was upon the mining of natural resources, and their transportation and exchange, saw a corresponding rise in human movement and interaction. It is therefore unsurprising that many of the earliest and most diverse records of the opium poppy appear in the Bronze Age.

It is often stated that the Sumerians of southern Iraq were the first to use opium for medicinal purposes, since they were thought to have recorded it on cuneiform tablets, translated in the 1920s by historian R. Campbell Thompson. *The Assyrian Herbal* features the term 'HUL-GIL' repeatedly.[21] Later historians translated this as as 'joy-plant', and took it to refer to the opium poppy.[22] Were this accurate, it would date Sumerian use of opium to around 3000 BC, but more recent scholarship has debunked the Sumerian theory. HUL-GIL more likely means 'joy-cucumber', although, disappointingly, the surrounding context remains too vague to know what it was used for, and 'No word in Akkadian or Sumerian has definitely been identified as opium poppy'.[23]

So opium still hadn't quite reached the Near East even while it was being used by the, theoretically, more primitive Neolithic peoples of the western Mediterranean. But it was on the move, and archaeobotanical evidence proves that Late Bronze Age peoples in Greece and Bulgaria were growing opium poppies as part of another wave of new crops.[24]

The Late Bronze Age, c.1500 BC, was key in the use and cultural significance of opium in the eastern Mediterranean and the
Levant, but also because of the flowering of decorative objects
and art at the time. The Únětice culture in Czechoslovakia was
a dominant metalworking force, rather like the LBK had been
in pottery, and the British Isles may well have supplied them
with gold and tin from Cornwall, showing just how far the trading routes stretched.[25]

One important Bronze Age people, the Minoans, flourished
on Crete, Santorini and other smaller Aegean islands from
around 3650 to 1250 BC. They were badly affected around 1600 BC
by a mysterious natural event, possibly the eruption of the Thera
volcano on Santorini, and went into a decline they eventually
succumbed to, after minor periods of recovery.[26] The evidence of
the Minoans' sophisticated palaces and temples was only rediscovered at the beginning of the twentieth century. They were,
primarily, fishing communities, but grew varied crops, as well as
olives and vines up on the Mesara Plain in the interior. They
were also traders, as they were perfectly positioned between East
and West, both to replenish merchant ships with provisions,
and to buy and sell goods. By the time the Minoans were established as a civilization, international trade was already flourishing throughout the Near East. Crete had become a world sea
power, and so it is no surprise to find, around 1800 to 1750 BC,
Cretan tin traders living many hundreds of miles from home, in
the Syrian port of Ugarit, a major metal-trading centre. Not only
are they there, they are there in some considerable numbers,
enough for provisions to be made for both an overseer and a
translator.[27] And these traders were interested in more than basic
living: imports of familiar home comforts such as beer, oils and
weapons, as well as clothing and leather shoes, feature in the
records.[28]

Their distinctive goods appear along the early trading routes, and the Minoan jugs known as *lekythi*, with their small bodies and narrow necks, indisputably depict scarified poppy heads. Scarification – the gentle cutting of the poppy head – releases the milky opium latex, which drips down the outside of the capsule before drying to form the teardrops known as the Milk of Paradise. The decoration on these *lekythi* demonstrate that the Minoans knew how to harvest opium latex. In the Bronze Age Mediterranean, snakes symbolized the underworld, but also health and healing, and one Minoan jug combines that with the poppy, indicating a medicinal use for the contents. A small toilet box, known as a pyxis, shows a bird tearing into a poppy capsule, enclosed by the Cretan 'horns of consecration', signifying that what the box held was holy and associated with immortality.[29]

In 1937, in a Minoan cult house at Gazi in northern Crete, the Poppy Goddess was discovered. Now in the Archaeological Museum of Heraklion, she is seventy-eight centimetres tall and her head is dressed with three moveable hairpins in the form of poppy capsules: they have been slit vertically five or six times, mimicking the harvesting of opium latex. Arms raised, eyes closed and with a beatific expression, she appears to be in a drugged state; the 'passivity of her lips is also a natural effect of opium intoxication'.[30] She has been dated to 1300–1250 BC and represents the earliest depiction of human opium use, and is generally believed to represent a state of ecstasy induced for religious ceremonies.[31] Also discovered was a clay pipe, rather like a primitive Victorian ceramic steam inhaler, but with an open bottom and a hole in the side, so that it might be placed over coals and then opium gum held over them through the small hole, perhaps on a metal rod or stick. The size of it indicates it may have been communal, and used by the congregation during the ceremony, as well as the priest or priestess.[32]

At the same time as the Minoans held Crete as their stronghold, the Mycenae dominated the north-eastern Peloponnese. In their citadel, also called Mycenae, fifty-five miles south-west of Athens, bronze pins with brown crystal poppy heads have been found, overall too large for use on the clothes or in hair, but perfect for feeding opium into a pipe.[33] A gold ring, now in the National Archaeological Museum of Athens, was also found. It depicts a goddess of fertility, reclining beneath a tree, holding three poppy capsules in her right hand, as she is presented with gifts, the first of which is another group of three poppy capsules. The goddess, derived from the pan-European Great Earth Mother figure, is surrounded by cult Cretan images such as the double axe, the sun and the moon, and the tree itself, depicting fertility. The ring and the image of the three capsules corresponds to the three cult symbols and the poppies' symbolic meaning: wealth, health and fertility.[34]

The Mycenae and the Minoans represent the first concrete depictions of opium use, as well as strong evidence of early drug apparatus. They also show that opium had multiple meanings within early Greek culture, particularly medicinal, ceremonial and mystical. Both societies declined and disappeared at roughly the same time, but by then opium had already moved on.

Cyprus lies 783 km east of Crete, around seventy-one hours of constant pulling for a fully crewed and loaded Bronze Age ship of around 11 tons, depending on the weather.[35] The ancient city of Kiteon lay on the south-east coast, where modern Larnaca now sits. Kiteon was colonized by the Mycenae, then by the seafaring Phoenecians, with the Egyptians arriving in 570 BC, only to be supplanted by the Persians in less than three decades.[36] Five hundred years later, it was annexed by Rome, before earthquakes destroyed it in the fourth century. The first excavations at Kiteon were carried out in 1929 by the Swedish Cyprus

Archaeological Expedition, and work has been almost continuous since then. The city's immensely varied past is seen in the wealth of the archaeological finds: including the first known opium pipe.[37] The ivory pipe was found, with other ivory objects, in the *sancta santorum*, or holy-of-holies, of Temple 4, under a pile of red bricks beneath a Phoenecian wall.[38] This temple was dedicated to a goddess of fertility, and collapsed *c.*1190 BC during a raid by the Peoples of the Sea – the much-feared Aegean Sea Pirates – and the pipe, along with its compatriot pieces, has been dated to 1300 BC.[39] It is 13.75 cm long, with a small cup-like bowl displaying distinct burn marks and with the image of the mysterious dwarf god, Bes, carved upon it. Bes, an Egyptian god adopted by the Cypriots, and a consort of one of their goddesses, was often depicted wearing a bull mask during ceremonies, sporting a distinctly priapic posture, but he was also an attendant at childbirth and a guardian of mothers.[40] Bes was associated with the renewal of life, as well as humour and music, and was something of a domestic god whose image featured frequently on everyday items such as knives or furniture.[41] Soon though, the bright star of these early Greek Aegean cultures faded, yet almost 1,000 km to the south, Egypt had begun to venerate the poppy. The growing conditions in Egypt are particularly favourable to *Papaver somniferum*, with cold nights and long, consistent hours of sunshine. Egyptian opium, known as Theban, was soon the most desirable variety.

Opium had reached Egypt at roughly the same time as it reached Crete and Cyprus, around 1600–1500 BC. There was an unscored poppy capsule discovered in the Deir-el-Medina, the workers' village close to the Valley of the Kings outside ancient Thebes modern Luxor on the east bank of the Nile River. Tomb 1389 dates from 1500 BC and contained the coffin of an elderly 1.75-m tall man, although his wife's coffin was missing. Their grave goods, all the things it was presumed they would need in the afterlife, were organized neatly, and included scarab beetles, documents, a razor as well as Cypriot juglets.[42]

A small dose of opium for an elderly, possibly arthritic worker, of relatively high status, seems plausible, but the tainting of a disturbed gravesite is not impossible either, so it is other finds that locate opium more precisely within the culture. Two earrings, featuring rows of dangling poppy capsules, discovered in the tomb of the pharaoh Siptah and his queen Tausret, in the nearby Valley of the Kings, pre-date 1189 BC, the year she died, having ruled alone for a year after her husband's death.[43] A necklace of the same date featuring beads resembling incised poppy capsules and a vase of blue faience in the shape of a poppy capsule were found at Armana, 402 km north of Luxor, demonstrating the importance of the opium poppy in Egyptian daily life and death.[44]

Further proof of Egypt's full adoption of the opium poppy in the Bronze Age is offered by the Ebers Papyrus, which dates from c.1552 BC. It was discovered by notorious American tomb raider Edwin Smith, who lived in Egypt in the latter half of the nineteenth century. Smith allegedly removed the papyrus from between the legs of an unknown mummy and sold it to German egyptologist Georg Moritz Ebers, from whom it takes its name, in the winter of 1873–4. The Ebers Papyrus is most famous for its instructions to dose infants with opium: 'Remedy to stop a crying child: Pods of poppy plant, fly dirt which is on the wall, make it into one, strain, and take it for four days, it acts at once.'[45]

It is, at best, a contradictory recipe, yet its cavalier administration to small children reveals the humdrum reality that opium use had already attained.

The Graeco-Roman Empires

Opium is the Latin derivation of the Greek *ópion*, meaning
'poppy juice', although poppy preparations were commonly
known as *mēkōnion*, referring to Mekones, now Kyllene, where
according to legend Demeter – the Greek mother goddess of
earth and renewal – first discovered poppies.[46] The opium poppy
was sacred to Demeter, as it was to her Roman equivalent Ceres,
and they are often depicted holding wheat in one hand and
poppies in the other. Incarnations of Demeter and her daughter
Persephone are all part of the ancient European mother-goddess
tradition, deeply associated with health and renewal, and with
life and death. In Greek mythology, the poppy was also associated with Nyx, the goddess of night, Hypnos, the god of sleep,
Morpheus, the god of dreams, and Thanatos, the god of death.[47]

With the rise of the Greek and Roman empires, society moved
to a more patriarchal, warlike model. These new societies, with
their increased wealth, sophistication and urban way of life,
brought about an equivalent rise in art and science. The Greek
poet Homer's works were composed sometime between 1100 and
800 BC at the beginning of the period when ancient Greece and
Rome began their rise to prominence. Both his great epic poems,
the *Iliad* and the *Odyssey*, include references to the poppy,
although the latter is of most interest.

The *Odyssey* continues the story of the *Iliad*, after the fall of
Troy, and features Helen presented with a drug, believed to be
opium or possibly an opium/hashish mixture, by Polydamna of
Egypt: nepenthe. Homer describes Egypt as a place where 'the
earth, the giver of grain, bears greatest store of drugs, many that
are healing when mixed, and many that are baneful'. To help his
friends forget the loss of Odysseus, Helen 'cast into the wine of

which they were drinking a drug, to quiet all pain and strife, and to bring forgetfulness of every evil'.[48]

Helen's role as the bringer of both wine, and relief, in the form of opium, and Polydamna's knowledge of medicines are typically feminine attributes in classical mythology: a subtle thing, passed between women. Diodorus Siculus, Greek historian, noted of nepenthe that 'from ancient times only the women of Diospolis in Egypt were said to have found a drug against anger and grief'.[49]

Homeric references to the opium poppy are concerned with the need for emotional oblivion, but Greek scholars were also discovering its many medicinal properties. One of the outstanding early scholars was Hippocrates. Born c.460 BC in Cos, he is often referred to as the father of Western medicine. Around sixty medical works survive that are associated with him, although it is impossible to know for certain how many of them he actually wrote. The most famous, his Hippocratic oath, included injunctions against unskilled surgery, interfering with the 'tender fruit' in a mother's womb, and bringing early death, even to those who 'beg for it in anguish'.[50] The Hippocratic oath has been reworked enough times for it to be little use as a set of rules for doctors to follow, but it established a holistic way of looking at illness and the patient, and the collected works are a fascinating look at the foundation of early medicine. Hippocrates and his followers, for instance, used questions that led to an understanding of the patient's pain to both diagnose and monitor disease and injury, and the way that they did so was detailed and accurate. Hippocrates is also thought to be responsible for the 'four humours' theory of the human body: that it is made up of 'blood, phlegm, black bile and yellow bile'.[51] These humours correspond – with one extra, blood – to the three doshas in Ayurvedic medicine, one of the world's oldest systems. When the humours or doshas are in balance, then the body will be in balance. The unfortunate downside of the humours theory is that bloodletting was the commonest method used to restore this balance, and became a mainstay of many physicians' practices – one that would claim many thousands of lives over the coming centuries.

The Hippocratic texts show that ancient-Greek doctors knew much about what *could* go wrong with the body, but they often didn't know *why*, and their associated pharmacology is therefore often more than a little awry. For instance, the womb was increasingly considered to be 'an animal within an animal', capable of determining its own actions and of 'wandering' within the body, although these symptoms were most likely indicative of postpartum stress or prolapse, uterine cancer or disease. Twenty-one of the twenty-five uses of opium in Hippocratic texts are gynaecological, and mainly for a wandering womb.[52] While these conditions were no doubt painful and perhaps dangerous, it indicates that opium remained strongly associated with women and fertility.

However, opium was used for a variety of other conditions and especially to induce sleep. Aristotle himself wrote in his text *On Sleeping*, that 'poppy, mandragora, wine, darnel, produce a heaviness in the head'.[53] The number of early medical texts mentioning sleeplessness suggests insomnia is a timeless human disorder.

Another early mention of medicinal poppy use comes from Aristotle's pupil Theophrastus. Theophrastus, author of *Historia Plantarum* (*Enquiry into Plants*) and *On the Causes of Plants*, is credited as the father of botany. Intriguingly, Theophrastus does not mention the opium poppy in such a way that would firmly identify it. He mentions poppy remedies, but these are not for the uses associated with opium. Instead, he discusses three types

of poppy, all of which appear to be wild, including the alarmingly named 'frothy poppy' he recommends as a bowel purge.[54]
Theophrastus also mentions a *rhizotomoi*, or root-digger, who
mixed hemlock and poppy to bring about a swift demise. The
root-diggers were botanists, and an important social group in
ancient Greek culture. Their knowledge of plants, and poisons in
particular, was usually far superior to that of scholars. Perhaps
Theophrastus was simply being cautious and adhering to the
Hippocratic determination to prolong life. Or, he was avoiding
the potentially awkward mention of the Keian Custom, a political hot potato at the time he was writing.

Keos, or Kea as it is now known, is an island in the Cyclades
close to Attica, and by the time of Aristotle and Theophrastus
had seceded from Athens. This put food supplies to the island
under enormous pressure, but the population was healthy and
long-lived. The Keians were a determined people, and when
faced with this food shortage introduced a practical solution:
upon turning sixty each citizen was to consider whether they
were still of use to the state or not. If not, a small ceremony was
performed, a wreath donned and a mixture of poppy latex, hemlock and wine downed from a 'Keian Cup', thus staying true to
the Keian thinking of 'Whoso cannot live well shall not live ill'.[55]
Emphasis in the accounts is upon the selfless willingness of the
aged Keian to drink from the cup, with no small amount of
theatre. Theophrastus was writing at a time when funerary rituals and customs were changing, partly due to the Greek desire
to create laws for governing daily life and reinforcing social
status.[56] Accounts of the Keian suicides vary, mainly as to
whether the custom was compulsory or not, but the introduction
of condoned euthanasia did not sit well with Hippocratic thinking, and Aristotle too thought that suicide was unjust to society.
Attitudes to old age and the place of the elderly in society were

complex and varied in the ancient world, but the idea that older people had little to offer was a persistent one. The question of if there was a right time to die and, if so, when that time would be, and whether the state has any part in making that decision, was already a thorny issue.

At the same time as Aristotle and Theophrastus were writing, and elderly Keians were allegedly holding suicide parties, the opium poppy began to appear on coins. Coinage began around the sixth century BC in what is now Turkey, and in 330 BC in Şuhut the Romans minted a coin depicting a wheat ear and a poppy head. Other coins from Şuhut depict a goddess holding wheat, poppies and flax, indicating the poppy's status.[57]

The Roman coins of Şuhut coincided with the vast campaign of Alexander the Great (356–323 BC) sweeping across Asia. The Silk Roads already existed as a couple of thousand miles of caravan trading routes, although they wouldn't start to carry large amounts of silk for another century. Alexander, another pupil of Aristotle, is often credited with introducing the opium poppy to Persia and India; what is far more likely is that with him he took supplies for his troops, then traded it and other goods during the campaign, rather than made any conscious decision regarding opium.

By the first century BC, the poppy featured on money, jewellery, in art and literature, and in homes and gardens across Europe and the Near East. The presence of the opium poppy in gardens is confirmed by the wonderful *hortus conclusus*, or garden room at the House of the Golden Bracelet at Pompeii. Painted across three walls is a stunning fresco that would have been open to the elements, featuring all sorts of plants, including roses, lavender and opium poppies, which were trained up a frame around the roses.[58]

Pliny the Elder – who, like the family of the House of the

Golden Bracelet, was killed by the eruption of Vesuvius that destroyed Pompeii in AD 79 – made frequent mentions of opium in his myriad works. The majority of them are rather vague, but occasionally he focusses in detail on how to tell genuine opium from the fake product, such as trying to dissolve it, or heating it to appreciate the odour. He cites the use of opium to cure 'bowels, snakebites, the stings of spiders, scorpions, etc.', and also for the easing of dropsy.[59] Pliny also warned against henbane, which he mentions in the same passage as the opium poppy, writing that it puts men out of their 'right wits', so people were still using henbane to counteract the problem of digesting opium without cramps or nausea.[60] Pliny's warnings are valid as henbane is a psychotropic, capable of inducing disturbing visions and the sensation of flying.

In contrast, the works of Pedanius Dioscorides offer a comprehensive account of the early uses of opium. A physician and botanist originating from Anatolia, Dioscorides was born around AD 40 in Anazarbus, near Tarsus, which was a seat of pharmacological studies. His five-volume *De materia medica* is the defining work of pharmacology of the Graeco-Roman period, and remained influential for the next 1,500 years. His purpose was clear:

> Although many authors, old and new ... have put together books on the preparation, testing and properties of drugs, I shall try to show you that my undertaking in this purpose is neither idle nor absurd, for some of my predecessors did not give a complete survey, while others took most of their information from written sources.[61]

Dioscorides was referring to the incestuous group of early physicians who interpreted and picked over each other's works, rendering them all but incomprehensible. His work, however, was meticulous and wide-ranging. He did not rely only upon texts by other physicians, but also collected folklore remedies from oral traditions, one of which was that adding wormwood juice to ink would stop mice eating your manuscripts. Particularly important are his specific descriptions of medicines and complaints which make identifying the opium poppy and its applications far easier. Not for Dioscorides the vagueness of earlier authors' descriptions of how to administer medications, but rather, 'applied to the finger and used like a suppository, the latex induces sleep'.[62] He was also aware of the difference between the horned poppy and the opium poppy, and that the horned poppy was used for the purposes of adulteration, by mixing it with gum or 'juice of wild lettuce' to look like opium latex.[63]

The stabilization of trade routes over Asia Minor and the Mediterranean – and the manner in which Dioscorides dispensed his advice – indicates that opium was readily available, and sold by herbalists who gathered together in dedicated quarters of larger towns and cities, such as off the Via Sacra in Rome, but Dioscorides drew a distinction between 'shop-bought' opium gum and poppies he had harvested himself. He also described in detail how to scarify the poppy head to obtain the opium latex:

> after the dew-drops have become well dried [the] knife must be drawn round the crown without piercing the fruit within; then the capsules must be directly slit on the sides near the surface and opened lightly, the juice drop will come forth onto the finger sluggishly but will soon flow freely.[64]

Detailed instructions such as these, the myriad references throughout classical literature, and the archaeological evidence, all prove that people were becoming more aware of the way in which opium could be used, and the way it affected the body over time. Herbalists noticed that those treated with opium could develop a tolerance to the drug, and graphic warnings against overdosing began to appear, where patients would display 'chilled extremities; their eyes do not open but are bound by their eyelids ... and through the throat the laboured breath passes faint and chill'. Should this happen, the patient should be made to vomit and kept awake. Yet, despite all this, there was little mention of the dangers of long-term use.[65]

Galen of Pergamon (AD 129 to after 215) was Emperor Marcus Aurelius' doctor, and the leading physician in Rome. Despite his blustering tones and occasionally suspect methodology, he adopted a pioneering stance on the crossroads between philosophy and medicine; between moral health and physical health. He was a keen observer of his surroundings, and subjects, and wrote extensively on his experience of dissection and vivisection.[66] Galen's *On the Dissection of Living Animals* has been lost, but he referred to it himself in his *Anatomical Procedures*, and gave demonstrations of how to effect paralysis, and performed trepanation in front of audiences.[67] His subject of choice was 'an ape', thought now to be macaques or rhesus monkeys, which he chose for their rounded faces, as they were 'most like humans beings'.[68] Galen's grisly work may seem like a barbaric sideline, but it is one that set the tone for medical and particularly surgical writing until the mid seventeenth century. In his rational observations of removing animals' ribs while they are tied down to boards, their distress is not reported, even as their heart is laid bare, still beating. The potential for struggle is inferred from the levels of restraints required, rather than a description of suffering.[69] This necessary separation between surgeon and subject is a pivotal moment in the history of medicine, and in the history of opiates.

Marcus Aurelius (AD 121–80) spent a decade on campaign, during which he wrote *Meditations*, dealing with the responsibilities of his role and the importance of duty and service. Galen dosed his star patient with detached precision. On an almost daily basis, he administered *theriac* (from the Greek word for treacle) to Aurelius, containing a number of different ingredients, including opium, although the 'poppy-juice' was removed from the compound when the emperor appeared to be 'getting drowsy at his duties'. Without the opium, this drowsiness was replaced by insomnia.[70] Theriac was a version of a 'mithridate' or universal antidote, allegedly created by Mithridates VI, king of Pontus, who feared poisoning to such an extent that he took a mixture of poisons each day, including opium, to make himself immune to them. Mithridate concoctions, some containing up to seventy ingredients, became almost compulsory among those in powerful positions until the Renaissance. On campaign on the Danube, Marcus Aurelius had to go without his theriac after a period of heavy use, and the nervous symptoms he displayed were those of a regular opiate user, 'So,' Galen noted, 'he was obliged to have recourse again to the compound which contained poppy-juice, since this was now habitual with him.'[71]

The emperor is often cited as one of the earliest documented drug addicts, but addiction was a concept unknown in the ancient world. Galen's enthusiastic endorsement of opium, and imperial associations, as well as his undeniable success as a physician, meant that it became a popular and desirable medicine in Rome, bought from druggist-stalls at the market.[72] The Roman appetite for both drugs and luxuries meant that most theriacs were exotic mixtures of genuine medicines and ingredients such as cinnamon and rare honeys. The spectrum of Roman life and ordinary medical knowledge is seen in the variety of people who supplied Galen with drugs or with recipes for cures. He credited those who gave him information, and some of them appear to have occupational links such as Celer the centurion with his cure for arthritis and tremors, and Paris the actor with an eye-watering recipe for hair removal, and a Bythian barber with a concoction for sciatica. Opium remedies included Flavius the boxer's dysentery medicine, and *acopon*, or painkilling recipes, from Orion the hairdresser and Philoxenos the schoolmaster.[73] A woman, Aquillia Secundilla, is credited with her recipe for lumbago.[74]

Even as Greek dreams of Troy were replaced by the bureaucratic realities of Rome, which thrived on taxation, war and trade, the Romans were feeling the curtailment of their boundaries. Hedged in by North Africa, seeing scant bounty to be had in the far north of Europe, they were instead looking east, back towards the Fertile Crescent, full of people, goods and money, all of which could be either sold or taxed. It was not a place without its perils. The Persians had proved mighty enemies, and the Arabs were deemed to be feral and dangerous. But the strategic trading stronghold of Byzantium was a prize that Rome had long eyed from afar.

In AD 312, Emperor Constantine, on campaign, saw a vision of a cross in the sky and heard a voice say, 'By this sign, conquer.'[75] He converted to Christianity, hitherto a proscribed and persecuted sect, and captured Byzantium. There, he would create a new Roman capital in the East: Constantinople. The Roman Empire was on the rise again, and with it, a new religion. Constantine's conversion soon spread Christianity far into the western reaches of the empire, but there, the trail of opium in Europe is lost, and the Iron and Dark ages show little evidence for its existence in the West. For our purposes, the history of opium continues in the East.

Chapter Two

THE ISLAMIC GOLDEN AGE TO THE RENAISSANCE

Silk and Spice

The history of opium in the East does not start with the drug itself, but with the infrastructure that allowed its introduction, then gave it the opportunity to flourish. The foundation of the Silk Roads of China and the maritime spice routes to southern India put in place a transport network between East and West that dominated trade until the opening of the Suez Canal in 1869.

Opium is associated inextricably with the history of China. Yet at the time of the Roman Empire, there is no evidence that the Chinese used opium at all, but rather, cannabis. The *Pen Ts'ao Ching*, or *Divine Husbandman's materia medica* from the second century BC, listed over 300 different plant and mineral remedies, including the first known mention of the use of *Cannabis sativa*.[1] Famed Chinese physician Hua Tao (*c.*AD 145–208) performed extensive surgeries after sedating the patient with a mixture of cannabis resin, datura and wine.[2]

China is also home to the history of one of the most extraordinary trading networks in the world, and one that became essential to the history of opium. The Silk Roads were a set of routes covering much of Eurasia and some parts of Africa. The name arises from the large-scale movement of silk west, and goods east, by the Han Chinese 2,000 years ago. Comprising two main routes, north and south, their various branch lines expanded and contracted according to wars and famines; some were large highways carrying camel caravans hundreds of animals strong, and some were little more than mule tracks. They didn't carry only silk, but all manner of goods, including horses and spices, and they represent the trading not only of commodities, but cultural, social, economic, religious and political values.

The Greek historian Herodotus, born c.484 BC, noted that a road network already stretched from the coast of Asia Minor to 'Babylon, Susa and Persepolis' whose messengers could carry messages over 1,600 miles in a week, regardless of the weather. 'Neither snow nor rain nor heat nor darkness of night prevents them from accomplishing the task proposed to them with the very utmost speed,' he wrote in admiration, and explained how the messages were 'handed from one to the other, as in the torch-race among the Hellenes'.[3] This was the Royal Road of Persian King Darius I (550–486 BC), an efficient extension of earlier trading roads, which used their model of regular staging posts offering shelter and safety, as well as respite and information.

Far to the east lay the Warring States of China, occupying a far smaller area than modern China, and situated on its eastern coast. Sophisticated early towns emerged around the fertile Yellow River Valley and its extensive coastline approximately 3,000 years ago, and in the millennium before, they were already recording the histories of their various dynasties with an advanced system of writing. These Chinese had been creating beautiful silks for 2,000 or perhaps 3,000 years by the time of the Roman Empire, but constraints upon production and safe travel meant that they were restricted, mainly, to aristocratic wearers.

The Han dynasty emerged in 206 BC and lasted until AD 220, and was the first time China operated under a central government. It was a period of both peace and prosperity under which the people flourished. Han is a name used for the ethnic group of northern China, and remains in use today. The early Han emperors were concerned with creating a political, philosophical and universal order, which included the teachings of Confucius (551–479 BC).

Under the energetic and splendidly portly Emperor Wu (141–87 BC), the Han had made their greatest expansions. Wu, greedy for foreign goods and determined to find a magician who could grant him immortality, took on the northern nomad tribes of the Xiongnu and the Yuezhi. Both tribes were skilled horsemen, who used bows to fight and hunt from horseback, and were frequent raiders of Chinese traders and settlements. In 119 BC, after ten years of futile and expensive battling with the nomads, Wu succeeded in forcing the tribes back to the north and pushed west from Chang'an – now Xi'an – through the Gansu corridor towards Kashgar and the Pamir Mountains, forging the three main routes of the Northern Silk Road. At Kashgar, the road split into three again, towards the Black Sea, towards Merv in Persia and towards Balkh in Bactria.

The Bactrian camel, an animal astonishingly well suited to carrying large loads over long distances in extreme conditions, was the favoured means of transport over the Silk Roads. Originating from the wild camels near the 'great bend of the Yellow River in north-western China through Mongolia to central Kazakhstan', they were preferable to the Arabian camel because of their dual humps and superior hardiness, including the ability to close their nostrils in dust or sandstorms.[4] They could 'carry loads of 220–270 kgs some 30–40 kms daily, or 80–100 kms if pulling a loaded cart', the equivalent to half their bodyweight, on average, amounting to a colossal amount of pulling power.[5]

This new route west also allowed Wu's envoy, Zhang Qian (c.200–114 BC), to travel outside China, with his intrepid Xiongnu guide, Ganfu. It began badly in 138 BC when they were both captured by the Xiongnu and kept prisoner for ten years. After their escape, however, with the wife and son Zhang Qian had acquired during his captivity, they went on exploring the Tarim Basin, home to the deadly Taklamakan Desert. Qian and Ganfu returned to Wu's court in 125 BC, after another period as unwilling guests of the Xiongnu, bringing back tales of other peoples, such as the Dayuans of the Tarim Basin, who were farmers and made 'wine out of grapes'.[6] Their adventures further south are also the first recorded accounts of Shendu, or India, in Chinese history, which he describes as 'hot and damp' and whose 'inhabitants ride elephants when they go in battle'.[7] Their explorations laid the foundation for the Southern Silk Road, the branch line of which went off at Yarkand across the Karakoram Pass to Leh and Srinagar to reach northern India.

The Han period was also when Chinese craftsmen were creating silk of such beauty and desirability that, when coupled with the creation of stable trade routes, international demand flourished. But, as one contemporary historian noted, 'while Chinese silk poured out of the country, all that came in return was jewels and exotic fruits, luxury goods destined for the enjoyment of the rich alone'.[8] The Han Confucianists were unhappy with this seeming imbalance that new trade was bringing to China and called for a period of isolationism to restore balance to the country, a theme that persists in modern times.

Rome, meanwhile, increasingly greedy and sophisticated, was looking east for luxuries. It was already familiar with the delicious pistachios and dates of Persia, Indian spices, and cloth and essential oils from Africa, but as silk began to appear from China, they seized upon it as the newest luxury, although, for many Roman soldiers, their first sight of silk was associated more with fear than with pleasure. Roman historian Cassius Dio wrote that high-quality silk was first seen by the Roman army in 53 BC, as the stunning banners of the Parthian army unfurled at the Battle of Carrhae.

It was a terrible defeat for Rome, one of the worst in the empire's history, and it was not only Carrhae that meant Romans were mixed in their reaction to silk: some of the old guard saw it as an immoral luxury. For where the Chinese had used silk to make structured, elaborate and above all modest court robes, Rome had put it to an altogether different use. Seneca the Younger (3 BC to AD 65) was furious – 'Wretched flocks of maids labour so that the adulteress may be visible through her thin dress, so that her husband has no more acquaintance than any outsider or foreigner with his wife's body' – and Pliny the Elder raged, 'So manifold is the labor employed, and so distant is the region of the globe drawn upon, to enable the Roman maiden to flaunt transparent clothing in public'.[9] But the outrage of these austere philosophers meant nothing to the thousands of merchants already making their living on the Silk Roads.

It was not only goods that passed along these trade routes, but people too. African-born Roman historian Florus described how foreign envoys came to visit the first Roman emperor, Augustus, between 27 BC and AD 14. The Chinese came, and then the Indians, 'bringing presents of precious stones and pearls and elephants, but thinking all of less moment than the vastness of the journey which they had undertaken, and which they said had occupied four years. In truth it needed but to look at their complexion to see that they were people of another world than ours.'[10]

The Indian diplomatic mission was a grand undertaking, but many of those who travelled the Silk Roads did so involuntarily. Ten thousand soldiers were taken prisoner by the Parthians at Carrhae and sent to man the eastern frontier.[11] Roman inscriptions from the second or third century AD in a cave complex in eastern Uzbekistan, attributed to soldiers from Apollo's Fifth Legion, show just how far from home people found themselves, courtesy of this extensive road network.[12]

Like the Silk Roads, the spice routes to the east coast of Africa and the west coast of India opened up around the first century BC. Business between Alexandria and the East became extensive when the Roman occupation of Egypt in 30 BC caused a rise in trade with both Africa and India, the main commercial centres of which were 3,000 nautical miles away.

The Red Sea was tiresome to navigate because of the perilous shoals that meant ships could travel only by day, putting in at night for safety. Once at the Bab al Mandeb, the gateway to the Arabian Sea, they had a long, if straightforward journey down the east African coast. There and back, via Zanzibar, would mean they returned home in around two years, laden with tortoise-shell, ivory, pearls and incense, as well as spices. But western India's Malabar Coast was the centre of the spice trade, and the spices it produced were quickly in huge demand, particularly pepper. The ancient port city of Muziris, located near modern Cochin, was a centre of this trade, and contained small Roman and Jewish colonies. A guide for mariners which appeared around AD 60, the *Periplus of the Erythraean Sea*, indicated the scale of the trade: 'Muziris, of the same kingdom, abounds in ships sent there with cargoes from Arabia and by the Greeks.' The author of the *Periplus* credited first-century BC navigator Hippalus for finding the direct sea route to the west coast of India. Previously, sailors had hugged the coastline in dhows, putting in regularly to make trading stops, much like the Silk Roads traders, but the Hippalus route made it possible for the sturdy 1,000-ton Roman trading ships, with their short masts and large square sails, to hove straight across the Arabian Sea. The traders set out from Egypt to both Africa and India in July, when the south-west monsoon wind – also known as Hippalus – blew in. Pliny the Elder, though as dismissive of the goods available in India as he was of silk, recorded that, in good conditions, the journey could be done in forty days from the Gulf of Aden.[13] Modern maritime historians have calculated that it could be achieved in as little as twenty.[14] Despite this, the sailors would then have to wait until December to begin their return journey, when the north-west monsoon winds would be strong enough to carry them home. A round trip to Malabar or Gujarat took a year, but it was far more dangerous than the African voyage.

The maritime route across the Arabian Sea had one enormous advantage: it cut out almost all the middlemen. There were Jewish and Arab settlements on both the north and south coasts of western India, almost all of whom were merchants brokering and trading goods between Indians and the West, but the endless exchanges of the land routes, each with their added mark-ups, meant that although the sea route may have been riskier and required more initial investment, the returns were greater.

On land, the Romans traded with the Iranian Parthians, when not fighting them. After the Parthians, from 224 to 651, from the east of Syria and almost all the way to the Hindu Kush, and stretching far into both south and north, was the empire of the Sassanids. They were Zoroastrians and worshipped one god, Ahura Mazda, who had handed down his wisdom to his prophet Zoroaster. They prized urban life, and were together under the *shananshah* – the ultimate leader – who ruled absolutely, but with great style and charisma. They believed in the principles of *Humata, Hukhta, Huvarshta*, or 'good words, good thoughts, good deeds', and were keen to absorb both ideas and people from other cultures into their growing towns and cities. Personal dress was important to all but the lowest in society and textiles flourished, including, of course, exquisite silk garments. The Sassanids were perhaps the first truly international consumers: they had money, taste and style. They had already inherited a lucky break in terms of geography and a changing world order, and they knew it. The *Letter of Tansar*, a Sassanid propaganda document of the sixth century, states that their land lies happily 'in the midst of other lands, and our people are the most noble and illustrious of beings'.[15]

Many people of the Sassanian Empire were also shrewd. The Sogdians, an Iranian people whose territory within the empire centred on Samarkand, situated on the Silk Road from Kashgar to Merv, traded so extensively between Turkey, the rest of Iran and the East, that the word Sogdian came to mean merchant. The Uyghur people of China, originally settled in the eastern regions of the Tarim Basin, began to spread west along the Silk Roads, mirroring the Sogdian move east.

The silk and associated luxury trades had a huge effect on early Persia, but the opportunity for business was about to move westwards.

Byzantium, which became Constantinople and is now Istanbul, was about to fall to the Romans. Byzantium, built by the Greeks during a period of colonial expansion some 800 years before, was perfectly positioned for trade between the Mediterranean and the east, sitting as it did on the narrow strip of land joining Europe to Turkey. In 324, Emperor Constantine, desperate to rejuvenate the Roman Empire, had conquered the city and renamed it Constantinople, rebuilding it over the next six years and consecrating it as a Christian city in 330. A combination of position at the crossroads between East and West, the opening up of the Silk Roads, and Roman organization and fortification resulted in Constantinople rapidly becoming one of the wealthiest and most powerful cities in the world. There were other cities with strong trading histories, such as Alexandria and Damascus, but they paled in comparison to the new imperial capital.

Constantinople merchants traded with the Sassanids in order to do business with the wider East. This is seen in coin distribution: no European coins have been found in China before the 530s and 540s, when Byzantine ones begin to appear. However, many earlier Chinese coin finds, sometimes numbering hundreds of pieces, were minted in the Sassanid Empire, and had probably been carried east by Sogdian merchants.

The Parthians were a people for whom self-improvement came not only through wealth, but also science, literature and art. Many of them spoke and wrote in Pahlavi, a prestige language of its time, and the ancestor of modern Persian, but they also worked with texts written by Coptic, Greek, Latin, Indian and Chinese scholars. The trading of goods with other peoples, their extensive travel networks and the confluence of international influences, both Western and Eastern, meant that during the Sassanid period, Parthia developed into not only a rich and cosmopolitan trading area, but also a centre for learning, and medicine.

In the *Avesta*, the sacred texts of the early Persians, there are three types of medicine: the knife, the plants and the sacred word. Adherence to the latter offered the best chance of avoiding the former. Running through the earliest Persian writings on medicine is a sense of wonder attached to their long history as a unique people and an ancient civilization, linked inextricably with their Zoroastrian beliefs. Early physicians attributed the introduction of medicine to the world to Jamšid, fourth of the old Persian kings, who reigned from a flying, jewel-bedecked throne that hurtled through the cosmos on special occasions. He ruled a 'rude and barbarous' land, but told the people to get out and build houses, and not to be content with cave-dwelling, and to organize themselves into professions.[16] His wife introduced alcohol to mankind, by mistake, after an accident with some bad grapes. Jamšid was also in possession of a holy cup containing a mysterious elixir of immortality, which when imbibed allowed the drinker to see the seven heavens of the universe, and to observe truth.[17] It may also account for the flying throne.

The recipe for this divine elixir, known as *haoma* in Persia and *soma* in India's vedic tradition, was supposed to represent a trinity of god, plant and drink. Botanical remains found in holy vessels and strainers indicate it was a decoction of either *Papaver somniferum*, or *Cannabis sativa*, mixed with the ephedra plant.[18] *Haoma* services were still carried out near the Iranian poppy-town of Yazd in the late twentieth century. Whatever the ingredients of these mystical solutions, they are a common element across European and Asian religions, and Persia was the place where these religions met soon after the fall of the Western Roman Empire in the fifth century.

By that time, Nestorian-Christian and Greek scholars, fleeing oppression east and west, came to Sassanid cities to study; one of their foremost subjects was medicine. By the sixth century, the city of Gondeshapur was the intellectual centre of Persia and home to the first medical school of the ancient world. There had been other academies teaching medicine, such as those at Nalanda in India from 427 and Nisibis in Turkey from 489, but Gondeshapur included practical teaching from practising physicians, rather than just studying texts. One of the first true universities, it accommodated students and teachers from Zoroastrianism, Buddhism and Manichaeism. Of all of these, the

Nestorian-Christians were the most influential before Islam. Each of their bishoprics contained a school, library and hospital, and there was a strong emphasis on teaching and sharing of knowledge. With its curriculum of astronomy, astrology, mathematics and science, as well as medicine, and its exiled Nestorian-Christian monk tutors, the Academy of Gondeshapur was the origin of the legend of the wise monk-teacher.

The Sassanid Empire was short, but in the nation of Persia it had established an elegant, lucrative and educated centre of exchange between East and West. But a transformation was coming, one that heralded the end of the ancient world: Islam.

Muhammad's Triumph: Islam's Golden Age of Learning

Hundreds of years of sporadic war between Rome and the House of Sasan came to an end in 629, when Emperor Heraclius overthrew the last of the Persian kings. Despite their constant squabbles, these two empires had divided the Fertile Crescent between them, and created continuity, if not stability. Into the breach created by their collapse came the Prophet Muhammad.

Born around 570 in Mecca, at the age of forty Muhammad was a merchant with a mediocre career behind him. He may or may not have been literate, and he was not rich. In short, he was the opposite of his wealthy and cultured Persian and Roman equivalents. Depressed, he went out and sought refuge in a cave, and was visited by the angel Gabriel. After three years, Muhammad began to reveal his revelations and preach publicly. The Arab tribes who worshipped hundreds of pagan idols, many of which adorned the Ka'aba in Mecca, had previously been regarded as the poor cousins of the East, 'of all the nations of the earth, the most despised and insignificant'.[19] Muhammad's teachings were not popular with many in Mecca, and at one stage he was forced to flee; this flight, known as the Hijrah, remains one of the most symbolic events in Islam.

Under Muhammad, the Arabs united in the worship of one god. In 629, just as Rome and the Sassanids had exhausted each other, the Prophet mustered an army to defeat the pagans of Mecca; by the time he died in 632, the majority of the Arabian Peninsula worshipped Allah. By 651 the Muslim conquest of Persia was complete. It was a gargantuan achievement: a religious event on a par with Alexander's military sweep across a continent. Muhammad's timing was perfect, and his legacy immense. His death allowed those men who had known him in life – the caliphs – to establish the first caliphate, and as the Prophet had left very few hard and fast rules for society, they quickly set about making their own. Muhammad's communes with Allah were written down as the basis of the Qur'an, and Islamic scholars began work on the Hadiths, meant to explain these communications in terms of Muslim daily life, comparable to the Jewish tradition of the Torah and the Talmud. (A brief reference to opium appears in an early Palestinian Talmud, c.400.[20])

The Christian ascetic tradition, particularly the stylites who lived on top of pillars, mortifying their flesh in the name of God, was influential in the Middle East, especially Syria, and associated piety with godliness in the strongest terms. Muhammad – drawing perhaps on his life as a merchant, and his time in the cave, as well as his perilous Hijrah – left an idea that the rich should not cheat the poor, and that equality should be promoted. The Qur'an also banned alcohol and other intoxicants.[21]

The first caliphs who succeeded Muhammad, the Rashidun caliphate, are often seen as overseeing a thirty-year golden era of both Muslim religion and government. Less successful were the Umayyads who followed them, who drank alcohol, and one of whom kept a pet monkey. Another Umayyad caliph hunted with a cheetah, which rode out sitting on the rump of its master's horse; the caliph's saluki dogs wore gold anklets and had personal human slaves. Things had gone horribly astray from the original preachings of Muhammad. After just under ninety years in power the Umayyad caliphate was toppled and replaced by the stricter Abbasids, who chose to create their own capital, Madīnat as-Salām or the City of Peace (now Baghdad), near the site of ancient Babylon.

The end of the Umayyads is the beginning of what is known as the Islamic golden age, which lasted over 500 years and spread rapidly as far as Central Asia, known then as Transoxonia. The acquisition of Transoxonia in the middle of the eighth century is traditionally associated with the introduction of paper to the Middle East, through the skills of Chinese prisoners of war kept at Samarkand. The fall of Samarkand to the Muslims in 712 also marked the movement east to China of many migrants who did not want to live under the new rule. The Tang dynasty of 618–907 controlled an expanded version of the Han territories during the peak of the silk trade, and despite a reputation for insularity in terms of immigration, these peoples from the west were absorbed into the Chinese population. This movement of Arab Muslims to China coincides with the first appearances of opium in Chinese writing, most particularly by the author of *A Supplement to the Pen Ts'ao*, called Ch'en Ts'Ang Ch'i.[22]

After Samarkand, Islam moved into the vanguard of science, medicine, civilization and thought. From the Iberian peninsula in the west, conquered in 711, to the Russian steppes in the east, the intellectual world was under Arab control. In Baghdad in 830, Abbasid Caliph Harun al-Rashid (*c*.795–809) created Bayt al-Hikma, the House of Wisdom, modelled on Gondeshapur, where scholars from all parts of the world were invited to come and translate all the knowledge that existed into Arabic. The intellectual and religious tolerance of the Abbasid court of Baghdad was an impressive testament to the new Islamic faith.

A series of scholars emerged not only in Baghdad but across the Arab world, whose contribution to medical knowledge seems rather like a checklist of all of the things it was possible to discover at the time, in anaesthesia, analgesia, surgery and pharmacology. One of the earliest of these scholars associated with the House of Wisdom was al-Kindi, a Basra-born philosopher who also wrote on medicine, and devised a scale for the accurate concoction of medicines, many of which contain opium, namely that of the white, or Egyptian poppy.[23]

Taking their lead from the Hippocratic corpus and Dioscorides, Muslim scholars combined them with Islamic instructions on healing the sick, and instructions for the afflicted to 'Seek treatment, for God the Exalted did not create a disease for which He did not create a treatment, except senility.'[24] Having access to so much written information, as well as the model of Gondeshapur and the Indian tradition of building hospitals, meant that medicine in the Arab world began to make strides forward, facilitated by the money brought in from a vast empire controlling much of the heartland of the Silk Roads. A Chinese visitor to the empire in this period could not believe the profusion of goods, where 'everything produced from the earth is there. Carts carry countless goods to markets, where everything is available and cheap.'[25]

From the ancient Silk Road trading city of Rey, near Tehran, Abū Bakr Muhammad ibn Zakariyyā al-Rāzī came to Baghdad. Known as Rhazes (865–925), he was one of the first recorded polymaths, and is often equated with Hippocrates in Arabic history. His two primary works were the *Kitab al Mansuri*, a ten-chapter book on temperament and physiognomy, and *Kitab al-Hawi*, 'the greatest medical encyclopedia produced by a

Moslem physician', which was influential until the Renaissance.[26] When Rhazes came to Baghdad and was working at
the Muqtadari Hospital, there were three forms of medicine in
operation: prophetic medicine, based largely on the teachings of
the Qur'an; folkloric medicine with its roots in Arab and Zoroastrian traditions; and Greek medicine. Druggists were becoming
respected professionals, and the state had stepped in to provide
regulation on weights, measures and qualities in the form of an
inspector, al-Muhtasib, and his assistants.

In Baghdad, opium – *afyūn* in Arabic – was already in use,
according to the methods of Dioscorides, in a decoction, a pill
or an ointment, either on its own or with up to dozens of different ingredients for diseases such as leprosy. From these
recipes, it often seems that the more terrifying the disease, the
more elaborate the treatment. Greek texts in the Hippocratic
tradition are patient-focussed and stress empathy as one of the
foremost tools of the physician, so it is not surprising that such
diseases merited 'special' medicines. Rhazes, however, was also an
intuitive physician who wrote accurate and nuanced works on
disorders as mundane yet distressing as bed-wetting in children,
and understood that smallpox could only be contracted once.
Like Galen, he continued with experimentation upon animals,
including testing mercury on a monkey.

Rhazes also wrote about surgery, on which the Arabic medical
community was making significant advances, particularly in pelvic surgery. He is often credited as the first physician to use
opium as a general anaesthetic, using the works of the prolific
alchemist and chemist Abu Mūsā Jābir ibn Hayyān, or Geber
(*c*.721–*c*.815), for guidance.[27]

An indication of how extensive surgical methods, particularly
those on the internal organs, had become is given by the works
on suturing created at the time, especially by Rhazes. Debate

among physicians was fierce: some recommended only cotton and silk to repair flesh, including notes by the Nestorian-Christian physician to the caliphs, Yūhannā ibn Māsawayh, known as Mesue Senior, about using strong silk to repair arteries.[28] Rhazes preferred to use the catgut strings favoured by lute players to repair abdominal walls, and also used horsehair sutures, which remained popular for centuries.[29] These writings suggest abdominal and arterial surgery was being performed, making anaesthesia of some kind compulsory. Although some simple, if relatively major, surgeries such as the removal of a bladder stone were achieved through heavy restraint of the patient, it seems highly unlikely that anyone could undergo abdominal or pelvic surgery, some of which details the joining of bowel sections, without having first been rendered insensible.

As surgical techniques progressed, Baghdad founded its own guild for making surgical needles, and often the physicians gave their own specifications as to what their needles should look like and what they should be made from, with gold and silver particularly popular. The finest needles were used for eye surgery, and a woman's hair used as sutures.[30] Ophthalmology was a preoccupation of the early Arabian physicians, and opium was a common ingredient in topical recipes for eye medicines. Al-Kindi's recipes contain a large number, proportionally, of eye remedies containing it, although Greek physicians had disagreed over whether it was helpful or harmful, because although it was a painkiller, it was also an irritant.

The famous Persian scholar Ibn-Sīnā, known as Avicenna (980–1034), was responsible for condensing a large amount of the theories we take for granted today. He named the five external senses, and some internal, such as common sense, which allows us to process external information and to understand how it will affect our welfare. His primary work was the *Kitab al-Shifa'* or *The Book of Healing*, a work not upon medicine but on science and philosophy, as well as early psychology. For Avicenna, as for many early polymaths, the separation between disciplines was tenuous, and he explored how we process thoughts and feelings, as well as astronomy. He was careful, with his medical works, to focus on the facts of his experiences as a physician rather than criticisms or opinions of other theories, representing an early and important move towards empiricism. Another of his works, *Al-Qānūn fī aṭ-Ṭibb*, or *Canon of Medicine*, was also central to the contemporary understanding of pain. Galen had described four different types of pain, and correctly located the brain as the organ which perceived it, but Avicenna identified fifteen different types.

Pain theory is central to the history of opium: understanding why and how we feel pain dictates how we try to relieve it. To illustrate how advanced Avicenna's understanding of pain was, the modern McGill Pain Questionnaire that is used throughout North America classifies twenty different types of pain, thirteen of which are in common with those in Avicenna's *Canon*. To relieve pain, he writes of the *taskin*, or painkillers, and *mukhaddar*, anaesthetics. Opium is listed as both a *taskin* and a *mukhaddar*, and its use as an anaesthetic is mentioned along with preparations for amputation. The dose mentioned for a painkiller is the size of a 'large lentil', but to induce 'a deeply unconscious state so as to enable the pain be borne' a 'half a dram' dose of opium is recommended, along with other narcotics including henbane, a dose that would certainly have put the patient at risk, as indicated by Avicenna's own terse warning of 'can kill'.[31] People with pain metabolize far higher doses of opium than people who are pain-free, something he had no doubt observed. He also found pigs' bristle efficacious for closing large wounds, but they were later banned in surgery by the strict Shafi'i school of Islam in the ninth century.[32]

Surgery was not the bulk of Avicenna's work, though. Like Rhazes, he was deeply interested in treating the patient as a whole. He was particularly interested in chronic conditions such as gout, for which he prescribed opium. He too recommends opium for insomnia, taken either orally or rectally, and the Arabs call it *abou-el-noum*, 'father of sleep'.[33]

The *Canon* has a whole chapter entitled 'Afion' in Book Two, and details an extensive knowledge in the management of patients using opiates, for everything from coughs and diarrhoea to headaches, but is particularly interesting on the dangers of opium and overdose, listing symptoms and the need to be aware that the patient may also be drunk. It also offers equivalent dosages of other medicines to compare with opium, such as cannabis seed, 'in triple weight' to the equivalent amount of opium.[34] The *Canon* advises, like the Ebers Papyrus, that opium can be used to stop a persistently crying baby. The seemingly endless list of ingredients for this infant medicine contains the key component in the last sentence:

Take bugle seed, juniper berry, white poppy, yellow poppy, linseed, celandine seed, purslane, plantain seed, lettuce seed, fennel seed, aniseed, caraway; some of each is roasted little by little; then all are rubbed together. Add one part of fried flea-wort seed which is not powdered. Mix the whole with a like amount of sugar and give two 'drams' as a potion. If it is desired to make it still stronger, one should add an amount of opium equal to a third part of it or less.[35]

Avicenna's life outside his studies is equally interesting. Typically dressed in a brocaded robe, leather shoes and a linen turban, he

enjoyed wine and female concubines, and a biographer noted
that of all his 'concupiscent faculties', his sexual capacity was 'the
most powerful and predominant' and he 'indulged it often'.[36]
Bearing in mind his startling intellectual abilities, one can only
imagine how powerful this capacity was. He never married, or
recorded any children, and died in 1037, a few years after going
on campaign with his emir Alā'-al-dawla Moḥammad, where he
suffered a serious illness in unfortunate and mysterious circumstances. A bout of colic laid him low, just as he and the emir were
retreating from oncoming troops. To try and cure himself, he
allegedly gave himself eight enemas in a single day, and continued rigorous purging, but his physician put far too much
celery seed into the mixture. When he became even sicker, a
servant, who was perhaps also a conspirator in his master's
intended demise, brought him mithridate, which induced a seizure. Although he nursed himself slowly back to health, he was
never the same again but continued to indulge in sexual excess,
and later died of an opium overdose.

Whatever the truth of his death, the truth of his career is that,
in terms of practical medicine and medical philosophy, he – and
the others like him of the Islamic golden age – provided the
essential bridge between the basics laid down in the Graeco-
Roman period and the Renaissance.

From the Dark Ages to the Crusades

Outside the Arab world and the Roman Empire, which had
receded from western Europe, things were not so enlightened.
After the Romans retreated from Britain in 409–10 and Christianity took hold, opium use also disappeared. This does not appear
to be any kind of religious statement, as the Coptic Christians of

Upper Egypt used opium, recorded by a papyrus of the seventh to eighth centuries requesting it for 'brother Paule', a poorly monk, but northern Europe had lost either the knowledge or the willingness to record the use of such a powerful drug.[37]

Most medical knowledge in the Dark Ages centred around the religious houses, mainly monasteries, where the Graeco-Roman teachings were still followed, and medicine was still based upon the humours. Ordinary people relied upon folk medicines, often in the control of a female member of the community, working from oral traditions.

Christianity arrived in Britain during the Roman occupation, and had mustered enough power to send a delegation to the Council of Arles in 314, and of Rimini in 353. But the Christians were under siege from the Picts, Scots and Britons, sending a message to Roman general Aetius c.446, begging for help: 'the barbarians push us into the sea, the sea pushes us back into the barbarians'.[38] 'Barbarians' is an appropriate term for some of these Celtic peoples, of whom the Greek historian Diodorus Siculus wrote: 'They are very tall in stature, with rippling muscles under clear white skin. Their hair is blond, but not naturally so: they bleach it, to this day, artificially, washing it in lime and combing it back from their foreheads. They look like wood-demons, their hair thick and shaggy like a horse's mane. Some of them are clean-shaven, but others – especially those of high rank – shave their cheeks but leave a moustache that covers the whole mouth.'[39] Many of these British and northern European Dark Age tribes were beer or wine drinkers, but others avoided intoxicants completely. The Nervii of Gaul and the Germanic Suebii did not import alcohol. Julius Caesar asked why and he was told, 'they allowed no wine nor any of the other appurtenances of luxury to be imported unto them, because they supposed that their spirit was like to be enfeebled and their courage relaxed thereby'.[40]

Queen Boadicea addressed her soldiers in AD 61 with a condemnation of their drunken foes: 'To us every herb and root are food, every juice is our oil, and water is our wine.'[41] But with such limited written records until the Norman Conquest, it is hard to obtain a clear picture of Dark Ages Britain in comparison with what was happening in the Fertile Crescent. Even in France, where the courtly King Charlemagne (c.747–814) was an avid record-keeper, there is no mention of opium or the poppy. In contrast, the opium poppy and the horned poppy were being cultivated in the elegant Moorish gardens of southern Spain.[42]

Some Vikings also cultivated opium poppies, high in the north of Denmark at Viborg Søndersø (radiocarbon-dated to 1018–35), as well as its boon-companion, henbane.[43] Neither are native to the area, and their presence together indicates they had been acquired from somewhere with a population that had knowledge of Graeco-Roman medicine. The Scandinavian seafarers, although they left no written records, were more than capable of travelling the world to trade.

As the Norman Conquest brought a uniform kind of Christianity to Britain in the second half of the eleventh century, back in the East, the Byzantines were facing the military might of the Turks, and in 1095 Emperor Alexios I requested help from Pope Urban II. Catholic Christianity was dominant in Europe, and Britain was drawn under Latin influence, not only in relation to the Conquest, but also the papacy's missions to rid the north of paganism. Jerusalem had fallen to the Muslims in 637, during their rule in the Levant between 632 and 661, and the Vatican was finally feeling strong enough to make an attempt to reclaim the Holy City.

Pope Urban's call to arms affected everyone from peasants hoping to be absolved of their sins, to aristocrats coerced into political and social alliances. The Crusades, which lasted, intermittently, until 1487, had a profound effect on European culture, literature, religious and military life, bureaucracy, and domestic life for the those left behind. Over time, the nature of these campaigns changed from pilgrimage to highly organized military campaigns led by the Roman Catholic Church. The lure of the East, across all social classes, also meant the Crusades heralded a West–East exchange on a mass scale, and brought the new wave of Eastern medicine, that of Rhazes and Avicenna, back to north and west Europe. But first, in the words of Hippocrates, 'He who desires to practise surgery must go to war'.[44]

Before the Crusaders ever saw a battle, their journey presented a particular set of problems to western and northern European pilgrims. Many of them were from agrarian backgrounds, with little or no experience of living in cramped situations where maintaining supplies of clean drinking water and food was difficult, let alone fighting and sustaining injuries. Diseases of the immune system, such as leprosy, were common, as was venereal disease. Other more mundane yet agonizing ailments, such as skin problems and haemorrhoids, occurred with tedious frequency, as in any population.

At the start of the Crusades, the most skilled physicians were among the Franks, the people united in western Europe under Charlemagne, in the area that would eventually become France and Germany. These men, each known as a *cyrugicus*, were more like general healers who could also operate. The medical schools at Salerno, Montpellier, Bologna, Padua and Paris were already established, and provided expensive though comprehensive education for those who could afford it. Graduates were called *medicus*, and they were few and far between on Crusade, but the written records that remain are associated with these high-status men. Later on, in the latter part of the thirteenth century, came the *physicus*, with a high level of theoretical knowledge, but mainly educated in the liberal arts, and many of the *physicus* on campaign were clergy. The rather more grisly *rasorius*/barber and *sanguinator*/bloodletter were numerous, and probably more useful. Apothecaries only appear on Crusade in the thirteenth century, meaning drugs would have been carried by the doctor, or purchased by troops along the route.[45] The evolution of this hierarchy in just over a century shows how Crusaders were rapidly understanding the variety of medical providers required by such a sustained campaign. The last such large-scale military movement across Europe had been by the Roman army, which maintained an excellent diet, high standards of personal hygiene, and a rigorous level of fitness. The Romans were also career soldiers, picked out at an early age, trained, and disciplined, bearing little resemblance to the tens of thousands of peasants and clergy, as well as the 'adulterers, murderers, thieves, perjurers and robbers . . . even the feminine sex' who set out from western Europe on the First Crusade in 1096–7.[46]

The trek across Europe towards Jerusalem, in the company of so many like-minded if occasionally shifty companions, must have been an extraordinary experience. Besides the sights and smells, the animals and sheer exoticism that abounded, there was also the reality that at some stage they would have to fight. Some of these battles were bloody, such as one in February 1098 during the Siege of Antioch: 'Wound after wound was inflicted and the fields were red with blood. You could see torn entrails, severed heads, headless bodies, corpses everywhere.'[47] These dramatic accounts were often written as religious propaganda tools, on both sides, but Crusaders did sustain serious injuries, such as blade blows amputating arms on the field, broken backs and jaw fractures.[48] For the doctors and surgeons working in these conditions, Galen's centuries-old work on dissecting pigs, dogs and monkeys came into its own. The weapons used at close quarters included swords, daggers and maces, and there were also bows and arrows, and crossbows, resulting in punctures and flesh wounds, with the attendant infections.

Extant accounts and medical texts from the early period of the Crusades indicate that European doctors used very few pain-killing agents or anaesthesia, and not that often. In the face of such severe wounds, the idea of no pain relief is horrifying, and the details of disease and afflictions suffered by the European pilgrims of the First Crusade leaves the impression of a dysentery-ridden, scurvied and scarred horde.

The Jerusalem-born chronicler William of Tyre (1130–86), who became ambassador to the Byzantine Empire, was certainly familiar with opium. In his *History of Deeds Done Beyond the Sea*, written towards the end of his life, he mentions the dominance of Egypt in terms of opium: 'the best opium ever discovered originated there and it is called "Theban" by physicians'.[49]

A contemporary of William of Tyre, the rabbi and doctor Moses Maimonides (1139–1204) was expelled from Spain as a child, and eventually settled in Fustat in Egypt. He became the personal physician to Saladin (1137–93), first sultan of Egypt and Syria, and founder of the Muslim–Kurdish Ayyubid dynasty. Maimonides wrote on the use of *diryaq*, an opium-based equivalent of theriac, in his *Treatise on Poisons and Their Antidotes*, which was used well into the Renaissance as one of the first works on toxicology. Maimonides' works also included a *Glossary of Drugs*, containing a comprehensive opium commentary, and the *Treatise on Asthma* in which an Almoravid ruler of Morocco dies when dosed inappropriately with *diryaq* during an attack.[50]

The issue of medical negligence was addressed in a ground-breaking set of documents written shortly after Maimonides' death, known collectively as the *Assizes of Jerusalem*. They were transcribed in Acre, and tell of a physician killing the servant of a client through ignorance. After a page or so of legalese, some sympathy is finally summoned for the lot of the servant's wounds, cuts, swellings, and broken head. A short passage refers to 'a powder or strong herb to drink' for the treatment of 'bowel disease', which if the servant 'drinks it and dies, reason judges him liable, in reason and law, to pay compensation'.[51] This is unlikely to be anything other than opium.

A New Centre of Learning: Western Europe

The 200-year period of the Crusades witnessed many changes in western European society. The thirteenth century was the start of a rise in Europe's high-status medical schools. Increasingly, medicine was a primary occupation for young men, rather than a secondary occupation for gentlemen, and occasionally women. Hersende, of Fontevrault Abbey in France, was appointed *maîtresse médecin* to King Louis IX on his Crusade to Egypt of 1248–50.[52]

Out on the Crusade route to Jerusalem, the hospitals that existed were used to cater more to the elderly and the chronically ill. The massive influx of exhausted, malnourished pilgrims, rife with sores, pests and stomach bugs, was a rude shock. Into this fray stepped the Order of the Knights of St John of Jerusalem, the Knights Hospitaller. The knights were a Roman Catholic military order, dedicated to St John the Baptist, based in Jerusalem, Rhodes and Malta. Founded around 1023, with the specific purpose of caring for the pilgrims who were flooding in increasing numbers to the Holy Land, the European recapture of Jerusalem in 1099 from the Muslims saw the order gain its own papal charter: charged with the care and defence of the Holy Land.

The Byzantines, meanwhile – in contrast to the monk-healer tradition of Gondeshapur to the east – had been severing the links between healthcare and religious obligation for some time, possibly as early as the sixth century, by removing monks from the wards and employing laypeople instead.[53] The secular doctors worked every other month, using their time off for private practice. The Pantokrator Hospital in Constantinople employed female doctors and nurses, and had a comprehensive staff including druggists, instrument sharpeners, priests, cooks, latrine cleaners and pallbearers.[54] These hospitals were working a scale unthinkable for the religious hospitals of western Europe. The collected Knights Hospitaller wards in Jerusalem could take 1,000 inpatients at a time, and 750 when it had to after a battle; their hospital even had an ambulance service, the ancestor of today's voluntary St John's Ambulance Service at community events in Britain.[55]

In contrast, the first recorded Crusader field hospital was at Acre, which in 1189–91 sustained the worst losses for the Christians in the history of the Crusades, and Germanic sailors assembled what was probably little more than a triage hut made from broken ships and sail canvas.[56]

No accounts of what went on inside these hospitals remain, but the things seen there – the surgeries and treatments – were taken back to the West by patients and doctors when they returned from the Crusades.

Scuola Medica Salernitana, the medical school at Salerno where both men and women attended classes, was founded perhaps as far back as the ninth century, at roughly the same time as the one in Baghdad. It had a stunning setting, inside the dispensary of a Christian monastery. In 1063, Alphanus of Monte Cassino, returning from pilgrimage to Jerusalem, arrived to teach there. Well connected and highly literate, Alphanus attracted a number of others who had also travelled widely in the East, and in Africa and India. They worked on translations of Avicenna and other influential Arabic writers, and on improving the teaching element of the school. Alphanus' *Premnon physicon* is the first surviving work in Europe that mentions opium.

In 1077, Constantine Africanus, a North African Muslim convert to Christianity, arrived at the school and began teaching students. His career there is now regarded as the start of Salerno's peak period. He translated works from the House of Wisdom in Baghdad, which were then sent to the schools at Bologna, Padua and Paris, as well as Oxford and Cambridge. One of the most famous is the *Liber isogogarum*, containing instructions for identifying opium overdoses. At a similar time, Trotula, later known and referred to by Chaucer as 'Dame Trot' in 'The Wife of Bath's Tale', was working on obstetrics at Salerno. She advocated the use of opium for various female complaints, including childbirth, and after childbirth if the womb ached, and the direct application of opium to the vagina in cases of sexual frustration.[57]

Salerno's combination of surroundings, religion and medical treatment meant that many sick and disabled people made pilgrimages to the school, and a series of scholars elevated the practice of medicine there. The school's most famous teacher is Theodoric Borgognoni (1205–c.96). Theodoric's father, Hugh of Lucca, was a well-known surgeon who had served in Egypt on the Fifth Crusade and tutored his son in medicine. Theodoric came to Salerno, and was certainly there in the 1260s, where he worked on perfecting anaesthesia using the *spongia somnifera*, or soporific-sponge method. In his most important work, the *Cyrurgia*, he includes the recipe, again including *Hyoscyamus niger*, or henbane, and credits his father, so it's possible that Hugh learned of the technique while in Egypt.

take of opium and the juice of unripe mulberry, Hyoscyamus, the juice of spurge flax, the juice of leaves of mandragora, juice of ivy, juice of climbing ivy, of lettuce seed and of the seed of lapathum which has hard round berries and of the shrub hemlock, one ounce each. Mix these together in a brazen vessel then put it into a new sponge. Boil all together out under the sun until all is consumed and cooked down onto the sponge. As often as there is need, you may put the sponge into hot water for an hour and apply it to the nostrils until the subject falls asleep. Then the surgery may be performed and when it is completed, in order to wake him up, soak another sponge in vinegar and pass it frequently under his nostrils.[58]

Theodoric Borgognoni also believed that a wound generating pus was unhealthy, and that instead of sticky poultices and ointments, wounds and sores should be washed with wine and kept dry. He wrote on elective surgeries, such as the procedure for haemorrhoids. The repeated mention of this awkward subject in medical texts throughout the centuries seems something of a preoccupation, yet for the sufferer of this common malady, the difference between a successful operation and a botched one is incalculable. The Arab surgeons had dwelled upon it, and al-Zahrawi, known as Abulcasis (936–1013), had devised a technique perfected by Theodoric 300 years later. The account is, quite simply, agonizing, as Theodoric explains in detail the way to grapple, literally, with these painful nuisances. Yet it is also an illuminating account of what it was like to be a patient undergoing elective surgery in the late twelfth century.[59] Borgognoni is the father of evidence-based medicine, a modern term for a very old concept. For the Graeco-Roman doctors such as Galen and Hippocrates, the philosophy of medicine was as important as the practice of it, but for men such as Rhazes, Avicenna and then Borgognoni, emphasis had clearly shifted to empiricism and the long-term welfare of the patient, something that began in the Islamic golden age. This rational, practical approach became widespread across Europe

with the many translations of Theodoric's *Cyrurgia* into vernacu-
lar languages such as Catalan.[60] The Salerno school also published a small manuscript called the *Regimen sanitatus salernitan-
um*, or the *Salerno Regimen of Health*, which was written in simple
rhymes and aphorisms, so that people could remember the recipes for medicines, and contained a variety of uses for opium. It
was still in use 200 years later when printing presses meant that
it could be distributed even further, with translations into Latin,
Hebrew and Arabic, by which time the power balance in the
exchange of knowledge shifted.

Salerno was rapidly superseded by Bologna, Padua and the
new medical schools at Paris, where medicine was studied as
part of an instruction in the liberal arts, and at Montpellier,
where a medical school opened around 1220, and which by 1300
was one of the most important teaching centres in the world.

Merchants of Venice: The Travels of Marco Polo

By the latter part of the thirteenth century, much of western
Europe had tired of the Crusades disrupting their lives and revenues, let alone that of their workforces. The emphasis had
returned to trade, and the city states of Italy, such as Pisa, Genoa
and Venice, were rising to dominance.

Italy's city states, while not unique in Europe, together consti-
tuted a power unrivalled anywhere in the world. In part, this was
a legacy of the order put in place by the Romans, which allowed
the administration of large cities; part of it was due to an improvement in farming and climate, meaning there was sufficient food
to supply these urban centres; and part of it was a rise in trade
and commerce. Instead of the absolute monarchies elsewhere in
Europe, these city states were merchant republics, home to mobile,

adaptable and commercial people. One of the great strengths of these city states were their guilds. Focussed on the prominent trades of the time, such as goldsmithing, spices, fishmongery, salt and iron, as well as painting and drapery (cloth and silk-working), the guilds provided protection for their members, as well as for the consumer, stabilized urban markets and provided a close-knit network from which lines of credit could be extended to guilds or merchants in other cities. In the earliest guild records, opium falls under the category of a spice, and was dealt with by guilds who called themselves grocers. Venice had a particularly strong and early guild system, with a very different set of merchants than other city states, with some fifty separate guilds by the late twelfth century, reflecting the diversity and quantity of the trade there.[61]

Some of these merchants were also adventurers, such as the Polos of Venice. They are certainly the most well documented, with over 150 early manuscripts of Marco's tales of his travels and some 2,000 devoted to the family as a whole. Niccolò and Maffeo Polo were brothers and merchants from Dalmatia who came to Venice, where Niccolò's son Marco was born, before they embarked on an epic journey east in the late 1250s. As Italy's city states had organized themselves into individual, closeted republics, in north-east Asia Genghis Khan (1162–1227) had trampled all those who stood in his way to create the Mongol Empire, which covered most of Eurasia. Various accounts of the travels of the senior Polos cast them as diplomats and missionaries as well as merchants, but what is certain is that they were determined to make their fortunes. They lived for a time in the Venetian enclave of Constantinople, taking advantage of the quasi-diplomatic immunity of its guild system, before moving to Sudak in Crimea in 1260. Sudak at the time was part of the newly formed Mongol kingdom of the Golden Horde, and in time proved dangerous, so the brothers decamped for Bukhara, in what is now Uzbekistan.

Three years later, they joined a diplomatic mission from one grandson of Genghis Khan, Hulagu, to his cousin and another grandson, Kublai, the Great Khan (1214–94) at Cambulac, now Beijing. The grandsons were dissolving the empire of Genghis into rival khanates, which made the east of Asia lucrative, if also dangerous and not a little confusing at times, but the Polo brothers spoke Turkic and possessed steady nerves.

Hulagu's diplomatic party took the Polo brothers through Samarkand, then the Pamirs to Kashgar, and through the Gansu corridor to Changdu, the Great Khan's summer palace, known as Xanadu to later Europeans, where they were allegedly the first Italians to meet Kublai Khan, in 1264. The khan asked them to return to Italy with a Mongol ambassador, Cogotai, as envoys to the pope, to ask for oil from the lamp of Jerusalem's Holy Sepulchre, and a hundred men 'acquainted with the Seven Arts' – grammar, logic, rhetoric, arithmetic, geometry, music, astronomy – who could teach his people about Europe. Like many of the Mongol rulers he was largely indifferent to religion, but recognized its importance in bringing as many people and as much territory under his control as possible. This is reflected in his choice of Uyghur, the tongue of his most wide-ranging ethnic group, as the written language of his empire. The brothers were given some asbestos cloth as a gift for the pope, which could only be cleansed by fire, and a *gerege*, a tablet of gold one foot long by three inches wide, bearing the inscription 'By the strength of the eternal Heaven, holy be the Khan's name. Let him that pays him not reverence be killed.' In what became trademark Polo family style, they managed to shed the burden of ambassador Cogotai in some nameless town when he apparently became too ill to travel, and continued back to Venice as the khan's envoys to the pope. They arrived in 1269, having shown the *gerege* to ensure their safe, and fully expensed journey, and pausing to transact business along the way. What happened to the valuable asbestos cloth is unknown. In Venice they collected Niccolò's teenage son Marco, and then set out for China once more, this time as envoys of Pope Gregory X to the Great Kublai Khan.

There was often little distinction between diplomatic, religious and commercial missions to the steppes – a significant amount of the earliest Polo manuscripts are bound with Crusades treatises, for example – but the Polos were still opportunists of the first order and their ability to piggyback onto any useful party heading in the direction they wanted to go was remarkable. Marco was no different, and spent twenty-four years in the East, building a successful career for himself as 'the Latin' for Kublai Khan. He is frequently described as a provincial tax collector in later accounts, but it is more likely he ran some sort of salt monopoly and spent the majority of his time travelling to and from India on behalf of Kublai Khan. His descriptions of his time in service in China, though, are of less relevance to the history of opium than his journey through Central Asia, where he met a hundred-strong camel caravan carrying opium back to the West, and went on to relate the tale of the Old Man of the Mountain in the country of 'Mulehet', a story that he had heard from 'several natives of that region'.

The Old Man had 'caused a certain valley between two mountains to be enclosed, and had turned it into a garden, the largest and most beautiful that ever was seen ... for the Old Man desired to make his people believe that this was actually Paradise'. In this garden ran milk, honey and water, and young maidens played musical instruments 'for the delectation of its inmates'. At the entrance to this garden was a fortress, 'strong enough to resist all the world', and there the Old Man entertained 'a number of the youths of the country, from twelve to twenty years of age, such as had a taste for soldiering, and to these he used to tell tales about Paradise, just as Mahommet had been wont to do', but 'no man was allowed to enter the Garden save those whom he intended to be his ASHISHIN'. Those chosen were given a 'certain potion which cast them into a deep sleep, and then causing them to be lifted and carried in. So when they awoke, they found themselves in the Garden.'

As the Old Man had promised, life in the garden in the valley was very fine indeed, and all continued well until the Old Man needed an enemy dealt with, when 'he would cause that potion whereof I spoke to be given to one of the youths in the garden, and then had him carried into his Palace. So when the young man awoke, he found himself in the Castle, and no longer in that Paradise; whereat he was not over well pleased', which is understandable. The Old Man would then deliver the youth a promise: 'Go thou and slay So and So; and when thou returnest my Angels shall bear thee into Paradise. And shouldst thou die, nevertheless even so will I send my Angels to carry thee back into Paradise.' A ceremonial dagger was presented and the dutiful youth despatched to the target's, and usually his own, death.[62]

The Old Man of the Mountain legend is an early mention of suicide-terrorism, and its inclusion in Marco Polo's accounts of his travels meant that it spread rapidly far and wide, even before the age of print. Like almost all legends, Polo's Old Man is a scrambled version of fact and fiction. Hassan al-Sabbāh, a religious fanatic of the Nizari Ismaili sect – a branch of the minority, Shia Islam – is believed to have been the Old Man of the story, and from 1090 onwards in Alamut Castle, around sixty miles from modern Tehran, he created a fertile, terraced garden within a defendable valley from which to attack the Abbasid Caliphs and the invading Seljuk Turks. Polo's Mulehet was in Lebanon. Al-Sabbāh did indeed surround himself with young, male acolytes, a group of *fedayeen* willing to die for their beliefs at his order, but once inside the castle itself, there was little of paradise to be had. 'Ashishin', now taken to mean that the potion the youths drank to put them to sleep was made up from *Cannabis indica*, at the time often meant little more than lowlives.[63] Cannabis was widespread throughout Egypt by the ninth century and the Arab world by the eleventh, much to the disgust and fury of stricter members of the faith.[64] The transportation to paradise the youths felt is more akin to the opium experience than to that of cannabis, but a mixture of the two would have induced both visions and then a deep enough sleep to have allowed bodily transportation to some other place. It is strongly reminiscent of Jamšid's ancient *haoma*. They were also drugged when they went on their missions: a mixture of cannabis steadied them and an ephedra element kept them alert.

Owing to the inclusion of such legends, and frequent missteps and confusion, there is a great deal of speculation about how far Marco Polo actually journeyed. Some believe he never made it further than the Black Sea, that his travels are a compendium of his father's and uncle's adventures, and certainly there are inconsistencies, exaggerations and downright fabrications in his *Travels*.[65] Yet his description of Central Asia and the East is consistent both in terms of landscape and in what he met with there, and there are too many everyday details of life in the East for it to be a pack of lies. In particular, his detailed description of the paper money the Chinese used in larger trade transactions feels authentic, with his Venetian soul perturbed by such notions of trust and lack of coin.

His absence from extant Mongol texts may well mean he wasn't quite as important as he made himself out to be, and his absence from Chinese records is attributed to the tendency to lump the *Hsi-yu*, Westerners, together. Among those who believe the travels were genuine, the theories that Polo spent his time in Badakhshan, then as now a poppy-growing centre, as an opium addict seem improbable. His account of the clean air on the Roof of the World – and how 'men who dwell in the towns below, and in the valleys and plains', upon suffering a fever would come into the mountains for two or three days, and 'quite recover themselves through the excellence of that air' – fits entirely with his own experience of feeling well 'at once' after suffering for a year with a weak strain of malaria picked up on the journey.[66] It could also be that in an area already dominated by poppy-growing the local herbal medicines contained opium latex which stopped coughing immediately, thus effecting what seemed like a miraculous cure.

Most importantly, Marco Polo's stories may have been lost entirely, had he not on his return to Venice in 1295 involved himself in Venice's naval battle with Genoa a year later. Held prisoner until 1298, he is said to have formed a friendship with a fellow prisoner, the writer Rusticello, and after sending off to Venice for his travel notebooks, recounted the story of his, his father's and his uncle's travels. Upon his release, he married, had three daughters and died in 1324, a legendary adventurer in his own lifetime.

The Polo family's journeys also demonstrate the extent to which it was possible to travel the world, even in the thirteenth century, by both land and sea. Despite many diversions caused by war or shifting political alliances, they still managed to roam Central and South-East Asia, as well as Egypt and Turkey, using reliable and well-known, if perilous, routes. In the next three centuries, these routes were expanded to include a continent of such riches even the Polos would not have believed, triggering a lift in global trade that truly did raise all ships, but there were many disasters to be overcome first – not least a scourging angel.

The Age of Discovery: Part One

Acre had fallen to the Muslims in 1291. The Crusades were over, and Europe stabilized quickly, allowing a new period of intellectual life to flourish. By the time Marco Polo died in 1324, Europe was looking forward to a period of prosperity. But the Silk Roads the Polo merchants had traded upon so successfully were harbouring something else that was eager to do business: plague.

The Black Death of 1346–53 killed anywhere between 30 per cent and 60 per cent of the European population, and estimates of the total deaths vary widely, from 75 million to 200 million people. *Yersinia pestis* came out of Central Asia in the early 1340s and swept west along the Silk Roads, and then covered almost all parts of western Europe by the mid 1350s.

The plague was devastating, but the sheer number of deaths had unexpected results. For many it raised wages and standards of living, and moved them off the land to towns and cities. The feudal system was challenged by the fact that suddenly it needed workers more than they needed it. The seeds of the middle classes were already starting to grow, particularly in the northern Low Countries, where the merchants of Antwerp and Amsterdam were becoming increasingly powerful. London, which had been a backwater in terms of European trade, was coming to prominence thanks to its busy port.

Opium, in the form of theriac and mithridate, made a return as one of the prime treatments plague doctors used to try and both guard against plague and to treat wealthier patients. As previously seen with the complicated leprosy medicines, how frightening a disease was can be measured in some sense through the number of ingredients in the medicine used to treat it. One plague theriac lists over seventy rare and expensive items, including 'viper's flesh, ground coral, balsam, pepper, rose water, sage, cinnamon, saffron, ginger, parsley, gum arabic, nasturtium, centaurea, storax, myrrh, and anis seed'.[67]

Because plague was so vicious, and struck so fast, theriac – with its preventative properties against poisoning and other ailments – underwent a revival. Its opium constituent was also effective against three of the main symptoms of plague: pain of the buboes and joint pain, coughing and purging diarrhoea. The preoccupation with health that was spurred by the Black Death brought in a new wave of interest in pharmacology and the work of the apothecary. In the great medical school of Paris, trade was highly regulated, which in turn spread out across France. In Europe in general, opium was regulated as early as the thirteenth century, and a study of the few existing inventories of apothecary shops showed opium was dispensed from fourteen out of twenty-four shops in Provence, three out of five in Aragon and seven out of eighteen in Italy.[68]

Papaver somniferum had become a fixture of the medieval herbarium, and was grown, often in some quantity, in the gardens of religious and private houses. Merton Priory in south London grew opium poppies, as well as other medicinal drugs including henbane, black nightshade and hemlock.[69] And in Oxford, the head of Merton College had a medicine garden by his house which grew opium poppies, and possibly also cannabis. Cannabis seeds, shattered as if to prepare them for use, were found when the site was excavated, along with greater celandine, hemlock, henbane and mint. The garden also contained a wide range of decorative shrubs and plants, reminiscent of the beautiful garden of the House of the Golden Bracelet in Pompeii. Opium poppy and hemp seeds were also found in the rubbish pit of the thirteenth-century house, showing that they had actually been used. The same plants, particularly the opium poppy, greater celandine, hemlock and henbane, were discovered in the garden of the nearby Dominican priory.[70] Opium even formed part of the gardens of the Fleet Prison in London, along with cannabis.[71]

Plague also had the effect of increasing demand for doctors. There were some superb doctors working at the time of the plague, such as Frenchman Guy de Chauliac (1300–68), who studied in Bologna and practised in Lyons. Deeply influenced by the works of Galen and Avicenna, Chauliac was based in Avignon when the plague swept across western Europe. Unlike many other physicians, he chose to stay and attempted to treat the sick. His accounts of the plague ravaging the population divide it quite clearly into two different types: pneumonic 'with continuous fever and spitting of blood; and death occurred within three days'; and bubonic, 'with continuous fever, and with ulcers and boils in the extremities, principally under the arm-pits and in the groin; and death took place within five days'. Chauliac wrote that he had caught bubonic plague himself but recovered, 'by the Grace of God'. He is also known for inducing unconsciousness in patients about to undergo surgery by compressing a nerve trunk in the neck. However, he was aware that this method wouldn't work in all cases, and that if the surgery was so painful it would put the patient's life at risk, then they should be medicated with opium first. A modern experiment to recreate Chauliac's anaesthetic showed that if he were using *Papaver somniferum* latex of the same strength, his dose would have been 194 mg, which would have rendered the patient unconscious for some considerable time, and could easily have overwhelmed an unaccustomed user or a child.[72] He did, however, have great success with anaesthesia, although his recipe for sore eyes – opium mixed with 'womanis mylke' – was perhaps less effective.[73]

Method of delivery was pivotal in early anaesthesia. The somniferous sponge required a delicate touch to avoid suffocating the patient with a mixture of drugs that would make them stop breathing, giving the anaesthetist's role a prominence it retains today. English medical texts of the period, and up to the time of Shakespeare, refer to an anaesthetic drink 'that men call *dwale* to make a man sleep whilst men cut him'.[74] Dwale was a recipe that, unlike European sleeping draughts, remained remarkably consistent in terms of ingredients, which can be divided into two groups: harmless, and potentially dangerous. Pigs' bile, bryony root, lettuce and vinegar added a herbal aspect and bitterness, while hemlock juice, opium poppy latex and henbane were the active ingredients. Small amounts of these potential killers were boiled up with half a gallon of wine and bottled until needed. The dwale recipe is of particular interest because of its inclusion of the large amount of wine that the patient drank, sitting next to a good fire until they fell asleep. The wine would have been rendered foul by the bile, bryony and vinegar, and most of the alcohol boiled off, so the effects were narcotic rather than alcoholic. The combination of hemlock with opium and henbane in half a gallon of wine would probably have proved fatal to patients on a regular basis, but the unpleasantness of the medicine, coupled with the rapid effects of hemlock and the more lasting effects of opium and henbane in the case of dwale, would have put them into a state of unconsciousness relatively quickly. Most importantly, the dwale was self-administered and the patient was controlling the dose. Probably for this reason, dwale was relied upon not only by physicians, but also as a folk remedy.

An almost exact contemporary of Chauliac, John of Arderne (1307 to after 1377) was an English physician who used a version of the dwale recipe to become one of the most influential surgeons of the age. England was lagging behind the rest of Europe in terms of medicine at this time, and relying heavily on the moralistic teachings of the early Christian church with regard to medicine. Ill health was caused by moral failings, and such non-sensical statements as 'Every cure is brought about either by the use of contraries or by the use of similars' were accompanied by 'as a chilling disease is treated with heat, or a dry one with mois-ture, just as also it is impossible for pride to be cured except it be cured by humility'.[75]

Arderne, although very much a man of his time in terms of politely crediting God for his success, was a shrewd political and financial operator as well as a practical surgeon. His speciality was treating the anal fistula, an exceptionally painful and debilitating condition for anyone, especially for a society of businessmen and aristocrats who spent a lot of time in the saddle. The surgeries he describes in his masterwork *Fistula in ano* (1376) are painful to read, let alone undergo, but again show the importance these elective procedures had acquired. Arderne had spent time at the Siege of Algeciras against the Moors (1342–4), where gunpowder and cannon had been used against men for the first time, and the horrors that he saw there were still impressed upon his mind thirty years later as he collated his masterwork. Such wounds, as well as the day-to-day miseries of men on the march or in the saddle, inspired him to find effective methods of pain relief. His anaesthetic for surgery contained mandragora and Egyptian opium, when it was available, rendered down into pigs' fat and then rubbed on the patient's palms, temples, chest, armpits and soles of the feet. He lost around half of his patients during or after surgery, due to his ointment, shock or post-operative infec-tion, but when he effected a cure he was so successful he was in great demand. His charges for surgery were on a sliding scale: for the wealthy, he charged £40, almost £30,000 in 2017, and for middling people, a hundred shillings, the equivalent of about £3,500.[76] Arderne is most famous for anaesthesia and proctology, but along with his mandragora and opium recipe is a note for an

insomnia cure, featuring pills made of opium and rosewater, 'and
he þat takeþ þem shal slepe for certayne'.[77]

The early part of the Renaissance, from 1300 onwards, brought
men such as Arderne to the fore of medicine and a new, practical approach to medicine and pharmacology, as well as pain
and surgery, had arrived. The old superstitions regarding the four
humours still persisted, but the new bourgeois classes of Europe
were increasingly looking for answers as to what ailed them,
and medieval surgeons knew that if their profession was to make
significant progress, they needed to study anatomy. Galen's monkeys would no longer do. Secular dissection appears first in Italy
and dates from 1286, when an outbreak of avian flu killed large
numbers of hens and people in Cremona, Piacenza, Parma and
Reggio, and the authorities wanted to know why. By 1300, the
university at Bologna had added dissection to the curriculum,
although private autopsies in the subject's home were more common. The prevailing view has long been that people before the
modern era had an overwhelming disgust and fear of having
their bodies analysed post-mortem, but records from Italy indicate this isn't necessarily true. In medieval Florence, Bartolomea
Rinieri's husband recorded that she had died in the morning
aged 'forty-two or thereabouts', of a diseased womb, and had asked
him 'to have her autopsied so that our daughter or others could
be treated'.[78] Bartolomea's request was not as unusual as might
be imagined, and as long as funerary rites were respected, the
body would be accepted for a church burial. The church was
slowly having to relinquish its hold on medicine.

When Marco Polo died in 1324, he willed '5 lire to every Congregation in Rialto, and 4 lire to every Guild or Fraternity of
which I am a member', finally putting God a whole lire above
business.[79] This is a simple demonstration of how important the
guild system was to Venetian merchants, and not just in Venice.

Across Europe, the commercial guilds that began to coalesce in ports and cities in the twelfth century had become forces to be reckoned with in all spheres of urban life. In Florence, nuns and monks, such as those associated with the Farmacia Santa Maria Novella (founded 1221), dominated in the thirteenth century, creating and selling herbal medicines and medicinal secrets, but in 1313, the Arte dei Medici et Speziali – the Guild of Physicians and Apothecaries – was formed to regulate its members and promote their own interests, pushing the religious houses to the edge of commercial life. They were soon dominating town councils and church congregations. Committed to bettering themselves, their trades and their neighbourhoods and cities, they were the beginning of the urban middle classes. For physicians and apothecaries, the guilds were particularly important: they not only regulated and promoted the trades, they served to disseminate knowledge and raise standards internally. Quality spot checks were not unusual, such as the testing of merchandise and calibrating of scales for apothecaries. In terms of opium, the guilds were a vector for keeping high-quality Eastern opium latex in demand, thus ensuring supply. The Medici family made sure their own needs were met by having a retail druggist's shop of their own, fittingly also called Medici, specializing in opium and other prestigious preparations, and run by Piero de' Rossi & Co.

As the careers of physicians and apothecaries became more clearly delineated, more regulated and highly respected, the moveable-type printing press was developed in Strasbourg by Johannes Gutenberg between 1440 and 1455. This led to a rush of manuals, dictionaries and treatises on medicine, as well as every other subject of interest in the Renaissance. *El Ricettario* (1499) was Florence's famous contribution to medical recipe books, and it was declared to be a book that 'no household should be without'. Such publications in turn led to more interest in all of these subjects from both professionals and literate laypeople. More students pursued a medical career, creating a shortage in cadavers available for study, leading medical establishments and physicians to request the bodies of executed criminals to further their studies.

Gabriele Falloppio (1523–62), one of the finest anatomists of his time, euthanized at least one criminal in order to dissect his body, the details of which are not only grisly but central to opium's mechanism: 'The Grand Duke of Tuscany ordered a man to be given over to us, for us to kill as we wished and then dissect. I gave him two drams [i.e. drachm] of opium, but he suffered from quartan fever, and its crisis halted the effect of the drug. The man, exulting, asked that we give him a second dose, so that if he did not die, we would intercede for a pardon with the duke. I gave him another two drams of opium, and he died.'[80] The bout of malaria the subject suffered had halted the effect of the drug, indicating that the body had metabolized the opium thus preventing an overdose, but two drachms – a quarter of an ounce – is a huge single dose, and four fatal.

The Swiss-German philosopher and chemist Philippus Aureolus Theophrastus Bombastus von Hohenheim, or Paracelsus (1493–1541), was active at almost the same time as Falloppio. After an extraordinary youth during which his physician father educated him in medicine, botany and natural philosophy, he became an army surgeon and travelled Germany, France, Hungary, Scandinavia and Russia, and possibly made it as far as Constantinople.

Paracelsus was one of the foremost minds in an age of polymaths such as Vesalius and Leonardo da Vinci; his lasting legacy has been in mineralogy and chemistry rather than the medicine he practised in his lifetime. He was also condemned as a quack and a sorcerer who was in league with the Devil, comparable to Faustus. However, his medical legacy was to change the use of opium in western Europe forever. He introduced a preparation of the drug known as *laudanum*, or tincture of opium heated with alcohol, from the Latin *laudabilis* meaning 'praiseworthy'. Evaporated and made into pills, he called it his 'stone of immortality'.[81] He referred to laudanum as an arcanum, or secret, to be relied upon over all other drugs to cheat death, playing on opium's ability to relieve both pain and fear.

The combination of opium with alcohol was nothing new. From the ancient world to the dwale recipes, they were commonly used together, but owing to his expertise in chemistry, Paracelsus enhanced opium's effects through heating it gently in alcohol. The pills he created were soon in great demand, and played into the revival of mystery of alchemy that was underway in the sixteenth century. He combined sophisticated chemistry with contemporary superstitions to create a medicine that became a legend. Laudanum marked a moment of huge change for opium consumption. It made the product more reliable and effective, and for the first time, moved towards standardized doses that could be prepared by an apothecary. With the proliferation of print culture at the same time, it was soon featuring in catalogues, medicine treatises and handbooks.

The demand for opium in Europe was firmly established by the middle of the sixteenth century, and not only among the elite classes to which it had previously been prescribed by physicians. But supply lines from the East were increasingly shaky, as the rise of the Ottoman Empire dominated and disrupted overland routes into Europe. Further east, the Indian Mughal Empire was starting to expand, causing even more trouble for the old Silk Road traders. To meet Europe's demand for the exotic, merchants had to find a new way to trade with the East; and they took to the seas.

Chapter Three

THE SILVER TRIANGLE AND THE CREATION OF HONG KONG

The Age of Discovery: Part Two

The progress made by science and medicine in the late medieval period was matched by achievements in seafaring, navigating and exploration, and international trade. The Hanseatic League was founded in Lubeck in 1159 by a group of like-minded merchants with interests in the Baltic, where Germany's sudden dominance of the northern seas in the thirteenth century achieved great importance in such a short time that it surprised even its own members. Initially, the goods the league dealt in, primarily timber, hemp, resin, waxes, furs and basic crops such as wheat and rye, were profitable but limited. *Kontors*, or offices, for the Hansa were formed in London, Bruges, Bergen and as far away as Novgorod in Russia. Despite a conservative outlook and constant infighting, the league and its associated guilds established a strong and far-reaching interdependent trade network in the north that would come to fruition in later centuries.

In the southern Mediterranean, the importance of sea trade to the city states was already well established and the maritime republics of Italy held the monopoly over trade with the East. A new age had begun, that of discovery, when various European countries including Portugal, Spain, Holland and England used new sea routes to explore and subsequently control vast territories. Goods, however, still made relatively short journeys before they were exchanged and further profits added by middlemen. The Ming dynasty came to power in China in 1368, and began to shut down the borders with their parts of the Silk Roads network as they pursued, once again, isolationist policies, and a revival of what they felt was the cultural heritage they had lost under Mongol rule. In eastern Europe, the Ottoman Turks had overcome the Balkans at the time of the plague to become the dominant force both there and in the Levant. European merchants, if they were to thrive, needed to establish the most direct routes to the luxury commodities their markets still clamoured for.

Advances in shipbuilding and design, as well as navigation, came suddenly but not out of the blue. The galley trade of the Mediterranean was all very well over short distances, as it allowed independence from the wind, but the ships were unwieldy and feeding the large number of men they required was unsustainable over long distances. The Portuguese, in the course of fighting with the Moors of North Africa, had become increasingly familiar with middleweight, nimble craft and so they looked to the East for a new way to build.

The ships that had plied their trades across the Indian Ocean to Egypt for centuries were called dhows by Europeans (the Arabs called them *baghla* or mules), and they came in many forms and sizes. Built mainly from teak, and weighing up to 200 tons, they had a deep keel and were held together tightly with nails, an idea they had borrowed from European ships. The largest cargo dhows had a double keel filled with lime and crushed coral which set like cement to provide ballast. Sturdy and fast, they were rigged with lateen – triangular – sails and could, to an extent, beat into the wind, unlike European ships. By the early fifteenth century, the Portuguese had created their own hybrid of the European galleon, the African fishing boat, and the dhow, called the caravel. With a low bow, no clumsy castle structures fore and aft, and lateen-rigged throughout, it was the perfect ship for exploration and coasting. It could navigate the open seas to open up new trade channels, and could also access estuaries and inlets in order to actually make the trades. The Infante Dom Henrique, later better known as Henry the Navigator (1394–1460), was also obsessed with finding the kingdom of Prester John, which had eluded Europeans in India, and was subsequently thought to lie somewhere in Africa. Henry was twenty-one when in 1415 the Portuguese took their first colony, Ceuta, on the North African coast opposite Gibraltar. The gold that arrived there on trans-Saharan caravans was of great interest to the Portuguese.

Portuguese caravels, swiftly copied by the Spanish, began to explore the seas surrounding them. Portugal quickly found Madeira and the Azores and began to work down the west coast of Africa. Iberian trade with Africa had been firmly established since the Middle Ages: the *Catalan Atlas* of 1375 was created by Abraham de Cresques of the Mallorcan Jewish community, and shows detailed knowledge of these Saharan trade routes, which worked on complex commodity exchanges of gold, slaves and Maldivian cowrie shells in place of coin. Because the trans-Saharan routes worked in such a long and convoluted way, by the time goods found their way to West Africa from the East African coast, there was little the Portuguese could offer that the West Africans wanted, so they had to find alternative ways to make their maritime adventures down the coast pay, and in capturing back their own men who had been taken by pirates and then sold to African slave merchants, they were introduced to a new large-scale commercial proposition altogether. Slavery, it became apparent, was very profitable.

The early fifteenth century was a time of sea exploration not only for Portugal and Spain, but also for China. From 1405 until 1433, the Chinese-Muslim military commander, admiral and eunuch Zheng He explored the routes to India, Indonesia, Egypt, Arabia and the east coast of Africa. He did so with a massive fleet numbering 317 ships and some 28,000 crew, by the command of the Yongle Emperor, who wished to impose Chinese control over the Indian Ocean trade.[1] The ships included some up to 400 feet long, as well as specialized water-carriers and others that were floating stables for the cavalry, one of which ended up housing giraffes brought back from Africa.[2] Although he was not a true explorer, one of Zheng He's most significant legacies was the opening up of Malacca in Malay. He died at sea on the 1433 voyage, and the successor to the Chinese Empire, the Xuande Emperor, stopped the expeditions as they did not sit well with isolationist policy. Zheng He's missions were largely erased from Chinese historical records and the Confucianist bureaucrats regained control from the powerful faction of eunuchs at the Chinese court. The very real potential for complete Chinese dominance of the eastern oceans was no longer a possibility.

Meanwhile, the Portuguese were making huge progress. In 1434 they succeeded in rounding the dangerous Cape Bojador on the West African coast, and started to bring back gold from Guinea, boosting their economy and that of neighbouring Spain. Making sure to build coastal forts to protect their new interests, they continued to explore and in 1444 navigated Cap-Vert, meaning they had managed to bypass the Sahara, a perilous overland obstacle. These longer journeys required bigger ships, more men and artillery, prompting another redesign of the fleet.

On caravels ordinary sailors slept on deck alongside a firebox for cooking and any artillery that was aboard. Placing heavy guns below deck was efficient, but reduced cargo capacity and slowed the ship down. The large three-masted caravel redonda emerged, as well as naus or carracks (which were slow but could carry large cargoes and were better at defending themselves than caravels) and, later, galleons for fighting pitched sea battles. This rapid evolution, copied immediately by the Spanish, ensured Iberian dominance of the oceans for a century.

In 1453 the Ottomans took Constantinople, and their control of the best East–West land route into Europe was complete. Yet after Henry's death, the African explorations fell into a slump through lack of funds, and the Crown sold off the interests to a group of merchants from Lisbon who were more than happy to exploit the trade in gold dust, ivory and slaves, and expanded the African trade privately. When John II, the Perfect Prince (1455–95), came to the throne in 1481 he was determined to retake the advantage for the Crown, and the following year established the Portuguese Gold Coast colony in 1482. He also invested in maritime expeditions and, in May 1488, Bartolomeu Dias rounded the southern tip of Africa, what he called the Cabo das Tormentas, or the Cape of Storms. The name was changed to the Cape of Good Hope, to represent the gateway to trade with the Indian Ocean, and the search for the ever-elusive Prester John. Returning home after a voyage of sixteen months, Dias helped design two ships, the *São Rafael* and the *São Gabriel*, that would change the history of the trading world. Across Europe, the race to reach the East by sea was underway.

Meanwhile, a westward route to the Indies was suggested in 1470 to the Spanish king, Alfonso. He rejected it, but a successful Genoese sailor picked up on it. After lobbying the various courts of the maritime nations, the enterprising Christopher

Columbus (c.1451–1506) finally secured support for a westward journey to the East Indies from Queen Isabella of Castile in 1492. Columbus, famously, had vastly underestimated the distance to Japan, and was unaware of the fact that the Americas lay in his path. He set out on 3 August 1492 with three ships and ninety men, and reached the Bahamas on 12 October. Columbus was, of course, an unmitigated disaster for the First Nation peoples he encountered, the people who 'got into the sea, and came swimming to us', each carrying a gift, but Columbus's tremendous miscalculation was the first of a series of events that changed the world.[3]

As Columbus sailed for Japan, sailor and navigator Vasco da Gama was defending Portuguese ships against the French. Portugal, at the behest of its king, John II, had been sending spies overland to Egypt, Africa and India to scout possible new trade routes. Coupled with what Dias had discovered on his 1488 expedition, the Portuguese were confident they could find a way to connect the two and bypass the troublesome Ottoman Turks. In the *São Rafael*, the *São Gabriel* and three other ships, da Gama set out for India on 8 July 1497 with 170 men, including his brother and the best Portuguese navigators of the time. They reached Calicut, India on 20 May 1498. On reaching the Malabar Coast, they were treated to the traditional lavish hospitality, upon which da Gama scraped together 'twelve pieces of lambel [a striped cloth], four scarlet hoods, six hats, four strings of coral, a case containing six wash-hand basins, a case of sugar, two casks of oil, and two of honey'.[4] The Malayali were distinctly unimpressed with these offerings, and the local, established Muslim merchants branded the Portuguese as opportunistic pirates rather than trade envoys. The return trip, badly planned and unlucky, saw the loss of half the hands, da Gama's brother amongst them, and two vessels of the fleet. Nevertheless, da Gama had

managed to purchase enough spices, including opium, to allegedly make a gross profit on his return to Portugal. Sick and
grief-stricken, it was four years before da Gama ventured to the
East Indies again.

Venice, tracking Spain and Portugal's movements closely, was
terrified that its control of the Levant would be undermined; as
the Venetian ambassador to Cairo said, da Gama's voyage would
be the 'causa de granda ruina del Stato Veneto'.[5] In 1502–3, da Gama
returned to India, and was far more successful commercially,
returning with 1,700 tons of spices, equivalent to Venetian
imports for an entire year.[6] But da Gama's second voyage was one
of conquest, with the intention of clearing the Indian Ocean of
Muslim competition for the spice market, and creating a Portuguese colony on the Malabar Coast. He failed, but the brutality
meted out to the Muslim populations he encountered made him
infamous in India, and unpopular in court circles on his return
to Portugal. The majority of Muslim merchants trading across
the Indian Ocean retrenched to Aceh, Sumatra, where they had
already established a stronghold.

In a state of near panic, Venice proposed building a Suez
Canal in 1504. It went nowhere. Although complicated navigable
networks had existed between the Red Sea and the Mediterranean before 1000, they'd fallen into disrepair because of the
territorial disputes over such a valuable tract of land. In the face
of Portuguese dominance, Venice was on the wane, and would
not be able to compete again for the best part of a century. The
decline of Venice profited one European city over all others.
Antwerp became the centre for the drug trade, and also diamonds, which were an increasingly important commodity as
they began to appear in abundance from India. Amsterdam also
benefitted, and both cities emerged as centres of wealth and
trade in the sixteenth century.

Opium was now classed as a part of the spice family by the merchants who dealt in it. Spices were both medicinal and culinary, much as they still are in India, and they were part of a complex commodities market that included gold, silver and copper coins, silk and linens, ambergris, borax, saltpetre, sugar, oils, nuts, dried fruits and living plants as well as myriad other items. The sheer scale of the opium trade alone is demonstrated by a letter from a Portuguese factor, Gonçalo Gil Barbosa, based in Cannanur (now Kunnar), north of Cochin on the Malabar Coast. Barbosa was part of a family in the service of the Duke of Braganza and was writing in 1503, when da Gama was already on his way back to Portugal, and recorded that a ship belonging to Coje Camaçedim, a Moorish merchant, had arrived carrying twenty *bahares* of opium, amounting to 8,400 pounds.[7] The ship was one of five that had left Aden for Cannanur, of which two were lost and two more had been forced to stop along the way for repairs. Such losses were not uncommon, and the quantities involved in a single shipment of one commodity to one private merchant give an idea as to the amounts of not only opium, but cloves, nutmegs, cinnamon, ginger and other spices that were circulating between the Indian Ocean, Asia and Europe. Families such as the Barbosas are unusual in that they were 'not noble', but they kept eloquent travelogues of their time on the trade routes, offering insights into the societies they encountered. Duarte, Gonçalo's brother, travelled the Red Sea route to the East, and made numerous references to the importance of the trade in opium, particularly from Aden, whose merchants dealt in 'gold, opium and diverse other things'.[8] He noted soon after how, in Moorish parts of Abyssinia, infant girls had been subject to genital mutilation: 'in this land the custom is to sew up the private parts of girls when they are born, and thus they continue until they are married, and made over to their husband then they cut the flesh again'.[9] Discoveries such as

these strengthened the early Portuguese and Spanish ideas that
the people they were trading with were savages, and the initial
Portuguese forays into trading in the East Indies were followed
up rapidly by military expeditions to take advantage of what they
saw as weaker nations. Da Gama's forces attempted a Malabar
armada and failed, but they captured Goa in 1510, and in 1511 they
sailed into Malacca on the Malaysian coast with 1,200 men and
took it as a Portuguese colony after forty days of fighting. The
capture of Malacca was a coup. Although the fortified port itself
was a nuisance to maintain and under threat from the displaced
sultan, it was also one of the few large, year-round harbours in the
Indian Ocean, and so had a constant stream of revenue. But the
Portuguese aggression in taking Malacca had serious repercussions in terms of trade with China, prejudicing Chinese
authorities against any further Portuguese incursions. As far as
long-term trade with south China was concerned, Portugal had
made a terrible error.

The Portuguese pressed on with their aggressive expansion in
Indonesia. In 1511, the first official embassy from Lisbon headed
out to Malacca, via India. Heading it was Tomé Pires, an apothecary and 'factor of the drugs', born in Lisbon around 1465.[10]
Pires was charged with taking Portuguese medicines out to
Malacca, and then securing other medicinal supplies when he
reached his destination. Pires's detailed descriptions of the trade
carried out at each place he visited indicate that opium was not
only a medicine, but a currency. It is mentioned in the same lists
as gold and silver, mercury, vermilion, horses and slaves, the only
drug to feature in them. Places are noted down as importers or
exporters, and the many tiny kingdoms of Burma and India were
notable exporters, their kings spending most of their time in
their harems, 'stupefied with opium'.[11] The Pires travel journal
is the first by a European to describe the Spice Islands – the

Moluccas – which had been converted to 'Muhammadanism' thirty years before. The Portuguese were interested primarily in cloves, and the Moluccas produced millions of pounds of them annually, harvesting them every two months. It was a source of potential revenue on an unimaginable scale, if the local people could be won away from the Muslim merchants – although this might prove difficult, as the native people were heathens: 'They are at war with each other most of the time. They are almost all related.'[12]

The Portuguese foray into Guangzhou, which they called Cantão, in 1516 resulted in a predictable diplomatic disaster, with many of their number eventually dying decades later, still prisoners in Chinese gaols, including Tomé Pires. But Portugal knew it had to pursue these new routes, for the Ottomans had taken Suez from the Mamluks in the same year with the clear intention of pushing east.

The tortuous completion of the Portuguese Magellan–Elcano expedition of 1521–2 proved that it was possible to circumnavigate the globe under sail, although only eighteen of the original 270 hands survived the journey.

On land, as at sea, the sixteenth century was a time of extraordinary change and innovation. In 1557, the Portuguese managed to negotiate an unlikely lease on Macao, situated on the west side of the Pearl River Delta about eighty miles south-west of Canton, as it had become known to the Europeans. This was not secured by their clumsy negotiating abilities, but by the fact that the Chinese Ministry of the Public Treasury was caught in something of a dilemma. In 1552, 800 exceptional virgins had been selected for Emperor Jiajing, and in 1554, he was still in need of an aphrodisiac potent enough to render him fit for such a monumental task. His doctors prescribed a recipe calling for quantities of ambergris, of which very little is found in China, but the Portuguese dominance of the seas meant they held a near monopoly on the grey, greasy product of the sperm whale's digestive tract, so sought after as a medicine and perfume fixative. This put them in a strong position to bargain for the land lease in Macao.

By 24 June 1571, the Spanish had captured Manila in the Philippines, the point at which trade with the East became highly integrated. Opium is listed with many hundreds of different commodities, ranging from glass beads and shells to gold and silver bullion and slaves, all of which were circulating around the world by the end of the century. The barbarity meted out in both the East and West Indies by the European conquerors – the *conquistadors* – was 'cruelty on a scale no living being has ever seen or expects to see,' wrote one eyewitness.[13] Yet both Portugal and Spain were in the midst of building a new history for themselves, one of empire and glory, of 'Sailing from the end of the Occident to the end of the Orient without seeing more than water and sky . . . a thing never attempted before by mortal man, nor ever believed possible.'[14]

Tea, Tobacco and Opium

'It is at the end of the monsoons, where you find what you want, and sometimes more than you are looking for.'[15]

Tomé Pires

For the Iberian navigators who first set out in the late fifteenth century, China and Japan were the ultimate destination. Columbus even carried a copy of Marco Polo's *Travels* with him in 1492. China, however, had its own problems. The Ming paper money Polo had written about had suffered a series of failures and was in terminal decline by the middle of the fifteenth century. Currency was a thorny issue, and China did not have enough silver or gold to create the high-value money it needed to operate over its vast territories, in terms of both commerce and taxation. Copper was the staple, but it was unsatisfactory and bulky, particularly with a taxable population that was rising rapidly. In 1500, the Chinese population was 155 million people, comprising just over 30 per cent of the world's population.[16] At the same date, the population of the Spanish Empire was 8.5 million, and the combined population of England and Wales was 2.25 million. For many Europeans, the scale of China was almost impossible to comprehend, but it also offered excellent commercial opportunities for anyone with ready stocks of cash in bullion. The Chinese also had a long history as sophisticated consumers of art and luxury goods, the kinds of luxury goods that newly wealthy Europeans coveted. Many of the early visitors to the South China Sea were private merchants, inspired by the journeys of Columbus and da Gama, and determined to try their luck. Their successes and failures went largely unrecorded, but the existence of Muslim, and later Christian *fanfangs* – foreign streets – inside coastal towns and cities indicate a significant local existence. Many traders on the streets were from South-East Asia and had been established in China's coastal region for decades. They too had problems obtaining enough silver currency to trade and Portuguese money was welcome, even if its merchants were only just tolerated. The Portuguese and the Spanish quickly realized that their silver money was worth a lot more in the Far East than it was at home. As soon as this news filtered back, more European privateers set sail for the South China Sea.

In 1526, the Iwami Ginzan silver mine was discovered on the main island of Japan by merchant Kamiya Jutei. It was

enormously productive, although there are no accurate early
records. Japan used this new money to deal with the Baltic for
fur, and from 1540 onwards, with China and then the Portuguese.
They also exchanged silver for gold, further complicating the
already sophisticated commodity markets of the area.

In 1545, on the other side of the world, the mining town of
Potosí was founded high in Bolivia's tin-belt mountain range.
Using more than 50,000 native workers, imported African slaves,
and countless mules and llamas to trek the precious metal to the
Pacific, by the end of the sixteenth century Potosí was producing
more than half the silver in the world: 254,000 kg out of a global
production of 418,900 kg.[17] Coupled with enormous production
from the hills to the north and west of Mexico City, Spain was
amassing wealth on incalculable levels. This silver arrived in the
East Indies via Chinese merchants who shipped it to Manila,
fuelling trade with outside merchants at a speed never seen
before.

These sea voyages brought unspeakable horrors to the people
of West Africa, the West Indies and South America. Local populations were decimated by cruelty and disease. Further examples
of botanical imperialism show just how huge these changes were
in a few decades. Crops unknown in China before the discovery
of the Americas, such as sweet potatoes, peanuts and maize, rapidly became staples for China's poor agricultural labourers. By
1538, less than forty years after Columbus's first voyage, peanuts
were already listed as a local product of Chang-shu county, near
Suzhou, west of Shanghai.[18]

China wasn't only importing commodities. The country was in
the grip of a series of dynastic wrangles that changed the course
of its history. Geography and global events were conspiring to
thwart Ming isolationism, even as it faced challenges from

within China itself. Therefore, they were surprisingly tolerant when the Jesuits arrived in China in 1582.

The Society of Jesus was already established in Japan, despite only arriving there two years earlier. China's long history meant that religious and secular traditions were muddled, and the Jesuits were prepared to overlook customs such as the veneration of ancestors, whereas the earlier Dominicans and Franciscan envoys pronounced indignantly that these heathen customs should be abolished. Understandably, the Chinese people of all classes were indifferent to what Rome had to say about their centuries-old customs.

The Jesuits flourished in Asia through their policies of tolerance and non-interference. Some of them even adopted Chinese dress. Matteo Ricci (1552–1610), a Jesuit missionary to Macao and cartographer, used the model of the Jesuits in Japan to avoid forcing European ideas on the Chinese. Through the influence of men such as Ricci, the Chinese viewed the Jesuits as collaborators rather than interlopers. Like his Jesuit counterpart in Japan, Alessandro Vaignanol, Ricci made every effort to learn the language and writing, although he was initially daunted by the task in front of him. Twenty years later, in 1602, he produced the first true map of the world combining Western and Eastern knowledge, and the first featuring both China and the Americas: the *Kunyu Wanguo Quantu*, or *Map of the Ten Thousand Countries of the World*. Ricci put China at the centre of his map, a diplomatic relations coup, although he did also label northern Russia as the land where tiny men and women rode into battle on goats, and described North Americans as people who 'kill one another all the year round, and spend their time in fighting and robbery. They feed exclusively on snakes, ants, spiders and other creeping things.'[19] There is also a delightful, although almost certainly apocryphal, story of an early draft of

Ricci's map featuring Europe in the centre. After an official enquired why this was, when surely China was the Middle Kingdom, Ricci retired to alter his map with a hasty cut and paste, and re-presented it with China in its rightful place, much to the satisfaction of the assembled dignitaries.

The *Kunyu Wanguo Quantu*, and Ricci's memoir of the Jesuit mission to Macao, *De Christiana expeditione*, initially published in Augsburg in 1615 and then in Antwerp and Amsterdam, were widely disseminated throughout Europe and studied eagerly by merchants wishing to do business in the South China Sea. Ricci's measured, pragmatic writing gives a strong sense of how he operated in China. Even on the tradition of foot-binding amongst young girls and women, a subject that was rapidly becoming politically and socially inflammatory throughout China, he noted simply, 'Probably one of their sages hit upon the idea to keep them in the house.'[20] This practical priest had moved the centre of the world from Europe to the Far East in more ways than one, with astonishing consequences.

By 1600, fuelled by this new prosperity and in no small part the crop imports, China had a population of 231 million. Meanwhile, the Dutch and English took advantage of a period of stability and prosperity to embark on their own worldwide naval explorations. To this end, they sent a number of private operators east to assess the situation. Ralph Fitch was a London merchant born around 1550 who travelled widely through India, Burma and South-East Asia in the 1580s. He is remembered primarily for bringing back the tale of the king of Thailand's white elephants, who lived in gilded stables and were dressed in cloth of gold, giving rise to the association of a white elephant with an expensive burden. In Burma, Fitch recorded the ready market for decent opium, and from Agra in India he was part of a fleet of 'one hundred and fourscore boates laden with Salt,

Opium, Hinge [asafoetida], Lead, Carpets, and divers other commodities'.[21] Fitch arrived back in London in 1597, more than eight years after he had left. In his absence, he had been declared dead and his will proved, but a new career awaited him, as an advisor to the East India Company.

The companies were a compromise between private merchant trade and the state. Various trading companies had been formed in England in the sixteenth century, such as the Muscovy Company in 1555, the Turkey Company in 1581 and the Levant Company in 1592. As far as China and the Spice Islands were concerned, the East India Company (EIC), founded at the end of 1600, and the Dutch Verenigde Oostindische Compagnie (VOC), founded in 1602, were of primary importance. Both benefitted significantly from the far-reaching infrastructure, trading protocols and maritime knowledge accumulated by the Hansa over the previous centuries. Spain and Portugal, meanwhile, were no longer in the ascendant, as they wasted their stupendous wealth on war and ceased to innovate at sea.

Although the VOC was created as an official entity slightly later than the EIC, the Dutch merchants were already trading with Indonesia by the 1590s, and reached China earlier than the English, who were using the EIC to reach the spices on the west coast of India. In 1600 a Chinese merchant – Wu Pu – returned from the East to Holland on a Dutch trading ship, and allowed himself to be publicly baptized at Middelburg.[22] He returned to the East as a VOC agent. It was the beginning of a century of heavy Dutch and English involvement in Eastern trade, which set the trend for their relationships with China and Indonesia for hundreds of years to come.

The English and Dutch companies differed in purpose at the beginning: the EIC was a merchant trading company, and the VOC was also a military organization determined to establish monopolies and to crush their Spanish and Portuguese competitors. In the sixteenth century, Holland had experienced a golden age of cartography including, crucially, the work of Flemish cartographer and globemaker Gerardus Mercator, who published the Mercator projection in 1569. The Mercator projection is a cylindrical world map that, despite its inaccuracies at extreme latitudes, was effective as a marine chart, and well suited to use on board ships. This level of knowledge, coupled with their maritime power, meant that the Dutch established their trade networks with the East rapidly, after the foundation of the VOC. In April 1621, they arrived in the Banda Islands. The Portuguese had tried to do business with the Spice Islands for over a century, dropping anchor periodically beneath the smoking volcano of Gunung Api. They found the native people so difficult to deal with that in the end they contented themselves with buying their nutmeg from intermediaries in Malacca. Not so the Dutch. A group of five islands of the Banda archipelago were the only known producers of nutmeg and mace in the world, and the Dutch were determined to have the monopoly.

Nutmeg in particular was thought to have special medicinal properties, and it is a potent natural anti-inflammatory. In sufficient quantities raw, it is also a powerful hallucinogen, and by the early seventeenth century the rich opium eaters of Bengal were consuming cocktails of opium, nutmeg, mace, cloves, Borneo camphor, ambergris and musk to enhance the effect of their high.[23] Essentially, this was just a mixture of the most expensive things in the world, and a display of wealth and consumption. It must have been a repellent concoction.

The Dutch control of Batavia (now Jakarta), and of the Spice Islands from 1609, meant they had a near unassailable position in Indonesia during the seventeenth century. Backed by the government and long-term investors, they had a stable and efficient business model, if a brutal one. The EIC manner of trading was as an umbrella organization under which each expedition was crowdfunded. This had the dual effect of limiting the company's loss, and also compelling crews and captains to be successful on each voyage. The EIC deployed all manner of tricks to sail into quieter harbours in the Banda Islands, out of sight of the Dutch fort at Neira, such as buying nondescript junks and making secret trades of provisions with the Bandanese, whose food supplies were being blockaded by the Dutch. The Dutch, meanwhile, were furious because the English had sailed into the East on their coat tails, without putting in the money, men or ships necessary to break Spanish and Portuguese control. The year the VOC arrived in Banda, Dutch philosopher Hugo Grotius published *Mare liberum* (*The Freedom of the Seas*), stating that 'the sea is common to all, because it is so limitless that it cannot become a possession of any one', and that 'Every nation is free to travel to every other nation, and to trade with it.'[24] But it was the subtitle of *Mare liberum* that spelled out clearly Holland's assumption of their political and legal superiority in Asia: 'Or, The Right Which Belongs to the Dutch to Take Part in the East Indian Trade'. In 1613, a conference was called in London to debate the matter, and Grotius attended as spokesman for the VOC, putting forward the Dutch case for their rightful monopoly. The representatives of the EIC responded with what amounted to a rude 'So what?', and relations in the East Indies deteriorated rapidly until outright war threatened. To avoid it, in 1619 England and Holland formed a treaty of cooperation in Indonesia, although a treaty of mutual mistrust, deceit and manipulation was closer to the truth.

In April 1621, the Dutch were weary of sharing what they saw as their territory, and wary of England's conniving overtures to Spain, so they arrived in the Banda Islands with a group of

Japanese mercenaries, and over the course of the summer, slaughtered, enslaved or banished 13,000 people, 90 per cent of the native population. They also built an impressive fort. The Dutch stranglehold on some of the most valuable commodities in the world – nutmeg and mace – had begun, but the manner in which it was achieved did not go unnoticed. The Dutch use of force even shocked the English merchants, one of whom recorded in a handbook intended for colleagues working in the East Indies that 'it may be seen at what an Expense of Blood and Money the Company have secured to themselves this Branch of Business'.[25]

The English attempted, unconvincingly, to support this victory of their supposed allies, but the EIC were keeping one eye firmly on *mare liberum*, and any opportunity to widen their Asia business. Trading with the Dutch was too expensive, and the way the EIC was funded meant that cash was often in short supply. Over the following years they made trade deals with Spain that allowed them to visit and trade in Spanish-controlled ports, much to the disgust of the Dutch. Finally, in 1666, the VOC representatives on Banda received news of the Second Anglo-Dutch War, and promptly made war on the EIC's single small fort on Nailaka. It was handed over immediately in return for safe passage. The EIC was cast afloat on the free seas, but it had lost the spice trade for good. Something else was going to have to take its place.

Chinese lore dates the start of tea-drinking to 2737 BC, when Chinese emperor Shen Nung was boiling water to drink, and leaves from the nearby *Camellia sinensis* tree fell into the water. Inhaling the fragrant aroma, Shen Nung drank the infusion, and a noble tradition was born.

In reality, tea was probably first cultivated around the Yangtze River in about AD 350, and then spread through Yunnan province.

The Tang dynasty (618–907) promoted tea culture over alcohol as a civilizing force. By the time Lu Yu wrote *Ch'a Ching* (*The Classic of Tea*) in the eighth century, it was a staple of Chinese daily life. An attempt to tax it, in 780, the year of the *Ch'a Ching*'s publication, resulted in public outrage. Lu Yu's complicated explanations of the importance of tea to the Chinese, and the rituals that accompany it, formed the foundations for the highly structured and deeply significant Japanese tea ceremony.

The Mongols are not remembered for their love of tea, but rather their love of fermented mare's milk, which Marco Polo compared to decent white wine, but the higher-status Mongols were consumers of strong black Pu'erh tea, which they used as a digestive aid after eating their fatty meat diet. They liked it so much they were willing to trade it for their prized ponies, so desperately needed in China to keep the communications routes running. Tea meant for trade in this way was pressed into hard black bricks for ease of transport and regulation of trading, and the Department of Ministry and Horses was established to oversee it. A *pecul* (133.3 pounds) of tea was exchanged for the best horses. As the first Europeans began to visit China, it is surprising that tea took as long as it did to make its way to the West, and it was Giovanni Battista Ramusio, the Venetian writer and geographer, in his introduction to yet another version of Marco Polo's *Travels* in 1559, who made the first mention of tea in Europe. The Persian merchant Haji Mahomed had told him of how the Chinese 'take of that herb whether dry or fresh, and boil it well in water. One or two cups of this decoction taken on an empty stomach removed fever, head-ache, stomach-ache, pain in the side or in the joints, and it should be taken as hot as you can bear it.'[26] Tea's medicinal properties were almost miraculous, according to many accounts, which explains its habitual consumption at all times of the day by the peoples who adopted it:

'The Persians, Indians, Chinese, and Japanese assign thereto such extraordinary qualities, that imagining it alone able to keep a man in constant health, they are sure to treat such as come to visit them with this Drink at all hours.'[27]

Coffee, although well known throughout Ethiopia and the Arabian peninsula, particularly Yemen, had only reached the sultan's court at Istanbul in 1555, where it had been adopted with relish. It is likely that coffee and tea trading with Europe began at about the same time; they were just adopted differently by different countries.

By the time of the European Renaissance, tea culture was deeply embedded in all levels of Chinese society. Augustinian missionary Martin de Rada described in 1575 how esteemed guests were greeted with a ceremony where the tea was served with a morsel of sweet conserve, presumably fruit, put into the bottom of the cup and eaten when it had soaked up the flavour, then washed down with the tea. Although he enjoyed the sweet, 'we did not care much for that hot boiled water, yet we soon became accustomed to it and got to like it, for this is always the first thing that is served on any visit'.[28] Lower down the social scale, sedentary workers such as weavers kept a pot and cup next to them as they worked and sipped throughout the day, the pot refreshed by a teaboy with a kettle. Others took tea breaks at stalls or shacks where they could also pick up fruit or a snack, and those with more time went to a teahouse, where they would be served ritually and could choose not only the variety of tea they desired, but the type of water too. Connoisseurs prided themselves on their ability to identify the origins of both. In the teahouses, fruit and sweet delicacies were complimentary. With a rapidly growing urban population, water quality was a serious issue, and there was a thriving industry that specialized in importing waters for tea into towns and cities. This imported water was more expensive than water from local canals or rainwater, which was also specially collected for teahouses. Cheaper teas made with inferior water were flavoured with flowers, such as jasmine, and the green tea so popular today for its antioxidant properties was regarded as fit for only the basest labourer.

Europeans would certainly have been introduced to these teahouses by their Chinese counterparts, as they functioned as meeting places where sobriety was an important element of the atmosphere. This was a departure for European merchants, who tended to inhabit their warehouses or offices, and then frequent taverns with friends and colleagues. The teahouse was a civilized way to do business, and the model played an important part in the development of European financial centres over the next century.

Chinese and Japanese tea arrived in Amsterdam with Dutch traders in 1610, and coffee arrived in Venice in 1615. The ritual involved in the preparation of tea, and the paraphernalia required, kept it in a domestic setting initially, where teapots, kettles, caddies and special tables, chairs and cabinets were unveiled for guests before 'tea and saffron were served together, the tea being hot, sweetened, and covered in a cup to preserve its aroma'.[29] The Dutch marketed tea and teawares to their neighbours, but coffee was already becoming popular, and only the Frisians of northern Germany took to tea as the favoured beverage, drinking it strong, sweetened and thickly laced with cream. By 1640, for most of Europe, coffee had prevailed. The famous British love of tea came later. Samuel Pepys, a keen follower of the latest fashions of all kinds in London, had a cup of tea in his office on Tuesday, 25 September 1660: 'tee (a China drink) of which I never had drank before'.[30] Tea had appeared in an advertisement in the newspaper *Mercurius Politicus* two years earlier, on 23 September 1658, when it was announced that 'The Excellent, and by all

Physicians approved, China drink, called by the Chinese, Tcha, and by other nations Tay alias Tee . . . sold at the Sultaness-head, ye Cophee-house in Sweetings Rents, by the Royal Exchange, London.'

The explanation for this lies in the English political situation of the time, which had been subject to the Puritanical Commonwealth, when luxuries were denounced, so imports such as tea had not received the exposure that came when Charles II was restored to the throne in the year Pepys first tried tea. Coffee, a bitter, sobering and stimulating drink, was an acceptable and worthy beverage for the City of London's serious merchants, but tea, with its dab of sugar in place of conserve, still smacked of the exotic. In the late seventeenth century, middle-class English women took to tea, its ritual trappings, and all things *chinoise*, with alacrity.

Thus, in just those few decades to the 1640s, international exploration and trade had changed the world forever. Goods and habits that had been local became international, and the movement of people accelerated from a trickle to a surge. Even plants suddenly began to move across these maritime trade routes, and tobacco is a prime example of this botanical imperialism.

Spain and Portugal, united under one king between 1580 and 1640, filled their galleons with as much South American bullion as possible. In Spain, the counting house in Seville was receiving hundreds of cartloads of 'silver, gold and precious pearls' in a matter of weeks, to the point where it 'could not accommodate it all and it overflowed onto the patio'.[31] They were also embarking on a different kind of Triangular Trade, the slave trade of the West Indies, which was so lucrative it made them the dominant world power in just a couple of decades. With this money, they fuelled trade across the seas, and they were particularly interested in strengthening their bases in Indonesia and China, bringing with them a whole host of new and exotic goods to trade, including people, medicines and tobacco.

The Spanish are the most likely to have introduced tobacco to Indonesia, bringing it from Mexico to the Philippines in 1575.[32] Archaeological finds of clay pipes on the Guangxi coast of China, bordering Vietnam, date from at least the mid fifteenth century onwards, so this documented date is probably somewhat late.[33]

When the Dutch reached Java, they observed the persistent native habit of betel-chewing, used as a social interaction and a mild stimulant, as well as an appetite suppressant. For many labourers, it was little more than a quid of areca and lime wrapped in betel leaves, chewed at all hours of the day, allegedly to clean the teeth and freshen the breath. Despite the red-stained mouth and copious spittle that appalled the new European arrivals, betel was not simply a lower-class habit. In all but the very poorest houses, complicated equipment, referred to as a betel-set, was brought out and placed in the centre of the room when guests arrived, and a mark of social status was to have a betel-servant to accompany the man of the house when he went out on business. The endemic chewing of betel mixed with areca and lime demonstrates that Indonesia was a ready market for a new mild narcotic such as tobacco.[34]

Europeans introduced not only the finished tobacco product, which they smoked in long reed or clay pipes, but also plants or seeds. Java and the Philippines both had excellent climates for tobacco and it soon flourished, with the Dutch sailors readily taking up pipe-smoking in what had become Batavia in 1619. The early Portuguese in the East remained convinced of the benefits of snuff, and many Chinese mandarins adopted the habit in the seventeenth century, carrying it in elaborately carved jade and ivory bottles, but the Dutch were hardened smokers of tobacco. Chinese traders took a liking to smoking and introduced the practice to mainland China through their trading contact in Taiwan, and the author Yao Lu writes of tobacco farming flourishing in Fujian in his book *Lushu*, written in 1611.[35]

The Chinese love of tobacco spread rapidly, with the Manchus of the north and north-east becoming particularly heavy users, and the state stepped in to halt what they saw as a lapse in manners and morals. Unlike the Indonesians, who would chew tobacco by adding it to their betel wrap, the Chinese were keen smokers. This may be linked to the role of incense and smoke in various Chinese religious and cultural rites, particularly the veneration of ancestors, but China rapidly adopted the custom of what they called *yancha*, or tea and smoke. The rituals of both came to form the core of the Chinese opium smoking experience.

From 1636, a series of edicts prohibited tobacco smoking, but it was too late and even beatings and ear mutilations could not stop people smoking. When the Ming Empire fell in 1644 and the Qing dynasty began, they were indifferent to whether the populace smoked tobacco or not and the bans were revoked. In the middle of the seventeenth century, the first basic cigarettes appeared.

The opium habit spread among the ordinary people in south-eastern China at much the same time as tobacco, but China's working classes had not yet been exposed to it. The existence of the opium poppy and methods of producing opium, or *yapian*, were recorded by Ming writers in the mid fifteenth century, but it was not until 1589 that it attracted a customs tariff.[36] Many of the Dutch in Indonesia added to their pipes a little opium and a pinch of arsenic, the Dutch version of theriac in the humid foreign climate, which was believed to protect against malaria and cholera. These crude recipes burned unevenly in a pipe bowl, and the Javanese – already experts in the elaborate preparation of mild sedatives – were soon making a much more sophisticated product, that came to be known as *madak*. Opium was mixed with plant roots and hemp, finely minced, boiled with water in copper pans, then dried and mixed with minced tobacco. It burned relatively slowly, but evenly, and imparted a pleasant sense of relief from boredom and anxiety, or *xinjiao*. It's unclear whether Yao Lu (d.1622) was smoking tobacco or *madak* when he described the mechanics of smoking: 'You light one end and put the other in your mouth. The smoke goes down the throat through the pipe. It can make one tipsy, but it also protects against malaria.'[37] Either way, it is most likely that the Dutch introduced *madak* to China in the early 1620s, through Taiwan merchants, and it may well be that many who smoked it were not aware that *madak* wasn't pure tobacco.

In almost all literature, any new fad or craze in a society is espoused, initially at least, as medicinal. Chinese literature is no exception, and much of the early writing about the anti-malarial properties of *madak* attributes it to the tobacco content.

In Europe, James I had already denounced ordinary tobacco-smoking. His treatise of 1604, *A counterblaste to tobacco*, branded tobacco a 'filthy noveltie' that was 'lothsome to the eye, hatefull to the Nose, harmefull to the braine, dangerous to the Lungs'. But England too had acquired the tobacco habit, and as perceptive as James was on the damaging effects of smoking, his opinion was dismissed as zealotry. The people were quite convinced of the health benefits of the tobacco pipe, and demand continued to grow. Europeans rarely smoked *madak*, however, preferring to consume opium in liquids like dwale, or to eat it as pills or pellets.

Owing to the prevalence of private trade between European and South Sea merchants and China throughout the seventeenth century, it is almost impossible to calculate the true extent

of *madak* and then pure opium use, and it was almost five decades before government documents return to the subject with
the capture of Xiamen, or Amoy as it was known, in 1683. Six
years earlier, the VOC had organized its holdings in Bengal
around opium farming. The company exported it mainly to Java
and China, and it was only with the capture of Amoy that the
Chinese government realized how widespread the problem of
opium smoking had become along the south-eastern coast. The
scale of trade between West and East was revealed the same year,
when the directors of the EIC wrote to their man in Macao
regarding the 'loss of Bantam to the Dutch, and the "Johanna"
outward bound to your place [Amoy] with her stock of £70,000,
most bullion'.[38] The relative value of this bullion in 2017 is £1–1.4
million.[39] The sinking of the *Johanna* was a significant blow, but
bearable for a company trading on the level of EIC. Profits
varied, but the 400 per cent made by da Gama on his voyage in
1502–3 was not unusual for ships surviving the trip to the East.
The risks were significant: between 1500 and 1634, 28 per cent of
all Portuguese ships involved in merchant trading were lost at
sea.[40]

The capture of Amoy was a turning point in Chinese attitudes
to opium, and to the people of the south-east. Opium habits had
long been common among China's wealthier classes, but it was
taken in moderation, as part of a regular routine that included
exercise, healthy eating and the taking of tonics and medicines.
It was also taken inside the home, and often in a separate room
which, like the European parlour for taking tea, was equipped
with special furniture, smoking paraphernalia and other recreational kit such as a mah-jongg set. Women smoked tobacco and
opium too in these domestic settings, and the *Siku quanshu*, the
official encyclopaedia of China compiled in the late eighteenth
century, recorded that in 1701 'From officials to servants and

women, everyone smokes today.'[41] And it was precisely the 'everyone' that was the issue.

By the 1720s, the Chinese government had realized it had a problem on its hands, and this coincided with the emergence of the opium dens in Fujian, principally Xiamen and Taiwan. A memo sent to the emperor described the 'private run inns' where opium was consumed, a corruption of the traditional teahouse. They were equipped with couches rather than chairs, fruit and sweets were still served, but the behaviour was 'licentious' and the 'sons of good families' were being lured and corrupted.[42] Another account shows that the people of Guangdong were making their own *madak* by 1728: 'The opium is heated in a small copper pan until it turns into a very thick paste, which is then mixed with tobacco. When the mixture is dried, it can be used for smoking by means of a bamboo pipe, while palm fibres are added for easier inhalation.'[43] For the working-class Chinese who frequented these private houses, smoking *madak* was much the same as visiting a tavern or a teahouse after work, a social occasion. The pipe, made from bamboo with brass fittings, was passed around, and anyone wishing to lie down for a spell could take to one of the couches. This was in stark contrast to the upper-class male opium smoker, who would retire to his salon for a period of contemplation induced by opium fumes from his bamboo opium pipe with silver fittings, and was not to be disturbed during his ruminations. As with tea, the opium connoisseur could identify the source of the drug, preferring the superior production shipped from Aden or Bengal to that cultivated in Malwa (Punjab) or anything grown in China. As usual, such luxury was an import.

The working-class lack of civility was at the root of the problem. The century after da Gama had arrived in the East had been marked by a global surge in commerce the kind of which the world had never seen before. The Catholic sailors, followed by the Protestant merchants of Europe, were commanding trade so rapidly and on such a scale that it defied regulation. Like the ancient Greeks and Romans, many railed against this new, seemingly unctuous, way of living beyond the bare necessities of life. Britain, unified in 1707, suffered the Society for the Reformation of Manners in the 1720s, where people were encouraged to inform upon their neighbours and to entrap them into immoral behaviour so that they might be publicly reprimanded. In the eleventh century China had invented a comparable system, *baojia*, to encourage mutual surveillance throughout the kingdom and thereby reinforce imperial power. It was revived and unified with governance during the Qing period in an attempt to halt this slide into immorality, and at the urging of the mandarins, the Yongzheng Emperor (r.1723–36) passed the eponymous edict of 1729, banning the import of opium.

The Yongzheng Edict is famously cited as the first moment China stood up to the ruthless commercial barbarians threatening to ruin the country, but in the context of the problem they had at hand, it was little more than a bread-and-circuses gesture for the anti-opium fanatics. Official opium imports had remained low, about 200 chests a year in Xiamen, compared to the amount that was clearly smoked in the south-eastern provinces.[44] Only approximately one third of the ships that weighed anchor in the Pearl River Delta and Xiamen were government or company ships; the rest were merchant vessels, arriving from Indonesia, Taiwan, Japan, Britain, Holland, Spain, Portugal, Denmark and Sweden. For Guangdong, and its southernmost region, Bao'an County, the die was cast.

Captain John Weddell at the Tiger Gate

'The Celestial Empire possesses all things in prolific abundance and lacks no product within its borders, there is therefore no need to import manufactures of outside barbarians in exchange for our products.'[45]   Emperor Qianlong

On 27 June 1637, Captain John Weddell and his four ships anchored just south of Macao, ready to open negotiations for the first direct English trade voyage to China. The Portuguese there were trading extensively with Japan, and the atmosphere in Macao was unique: Muslim heritage meant that many women were lightly veiled in the streets, but they also wore bright colours and went about freely. They also wore Japanese kimonos when they were inside their own homes. The Portuguese had been tolerated by the Chinese authorities as they had been effective at keeping the Pearl River free of pirates, which had long been a problem. Robinson and Mountney, two of Weddell's fellow sailors, were sent up the Pearl River to try and bypass the Portuguese, but were rebuffed by local customs officials who told them that they must apply to the mandarins for the proper papers in order to trade. They returned to Weddell and gave him this answer, and his response was to sail all his ships straight up the Pearl River towards Canton, seventy-five miles to the north-west.

Travelling with Weddell was Peter Mundy. Originally from Penryn in Cornwall, as a boy he had accompanied his father, a pilchard fisherman, to Rouen, and in 1611 had been put aboard a merchant ship to start his career at sea. In his late twenties he began to travel, first to Constantinople and then on to India, where he went into the pay of the East India Company. A keen diarist, his blow-by-blow account of Weddell's attempts to begin trading with China on behalf of England provide an almost cinematic vision of how the catastrophe played out.

One of the problems the English had in trading with the Chinese was that, in Chinese eyes, they looked far too much like the Dutch, of whom the Chinese had formed a poor opinion, and were called 'red barbarians'. In 1635 an English ship, the *London*, had called at Macao and the crew identified as Dutch, and the higher Chinese authorities had imposed a fine upon both the mandarins and the Portuguese for trading with them. This united the Chinese and the Portuguese in wanting to be rid of Weddell as soon as possible, and with minimal fuss. And now, he had sailed straight up the Pearl River. Weddell passed two small Chinese junk fleets and reached the Tiger Gate, where he decided to put in and wait to assess the situation. When his men attempted to go ashore and secure some fresh food, they were driven back by the local villagers, who, aware of the fine, wanted no part in helping the red barbarians. Instead of retiring back to the ships and considering his position, Weddell instead put out a bloodied ensign and made preparations for war. Quite what was going through his mind at the time remains a mystery. A messenger was sent, along with an interpreter, to request that Weddell stand down and wait six days, after which his passes would be granted and the tiny fleet would be allowed to go up to Canton. The following day, some of the men went ashore carrying a white flag on a stick before them. This meant nothing to the rural Chinese villagers, who associated white with death and funerals. They at first refused to trade with the English, but then relented, and followed the party of foreigners around as they bought what they wanted and inspected the village.

Peter Mundy, probably the most well-travelled Englishman of the seventeenth century, was travelling with the fleet on behalf of the EIC, and went ashore out of curiosity. When the villagers offered him refreshment, he took it. 'The people there gave us a certain Drinke called Chaa, which is only water with a kind of herb boyled in itt. It must bee Dranke warme and is accompted wholesome.'[46]

Cha passed from there into the Indian languages, and is now usually written as *chai*, but apart from Mundy's early reference, Pepys knew the same drink as tea. This is because English merchants found themselves dealing largely with the merchants of Fukien province, where the same drink was known as *teh*.[47]

Weddell, meanwhile, waited out his six days quietly, and when the messenger returned to ask for another four, promptly discharged his guns upon the fort at Tiger Gate. The fort fired back, but as the English ships were so close, and they lacked the ability to aim at that angle, most of the balls rolled harmlessly out of the cannons' mouths into the grass. Only one shot connected with Weddell's ship, and none of the others suffered any damage. The soldiers from the fort promptly fled, and Weddell and his men went into the fort, took the bits of it they needed for repairs, some useful artillery, and went back to the ships.

When a messenger arrived again, and offered to take representatives to the commodore further upriver, Robinson and Mountney set out, bearing gifts. The commodore, suspecting that the English could offer a lucrative proposition, did not turn down their request for trading rights, but didn't grant it either. A Chinese intermediary who called himself Paolo Norette, but claimed to hate the Catholic Portuguese, acted as translator between the English party and the Chinese officials. Norette was what the Portuguese called a comprador, an agent who understood Chinese language and customs, and had a wide circle of local acquaintances harnessed to business acumen and specialist commodity knowledge. The compradors had become invaluable to trade in Canton, Macao and the south China coast; finding the right one was crucial. Mundy identified Norette's fluid role as a comprador succinctly when he described their new factor as 'a Mandareen who formerlie had bene a servant and broker in Mocao, whoe being abused by the Portingalls fled to Cantan'.[48]

The English petition, in which Weddell and company assured Norette 'wee were English men and Came to seeke a trade with them in a faire way of merchandizinge', was hastily drawn up by the nearest Chinese calligrapher and handed over to the commodore.[49] Presented by the commodore to his superior, the marine superintendent immediately rejected it and ordered the English ships back out to sea, on pain of death: 'you have shown great daring by attempting to trade by force with us, we having forbidden it; and in doing so you appear to me to be like puppies and goats who have no learning and no reason'.[50]

Norette, returning to the English ships with this response, translated this to Weddell as the marine superintendent having granted Weddell's request to trade and to establish a trading fort in the river mouth. He requested that three of the English party accompany him to Canton, and that Weddell return the guns he had taken from the fort at Tiger Gate.

Weddell, well pleased, began busily trading in sugar. The locals, seeing the business being transacted by the Englishmen on the banks of the Pearl River, reported to the marine superintendent, who sent three junks downriver, armed and impressive, to try and dissuade him. But Weddell was feeling confident – his translator had, after all, told him that he was permitted to carry out his trade. He responded to the official warning to desist with a curt reply: 'We have no leisure, at present, to answer your vulgar letters at more length.'[51] In the middle of the night of 9–10 September, the watch saw three small, darkened junks approaching, and when they were within range, let off a warning shot. The junks were crammed with fireworks, supposed to go off when they bumped into the English ships. Instead, they were now blazing yards away in the Pearl River, but drifting downstream towards the fleet. Weddell managed to manoeuvre his ships out of the way, but when dawn broke and they saw the burnt-out junks, they realized how close they had come to disaster. Peter Mundy recorded how worried they were about their men up in Canton. Robinson and his men had been seized and locked in an empty house without food, and Norette severely and publicly beaten. Norette had, of course, betrayed them. He became so notorious as a double-dealer that letters of warning reached London merchants and King Charles I less than a year later.

Weddell set about raiding local villages in revenge, and destroying the fort at the Tiger Gate. Then he withdrew to mountainous Lintin Island, populated mainly by goats, and wrote the captain-general of Macao a blistering letter about the treatment he and his men had received from Canton. At Macao, it took another three months for the Portuguese and Chinese alliance to drive Weddell out, but finally, on 27 December, they were hounded onto their ships 'by Fire and Sword' and left, as Peter Mundy recorded. Of the main group, the resourceful Mundy was the only one to make it back to England. Robinson died on Madagascar, and Weddell disappeared somewhere in the Arabian Sea after leaving Cannanore in India. It was assumed his ship was lost with all hands. Thus ended England's first attempt at trading directly with the Chinese merchants of Canton.

The Beginnings of Hong Kong and the Rise of Canton

Hong Kong island was originally one of many hilly islands just outside the Pearl River Delta. The good natural harbours and fresh water supplies of the islands were known to Western sailors from the early sixteenth century onwards. There were around twenty small villages and hamlets on the nearby coastline, with others living on houseboats.[52] Labourers came and went with the seasons, but the main industries were fishing, pearls, quarrying, and harvesting the *Aquilaria sinensis* tree for incense. Incense was an important part of Chinese funerary rites, as the semi-preserved bodies of family members were sometimes kept in the home for up to two years. This was the main trade until the coastal evacuation of 1662–9, which devastated the area economically.[53] *Aquilaria* grew on the barren, hilly landscapes where nothing else would, and was in high demand throughout first China, then further afield. The scent arising from the water-driven incense mills, grinding the dried *Aquilaria* into powder for *joss*, or good-luck sticks, led to the fishermen living in the hamlets calling one particular bay 'Hong Kong', the 'fragrant harbour', and its related settlement Hong Kong Village.

Twice during China's long history, the south-east and the South China Sea coastal regions have backed the wrong side in dynastic wrangles. The first time, while harbouring the Southern Song from the Mongols, they benefitted from a significant economic boost, not only in domestic but in international trade, as the imperial refugees brought with them a more sophisticated infrastructure than the primitive fishing culture already in place. The second time they supported a losing dynasty was a disaster for the area.

The Manchurian Shunzhi Emperor came to the throne of the new Qing dynasty in Beijing in 1644. The Southern Ming Emperor and the Ming loyalist Zheng Chenggong still opposed Manchurian rule and Zheng had been a particularly trouble-some agitator, bringing 100,000–170,000 men out of Fujian to fight against the Manchus. Fighting styles were particularly important, as the vastness of China meant military skills and preferences for fighting differed widely across the nation: the Manchus were Mongols and therefore had developed a strong cavalry base, whereas the Southern Ming of Zheng Chenggong fought on foot, and owing to a dense population, could ship in more soldiers by water to Zhejiang and Jiangsu as they needed them. Zheng retreated to Taiwan to consider his next move.

The Shunzhi Emperor died, and was replaced by the six-year-old Kangxi Emperor (r.1662–1722), whose regent, Oboi, fearing Zheng's ability to bring troops in by water, ordered the clearing of the coastal regions from Shandong to Fujian and south to Guangdong, so that there would be no support for Zheng should he try to return that way. This measure was understandable in the light of the new infant king on the throne, whose regents needed to impose stable rule, but the severity of the southern coastal clearances changed the economic and ethnic landscape of Guangdong forever. For the fisherman and tenant farmers of San On county, which included the island of Hong Kong, the evacuation meant they were relegated to living on the edge of the clearance zone, inland and homeless in an inhospitable landscape. Many of those without family in the interior died from starvation. The production of incense ceased, and Hong Kong was a fragrant harbour only in the memory of the exiled fishermen.

By the 1680s, the edict had been revoked and people had returned to the coast, and Hong Kong was inhabited once again. The first groups to arrive were poor, the peasant farmers and fishermen who had previously eked out a living there. The workforce was not large enough to be productive, so the government tried to induce migration by offering benefits to those willing to move there. A large number of China's migrant or Hakka people responded, including the two Zhu brothers. The new arrivals, euphemistically termed 'guest people' in Chinese, quickly found that, as poor as the island was, it was exposed to Japanese, Chinese and international pirates alike, so one brother took several families to settle in the safer environment of Kowloon Bay, and the other brother took families to Shek Pai Wan, or what is now known as Aberdeen Bay. There, upon a hill, they built a walled compound that became Hong Kong Village, and took in women of the *shuishang ren*, the Tanka water-people, to help them get established. The wall was still standing in 1957.

For a long time, Hong Kong continued as a poor, scrappy settlement made up of seven villages, exposed to the bandits of the sea, and looking on somewhat forlornly as the huge cargo ships of international companies and the yachts of the privateers sailed straight past them on the way from Macao to Canton. The friendly bays and good water meant that storm-damaged ships would put in for running repairs, but business was done elsewhere. And business was brisk: the eighteenth-century sea trade in Canton set the scene for trade between the British and the Chinese for the next two centuries. After Taiwan was captured in 1683, in 1684 the Kangxi Emperor issued an edict ordering 'I command you to go abroad and trade to show the populous and affluent nature of our rule. By imperial decree I open the seas to trade.'[54] Canton was decided upon as the funnel for trade. So, as Chinese ships rushed out towards Manila and Japan in their hundreds, European ships rushed up the Pearl River. In 1685, the people of Edo (now Tokyo), aware that they were almost mined out, issued an edict banning export of all precious metals from Japan. Canton was suddenly dependent entirely upon trade from Indonesia and the West. All along the Pearl River Delta, tiny settlements sprang up to service the incoming ships, called bankshalls, a corruption of bank-stalls, run by what the English called 'Sampan-Sams', taken from the little three-plank sampan supply boats the Chinese owners punted up and down the coast.

For European sailors who had spent months aboard ship surviving on salt beef, pork, beans, chickpeas and ship's biscuit, the sampans formed convenient floating markets of fresh fruit and vegetables, and even live pigs, goats and wild duck, as well as medicines and women. Bigger bankshalls were run by compradors, and provided more official services. All of them were known as the Cantonese by the Europeans. These compradors were particularly useful in dealing with on-board deaths, which were a common occurrence, as Europeans could not be buried in mainland China. The bodies of European traders from Macao were returned there, but those without ties were taken to Dane's Island, now known as Changzhou, or French Island, now known as Xiaoguwei. These islands belonged to neither the Danes nor the French, but the merchant ships of both nations camped out on them to perform repairs and gather themselves before arriving in Canton proper. Whampoa Island, halfway between Macao and Canton, was a convenient staging post for the largest bankshall depots and served as an administrative halfway house.

The late seventeenth century was a time of organized chaos in the Pearl River Delta, so Canton fell back on its own guild system to maintain control. Unlike European guilds, which brought together merchants from different places under the umbrella of a single trade, Chinese guilds were based upon what they called their 'native place', reflecting the deep Chinese attachment to their ancestry. More personal connections were often formed with secret societies which, although they had their roots in political movements, from the late seventeenth century onwards were an increasingly important part of business life in China, and particularly in the south. Like merchant guilds, they were patriotic, patriarchal and deeply loyal. They also retained the trappings of most secret societies, such as hierarchies, initiations, oaths and special systems of communication. These interwoven groups were difficult for native Chinese to access, and impossible for Europeans. They also enabled corruption and bribery to become endemic within the system, giving foreign merchants a way into the market. In Canton, Chinese merchants, or *hongs*, formed a trade monopoly from a series of warehouses called factories along the shore. Compradors worked as intermediaries between them and the Europeans, dealing with their opposite number on-board ship, known as the supercargo. Supercargoes were arguably the most important men aboard, and charged with finding out conditions on the ground as soon as the ship dropped anchor: many had set sail up to a year before, and prices and supply chains always changed in that time. Once business had been done, the comprador reported to the *hong* merchant, who attended the government trading house to pay the government taxes. Government supervisors were known as *hoppos*.

The *hong* merchants, the Cantonese, and the Europeans benefitted substantially from the opening up of trade coupled with the Second or Mexican Silver Cycle, which picked up at the beginning of the eighteenth century and lasted for five decades, until the Chinese demand for bullion levelled off once more. To put this enormous supply into context, the Second Silver Cycle delivered to China more than twice the silver bullion than the total supply of the previous two centuries, and made the Mexican peso the default currency for trading in the East Indies until the early nineteenth century. The EIC and the VOC struggled to raise the cash to compete in this market and Isaac Newton wrote in *Lords of the Treasury* in 1717 that the Chinese trade 'carries away the silver from all of Europe'.[55]

The traders as a whole also benefitted from the rapidly rising population in China's interior who were thriving on the new food crops imported from the Americas. In the second half of the seventeenth century, the Chinese population had reached

268 million, but unlike Europe, which was becoming increasingly urban, China relied upon the basic unit of the rural household in what was still an almost completely rural population.[56] In the first half of the eighteenth century China, fuelled by the money flooding in, population increase and a stable dynasty, almost doubled the size of its territory and the Han population boomed. The acreage under cultivation expanded by approximately half again. It was cultivated mainly by China's indentured labourers, the coolies, who mitigated their back-breaking and, in the case of rice farming, wet work with the trio of tea, tobacco and opium. The opium was particularly important for the rice farmers. It quelled the symptoms of the endless water-borne fevers and diarrhoea that plagued the rice paddies, allowing a steady but unremitting pace of work, as well as alleviating arthritic pains and boredom. Fevers and rheumatic problems were also endemic to the subtropical hills of southern China. The Chinese had also realized that unlike alcohol, such as the dangerous 'ardent spirit' and gin equivalent *samshu*, and other intoxicants, opium smoking did not create a tolerance, so the same effect could be had day after day with no increase in consumption, and thus spending.

By the beginning of the eighteenth century, the VOC was providing Canton with most of its opium out of Batavia. To put the importance of this opium trade into context, the detailed records of the VOC show that between 1702 and 1781 opium, mainly from Malwa, made up 52 per cent of its Batavian spice trade. Pepper, always perceived to be the giant of the spice industry, was a mere 12 per cent and beaten even by cinammon at 14 per cent.[57] This sort of trade dwarfed the French and English companies who sent one or two ships a year between 1699 and 1714. The EIC had adopted a more structured system of finance over the previous century and in 1714 took an office in Hog Lane,

Canton, a far cry from its vast bureau on Shoe Lane in the City of London. The following year, the pope issued another papal bull against Chinese funerary practices, still mistakenly under the impression that China was remotely interested in Rome's opinion on their centuries-old customs. China promptly expelled all Western missionaries not attached directly to court, and the mandarins became even more contemptuous of the greedy, insolent Western barbarians.

In 1720, China granted the monopoly on South China Sea trade to a group of *hong* merchants operating from the 'Thirteen factories' on the Pearl River at Canton. The Cohong, as they were known, became immensely powerful in one stroke, and held the monopolies on tea and silk, both now in high demand in Britain. The EIC was one of the first to react to this new development, and did so with surprising subtlety. Even with the help of the supercargoes and compradors, the *hong* merchants were hard to deal with. The discussion of facts and figures Europeans considered essential in the general course of business was viewed as distasteful conflict by the *hong* merchants, who were clannish and secretive.

These two events caused the EIC to reconsider how they did business in Canton. They had previously employed compradors who spoke Portuguese, but that was out of favour. Or, they had given French/Chinese-speaking missionaries free passage on their ships in exchange for translation services. With neither a viable option, the EIC began to train employees to speak fluent Chinese, rather than the 'chop' Chinese favoured by London business houses for the previous century. One of these employees, James Flint, was particularly successful in learning the language when he was abandoned in Canton in his mid-teens after sailing with the EIC ship the *Normanton* in 1736. Three years later, as a bilingual English–Chinese speaker with a Chinese alias, he was shipped to India on company business, before returning to China after a further three years, this time as a language student fully funded by the EIC. In 1741, he started work in the office in Hog Lane, and was soon the essential English linguist for all the EIC ships arriving in Canton. As Britain fought the War of Austrian Succession back in Europe, with Flint's help, and others like him, the EIC began to dominate trade with the Cohong. By the end of the war, the EIC had out-grown Canton and were looking to establish trade depots up the main south-east China coastline, beginning where they had left off an attempt in Ningbo some years earlier. Flint was integral to these machinations, and made direct overtures to Beijing, something utterly forbidden by protocol. After a messy squabble, the EIC were halted in their tracks in their attempt to open up Chinese trade; a Fujianese interpreter was publicly executed in Canton as a warning not to get too friendly with the barbarians, and Flint was imprisoned on Macao for three years. Upon his release, he went to America to farm soybeans and make soy sauce. He also introduced Benjamin Franklin to tofu.

Meanwhile, Flint and his actions under the aegis of the EIC had serious commercial consequences for European traders. In 1757, trade with foreigners was restricted entirely to Canton, strengthening the Cohong again, and delivering opportunities for huge amounts of smuggling and corruption. Foreign mer-chants were not allowed to be full-time residents in Canton, and it became illegal for them to learn or speak Chinese, making them even more dependent upon the comprador system, as well as sowing deceit and obfuscation. Worse, it was increasingly apparent to the mandarins that plenty of opium was still getting into southern China through smuggling, despite the 1729 restric-tions. There had been no slowing down of opium consumption in China, and prohibition had only seemed to speed up the smuggling, as an ever-greater proportion of the working pop-

ulation relied upon it as a panacea. The Chinese rightly identified the British merchants as the main culprits, but having
concentrated their authority so narrowly in Canton, they were
powerless to stop the endless covert offshore and coastal trading
that the British, and to some extent the Dutch and Portuguese,
used to offload their opium cargoes.

It can be safely said that British–Chinese relations were at a
low in 1757, yet elsewhere, the EIC was about to alter the course
of not only a nation, but a subcontinent. That same year, the
increasingly militarized EIC won the Battle of Plassey over the
Nawab of Bengal, putting them in control of India's cheapest
and best opium. The company knew precisely the market for it:
Canton, despite the ban on opium imports. Desperate for Chinese tea, and rich in opium, the EIC spent the next two decades
working their way around the problem. Their solution would
change the histories of India, China and Britain forever.

PART TWO

In the Arms of Morpheus

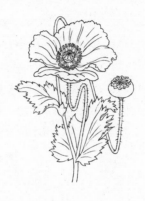

Chapter Four

THE ROMANTICS MEET MODERN SCIENCE

The Three Empires

'There is no supremacy and grip on the world without means and resources; without land and retainers, sovereignty and command are impossible.'[1]

Babur (1483–1530), founder of the Mughal Empire

The Battle of Plassey and the capture of Calcutta marked the consolidation of the British India that had been under construction since 1600, and established a British stronghold in the Mughal Empire that enabled them to bypass the Ottoman and Safavid empires that had dominated trade routes from the Balkans to the Bay of Bengal since the fourteenth century.

These three vast empires not only dominated trade, but they also became distant dreams, as tales of the wonders to be seen and had there finally made it back. Those who had returned from the Crusades had rarely spoken of wondrous places and gold-bedecked palaces, but soon, these three dynasties, covering combined lands almost too large to be comprehended in Western Europe, figured large in its imagination.

From 1520 to 1566, the Ottoman Empire was under the control

of Suleiman the Magnificent, who instigated a period of change for this vast area, transforming a turbulent, aggressive ideology into a more settled and urban way of life, which included the creation of a bureaucratic system to rule such a gigantic territory, from Istanbul. A new Ottoman identity as the protectors of Sunni Islam was also created. These amalgamated realms had long been plagued by bandits and warlords, and rebellions were common. Anatolia, where opium growing was a flourishing trade, was the site of persistent protests, such as the Celali Rebellions of the late sixteenth century. Most Ottoman protests were made up of farmers recruited as irregular troops during times of taxation or hardship, led by the local smugglers, trouble-makers and headmen. This period of the Ottoman Empire laid the foundation for modern organized crime in Turkey. Trafficking, in any kind of profitable goods and people, had been the business of these bandits since time immemorial and opium was widely exported along with other goods. In 1546, French naturalist Pierre Belon visited Asia Minor and Egypt and was stunned to see a fifty-camel caravan, packed with Turkish opium. He commented on the widespread use of opium amongst the Ottomans, writing, 'There is no Turk who would not buy opium with his last penny; he carries it on him in war and peace. They use opium because they think that thus they will become more daring and have less fear of the dangers of war. In war-time such quantities are purchased that it is difficult to find any left.'[2]

Ottoman sultans seem to have taken opium as a matter of course, and this was often attributed by witnesses to the fact they didn't drink, but the men in the street also took a range of narcotics freely and as part of their ordinary social interactions. Not only did they take opium, they 'smoked a green powder made from the leaves of wild hemp', from 'hookahs, the Turkish pipe with smoke inhaled through the water'.[3] Again, as in Marco

Polo's time, it was noted that it was the rougher sort of men who smoked hemp. Another drug popular in Istanbul was *tatula*, or *Datura stramonium*, best obtained from apothecaries, who had in turn obtained it allegedly from Jewish smugglers; it was deemed especially dangerous when smoked along with opium.

The Safavids, one of the greatest Persian empires, were also cultivating and using large amounts of opium recreationally, and all attempts to curb it failed, even when restrictions were backed by strict Shiite Muslim ideology. It became commonly associated with death in Persia in 1577 when Shah Ismail II was poisoned with it after a rowdy night out on the town. After 1600, when the East began to open up to travellers, tales of the wonders of the Safavid Persian court began to filter back to western Europe. From opposing sides, they shared the common enemy of the quarrelsome and overbearing Ottomans, and so the stories of high culture and the astonishing sight of Isfahan held even more appeal for readers in the West. A French jewel dealer, Jean Chardin, arrived in the royal capital for the first time aged twenty-two, and later wrote that it 'consists particularly of a great number of magnificent palaces, gay and smiling houses, spacious caravanserais, very fine canals and bazaars and streets lined with plane trees ... from whatever direction one looks at the city, it looks like a wood'.[4] He also observed that perhaps nine out of ten Persian men took opium pills. Another visitor related how the young shahs were raised in tents, guarded by 'black eunuchs within and white eunuchs without', taught only about religion rather than politics or statesmanship and that they 'abandon him to women and indulge him in every kind of sensuality from his most tender years. They make him chew opium and drink poppy water into which they put amber and other ingredients which incite to lust, and for a time charm with ravishing visions but eventually cause him to sink into an absolute insensibility. On the death of his father they seat him on the throne and the court throw themselves at his feet in submission. Everyone tries to please him but no one thinks of giving him any good advice.'[5]

The free availability of locally produced opium throughout these huge empires meant that it was not only an elite habit. Opium eating was particularly prevalent in all levels of Ottoman and Persian society. In the East Indies as a whole, opium eating had already become a generally accepted habit, even amongst the poor. As Portuguese writer Cristobal Acosta noted in 1592, they regarded it 'in the way that a worker looks upon his bread', although he thought the use of it as a sexual stimulant 'repellent'.[6] He also noted, on his return journey when in charge of sick Turkish and Arab captives on the ship, that they were habitual users and in danger of dying if he could not supply them with the drug. Instead they had to make do with large quantities of wine.

If even the most ordinary of men were enslaved to opium for survival, there were those who took it to new extremes, and to the east lay the most ostentatious opium eaters of all: the Mughals. The Great Mughal Empire of India was founded by Babur in 1526. The Mughals claimed ancestry to Timur and Genghis Khan, and were Muslims displaced from Central Asia. In creating a new empire, they retained some of their own customs, but also adopted those from elsewhere and their court culture was heavily influenced by the splendour of the Persians. Yet they kept their nomadic ways and never remained anywhere for too long. This had the effect of concentrating the notion of royalty in the personage of the emperor, and the Mughal rulers became ever more splendid in their personal appearance. They were both emperor, and capital of the empire embodied.

By the time the Mughals were established, the ruling classes of all three empires had cultivated a strong opium culture, but unlike the other two empires and despite their religion, the Mughals also liked to drink wine. A great deal of wine. This was not restricted to the men, and women were also allowed to join the royal parties, although it is unlikely that they were permitted to imbibe. The youngest daughter of Babur, Gulbadan Begim (*c*.1523–1603), described what it was like to attend the annual Mughal mystic feast, to celebrate their dynastic good fortune. Of all of the ninety-six well-born women who attended, she picks out two women, named Shad Begim and Mihrangaz Begim, who 'had a great friendship for one another, and they used to wear men's clothes and were adorned by various accomplishments, such as the making of thumbrings and arrows, playing polo and shooting'.[7]

From the tales of their feasting, carousing, eating and hunting, the Mughals were consumers on a tremendous scale. Humayun, Babur's son and Gulbadan Begim's half-brother, admitted freely to being an opium eater, as was his son after him. They paled in comparison to Jahangir, though, ruler of the Mughals from 1605 until 1627. Even the name he chose for himself, which translates to 'Seizer of the World', is a bold declaration of his intentions to enjoy life to the full. Both his brothers had died of alcoholism, and Jahangir was so inebriated by his wine and opium habits that from 1611 his wife Nur Jahan ruled almost in his stead, after his first wife Man Bai killed herself with an opium overdose in 1605. Jahangir lived in monumental style, and when the court was on the move, he was accompanied by a personal guard of 8,000 men, up to another 100,000 mounted warriors and hundreds of thousands of animals and people, with a procession stretching over a mile and a half.

Jahangir was the most mobile of all the Mughal emperors although, unlike his ancestors, this was probably more to do with evading any real responsibility than fleeing from the Uzbeks. His wandering progress was, allegedly, spiritual and there is no doubt he was educated in spiritual and religious matters and made genuine attempts to reconcile the diverse faiths of Hindustan with Islam. He was also a collector, naturalist and a keen observer of the country around him on his travels. He greatly expanded the royal library and kept his own inventory of books acquired, the first Mughal emperor to do so personally. In Gujarat and Portuguese Goa he had agents who were charged to source exceptional European artefacts, timepieces in particular, and he assembled an impressive royal menagerie, featuring a North American turkey, a zebra from Abyssinia and an orangutan. The memoirs he wrote himself are fine pieces of imperialist propaganda.

Meanwhile, the court enjoyed regular Thursday-night drinking parties in their lavish gardens, where everyone was to have exactly what they wanted in terms of alcohol and drugs. Taking the lead from the Persian court, where wine had been traditional for centuries, the Mughals wished to appear similarly sophisticated, but they also used strong spirits, and descriptions indicate they took their opium dissolved in cups of wine or liquor. One hopes these were not the 'spirit of mutton, spirit of deer, spirit of goat' distilled in Surat, as reported by one EIC agent, created by adding a portion of whichever animal 'spirit' was desired to the still.[8] When, in 1621, Jahangir's 'old and trusted servant', the keeper of the royal intoxicants, died, Jahangir appointed two in his stead, one for wine, the other for opium.[9] He was a man of tremendous appetites: at about the same time, he recorded that between his eleventh and his fiftieth birthday, he had hunted almost every day, and that he had seen 28,532 animals 'killed in my presence', of which over 17,000 were by his own hand, including birds, mountain goats, sheep and deer, but also eighty-six lions and ten crocodiles.[10]

Jahangir was also responsible for granting the opium trading rights to the EIC in 1617, as part of a package of trade concessions, and after repeated ambassadorial missions from England. As early as January 1613, the EIC had established a warehouse or factory at Surat on the coast of Gujarat, defending it against the Portuguese, and Sir Thomas Roe arrived in 1615, and spent three years at court drinking and waiting on Jahangir, to secure EIC interests. Roe's account of his time at the Mughal court was part of a collection of travelogues published in 1625, as *Hakluytus Posthumus* or *Purchas his Pilgrimes*, which became a touchstone for readers interested in the wonders of the East. Roe's descriptions of Jahangir's daily life are extraordinary, with mentions of 600 elephants and upwards of 10,000 horses all on the move at the same time, and dressed in finery of an almost unimaginable splendour. Roe found himself having to get on his horse just to be out of the crush of people. Jahangir himself wore a plumed turban, decorated on one side with a ruby 'as big as a Walnutt', mirrored by a diamond on the other, and at the front 'an emralld like a hart, much bigger'. And around 'his neck hee carried a Chain of most excellent pearl, three double; so great I never saw; at his Elbowes, Armlettes set with diamondes'.[11] Jahangir's court jeweller was, intriguingly, a Dutchman. The emperor's gloves, Roe was pleased to note, were English, but even the description of the dressing ceremony is exhausting and must have been tedious on a daily basis, and there is little wonder that Jahangir was often 'at Play' and 'fell to sleep'. There are frequent mentions of the emperor's women, and how much time he liked to spend with them. Although the European descriptions of the royal harem are less than romantic, the image of the emperor lounging among his female coterie is a powerful one. In reality, there were strong women in the harem, such as Nur Jahan, who built private palaces for herself along the route of her husband's processions, and who also had her own trading interests. Mughal women preferred to trade with English merchants rather than the Portuguese, after the

Portuguese captured a ship, the *Rahimi*, belonging to the emperor Akhbar's mother Maryam Makani, which traded spice, opium and textiles for export. Nur Jahan eventually acquired the title 'protector of English goods', indicating the strength of her position with the English, and as such it is unlikely that she did not play a part in the negotiations with Sir Thomas Roe.[12]

Jahangir died in 1627 in Kashmir, still on tour, but crippled by decades of intoxication. The tales of him and his court that had reached the West, however, were to have an immense legacy. He is the most famous of the opium-eating Mughals, and the descriptions of his court had particular importance for European readers. By contrast, in the Habsburg Empire and the rest of western Europe, opium was still regarded by most as an exotic import. The produce of the different empires was viewed distinctly and people argued over which was the superior article, and how to consume it. In England, where Turkish opium was still generally thought to be the strongest and most easily available, although Egyptian remained the finest, developments were about to take place that altered the consumption of opium in the West forever.

'Medicine would be a cripple without it.'
Thomas Sydenham,
*Medical Observations Concerning the History
and the Cure of Acute Diseases* (1676)

When, in 1603, Shakespeare had his villain Iago speak of the unhappy Othello's tormented state of mind, he referred to the classic recipe, 'Not poppy, nor mandragore, Nor all the drowsy syrups of the world, Shall ever medicine thee to that sweet sleep, Which thou ow'dst yesterday.'[13] As *Othello* was written, England was in the grip of another wave of plague, and medicine was the source of much renewed interest as part of the overwhelming wave of Renaissance humanism spreading throughout Europe. Philosopher and statesman Francis Bacon (1561–1626) called for a more empirical approach that would change the human condition for the better. He hoped that the world would profit from a continued age of discovery, and the title page of his masterwork *Novum organum scientarium, or The New Instrument of Science*, published in 1620, shows a ship passing between the Pillars of Hercules as it exits the Mediterranean for the Atlantic. Although Bacon had nothing new to say on opium in his quasi-medical treatise *History of Life and Death*, it is remarkable for its sheer humanity and breadth of influence, and he did hope that his work would be for the general good, wishing 'that through it the higher physicians will somewhat raise their thoughts'.[14]

In London, physicians were often seen as figures of fun, preferring to work in theory rather than practice, leaving most patients at the mercy of the barber-surgeons, apothecaries, midwives and, often, quacks. These London physicians were generally divided into two camps, that of Galen or Paracelsus. Galen's tradition was based on herbs and holistic medicine, whereas Paracelsus had of course favoured the alchemical or specific route to treating the patient. The followers of Paracelsus were regarded with disdain by the Galenists in the debates in London's Royal College of Physicians. For them, Paracelsus carried the brimstone whiff of Faust, but for others, his ideas still resonated.

London was an important intellectual centre in the seventeenth century, particularly for medicine. It was a time of war, both at home and abroad, but an overall rise in living standards meant that education, arts and sciences were becoming a priority as they had in other centres before. People were becoming more self-reliant and beginning to question the dogmas of the past, aided by instruments such as globes, telescopes, microscopes and barometers. A number of extraordinary minds across all fields acted as catalysts for chemical and scientific experimentation, not least the great polymaths such as William Harvey, who discovered how the circulatory system worked, and whose teachings inspired others like Christopher Wren, John Locke and Robert Hooke. A contemporary of these men, Thomas Sydenham was born in 1624, in Dorset, to a military family. His time at Oxford University was cut short by the English Civil Wars (1642–51), and he ultimately only qualified as a doctor at Pembroke College, Cambridge in 1676. He had, however, been granted a licence to practise medicine in London from 1663 onwards. It had been an impressive couple of decades for progress in all fields, and in 1657, Christopher Wren had conducted an experiment of utmost importance for the future of the history of medicine, when he administered the first recorded intravenous injection, to a dog.

Wren was helped in his endeavour by Robert Boyle, an Anglo-Irish chemist of wealthy background, who in 1655–6 took lodgings in Oxford in the apothecaries' quarter, so that he might easily practise his experiments. His apartments are now covered by University College. Wren, by this time aged twenty-four, was sitting with Boyle and others, discussing how poisons worked, when Wren declared he knew how to move liquid into the blood of a living creature. They obtained a dog and summoned assistants to restrain the dog to a table, and Wren used a lancet, followed by a sharpened goose quill, and an animal bladder to perform the injection, which he wrote about later, saying, 'I Have Injected Wine and Ale in a liveing Dog into the Mass of Blood by a Veine, in good Quantities, till I have made him extremely drunk, but soon after he Pisseth it out.'[5] He went on to say that he had tested 'the Effects of Opium, Scammony & other things' in the same way. The dog injected with a mixture of opium and white wine survived, because he was made to get up and move until the effects had passed, by being whipped around the garden.

Boyle, Wren and their friends continued with these experiments when the opportunities presented themselves, and Wren had little doubt that it could work on people, particularly 'Malefactors'. From 1660 onwards, men such as these were presenting their findings to the new Royal Society in London, which brought together the best minds working in the city at the time. One of those recording what the members of the Royal Society worked upon wrote of Wren's and Boyle's work with intravenous injection, 'Hence arose many new experiments, and chiefly that the transfusing of blood.'[16]

The restoration of King Charles II to the English throne, the founding of the Royal Society and the intellectual community that formed around the centre of London prompted many rapid developments in a short time, not least the work that Sydenham had busied himself with at the same time as Wren's and Boyle's experiments. He had been working with a great range of patients suffering different ailments, and was particularly convinced of the value of observing hospital patients over time. He was living and working in Pall Mall in premises next to an apothecary, Mr Malthus, whose shop was called the Pestle & Mortar. Doctors such as Sydenham were becoming skilled at devising medicines from old remedies as well as the ones that had arrived from the New World, such as ipecac and quinine. As with China, new foods were also arriving in Europe, such as potatoes, rice and corn, which allowed the working populations to grow, although some did come with attendant health diseases, like pellagra in corn. Sydenham promoted the use of opium strongly for many ordinary ailments, believing that 'Of all the remedies it has pleased almighty God to give man to relieve his suffering, none is so universal and so efficacious as opium.' Yet, only two years after Sydenham began to practise officially, the twin horrors of the Plague and the Great Fire saw he and his family flee to the country. There, he began to write up his observations, many of which – such as those on gout, which he admitted was largely suffered by 'bad-living and hard-drinking profligates', and mental health, for which he advised plenty of exercise such as horse-riding – are now seen as the beginning of the clinical age of medicine.[17] For this he is known as the English Hippocrates, but he did not receive much respect from the majority of the medical establishment in his own lifetime. His sensible works on fevers, gout and arthritis went against received wisdom and it seems that although he was never truly poor, he was not among the elite of London's physicians.

Sydenham, though, was truly most influential in the creation of a new form of opium, which also no doubt helped him with his pioneering works on fevers. As seen from Galen to Paracelsus and the habitual Persian user, pills made of opium had long been in use, and Sydenham experimented with the drug to try and create an improved form. Pills often gave users stomach cramps and sickness, and much depended upon the skill of the druggist in determining the dose. As with dwale and with Wren's white wine mixture, alcohol was frequently used with opium to mask the bitterness, to help with intoxication and also digestion, and because alcohol was used readily on its own as medicine.

Alcohol also has an effect on opium latex, making it feel more potent to the user, and so no doubt Sydenham had experimented enough to find the use of sherry, a premium fortified wine, beneficial in his recipe, which also included opium, saffron, cinnamon and cloves, which were mixed, macerated for fifteen days, and then filtered.[18]

Unlike Paracelsus, who kept the key to his Stone of Immortality a secret, in 1667 Sydenham shared his knowledge in the interests of his fellow man. The recipe was an instant success. It had all the positive properties of an ancient theriac, such as saffron, cinnamon and cloves, which made it reassuringly expensive, but then it was soaked in sherry, and it was much easier to take and gentler on the stomach. And as apothecaries and opium supplies both became much more reliable in the latter part of the seventeenth century, the dose was almost standard, and could be dispensed easily over the counter. For the apothecaries such as Mr Malthus, it was relatively easy to make up and not so time-consuming as pills. A rapidly intoxicating, fever-reducing painkiller that also calmed the bowels and the senses: Sydenham's laudanum recipe was disseminated rapidly through England, France and then on through western Europe.

From this point onwards, the way the East and West chose to consume opium would never be the same again. The West would always choose the faster route, whereas in the East, the biggest consumers, such as Persians and the Chinese, remained committed to opium pills or smoking. The sociability of smoking was an obvious draw for men in the East, and the pills a convenience they had been accustomed to for generations, particularly in rural areas. For the rising urban population of the West, where druggists were common and supply unrestricted, it was a simple thing to take a half-pint bottle and obtain a dose for the family medicine cupboard; because it was measured in drops, it was easier not to overdose a child. A new age in drug-taking dates from Sydenham's laudanum recipe, as made up by Mr Malthus. Apothecaries across Europe were achieving a new prominence through the creation of these new medicines, and it is a remarkable coincidence that, less than a year after Sydenham's publication, in Darmstadt in Germany, Bavarian apothecary Friedrich Jacob

Merck bought the Angel druggist shop, starting a pharmaceutical dynasty that is now one of the world's biggest companies.

Sydenham's generosity with his skill and time are shown in a case he assisted on almost a decade after he published his laudanum recipe. The physician and philosopher John Locke (1632– 1704) was a close contemporary and friend of Sydenham and had a thorough knowledge of medicine, although he ceased to practise as a doctor owing to his increasing political and intellectual commitments. In 1676, he made the first known report in Europe of the distressing and excruciatingly painful disorder trigeminal neuralgia, commonly known as *tic douloureux*, a disease that would go hand in hand with opiate abuse for the coming century and a half. The Countess of Northumberland was suffering a severe case of neuralgia of the nerves in her mouth and face. Her husband was the ambassador to France, but her French doctors had failed to cure her, despite even removing two of her teeth in a last-ditch attempt. This was also botched. She was left in a state of near-permanent nervous agony. Locke was called in to see if there was anything that might be done, and he wrote to colleagues, including Sydenham, with a detailed report of the condition and requests for advice. Sydenham, whose ideas were not particularly popular amongst the medical establishment, despite his success with laudanum, wrote back with what he would do 'were she one of those poor people my lott engages me to attend (for I cure not the rich until my being in the ground makes me an Authority)'.[19] It is clear from Locke's letters that he held Sydenham in high regard and valued his advice, which included, naturally, opiates internally and laudanum applied to the affected parts. It is also clear just how much pain the countess was in, and how quickly it was possible to become dependent on the medicine that brought such relief. Most of the other measures Locke and Sydenham discussed for her treatment, with the exception of hyoscyamine, were little more effective for neuralgia than the rosemary water or syrup of violets used to deliver them.

Locke's account of his treatment of the countess is no more than a foonote in the vast body of work he bequeathed to society, but it is a milestone in the history of opiate use to treat a nervous disorder. Laudanum and various medicines containing it rapidly became the standard treatment for neuralgia, and almost all nervous conditions.

In contrast to Locke, Sydenham may have felt that his influence in his own lifetime was limited, yet ultimately it was enormous. While he may have given away the secret to his laudanum recipe, therefore making it possible for any apothecary to concoct, he was also pivotal in the birth of proprietary medicines – something that was to become a cornerstone of opiate consumption throughout the eighteenth and nineteenth centuries.

At the house in Pall Mall, Sydenham took a pupil, one Thomas Dover, born in 1660 and educated at both Oxford and Cambridge. Sydenham treated Dover when the latter contracted smallpox, with what was then a modern treatment of confinement to a clear, well-ventilated room, coupled with 'cooling', including medicines containing opium to both bring on sweating and to calm the patient. Recovered, Dover married and returned to the country to oversee his sick father's farm in Warwickshire, hoping to continue as a doctor there. After his father's death in 1696, he moved to Bristol, where he became a volunteer doctor at the new St Peter's Hospital for the poor, following in Sydenham's footsteps. In the twelve years Dover was in Bristol, he built up a lucrative practice, but continued to see poor patients. His work ethic was remarkable, perhaps another trait he acquired from Sydenham, and during one typhus outbreak, recorded seeing twenty-five patients a day, taking breaks to meet with a surgeon and an apothecary in a coffee house to compare notes. This meeting of colleagues during a time of professional stress shows how important this triumvirate were. As with Sydenham and Malthus, the working relationship of a doctor with an apothecary was not only one of professional courtesy, it was a close partnership that required a high level of knowledge and trust on both sides.

The late seventeenth century was a time of change in the apothecary business. People had more money to spend on what they may previously have regarded as luxury items, and increasingly, self-medication was becoming part of the daily regimen of many. Drugs, then as now, required a trusted retailer and good apothecaries were valued members of the community, a far cry from the itinerant quacks of the quarterly fair. Their business, in many ways, was more reliable and safer than that of physicians, whose results were often decided more by luck than by their own skill. As Francis Bacon observed, the patient may be doomed from the outset and 'therefore many times the imposter is prized and the man of virtue taxed'.[20] The apothecary, however, had a much steadier business, often more concerned with the long-term management of chronic conditions, yet competition between the two factions, the doctors and the apothecaries, was fierce, as evidenced in a speech by Dr Samuel Garth at the Royal College of Physicians in 1696:

Medicine itself is sick. This Art, of all others the most useful, knows not how to help itself; while rather from mock Physicians, than diseases, this country suffers . . . Here an operator, mounted on his pyed horse, draws teeth in the streets; another is so obliging, as to be at home at certain hours to receive fools; another pores in urinals, and if he finds no disease there, he makes it . . . Yet not with weapons do these swarms of mountebanks inflict wounds, but with some nostrum more dangerous than any weapon.[21]

The nostrums he sneers at were a reference to the medicines available from the druggists and apothecaries that lined certain London streets, and dispensed medicines across the counter. The speech was a call for the Royal College of Physicians to bring the making and dispensing of medicines into the realm of the doctor, and remove it from the hands of the apothecaries. The suggestion was to sell medicine to the poor at cost price, but what seems like an early, positive attempt at regulation of medication in favour of the patient, was also a turf war. The London Dispensary opened in 1698 at the College near St Paul's Cathedral, 'where all sorts of Medicines both Chymical and Galenical are prepared of the best drugs, and with all the exactness imaginable' in an 'Elboratory' with two consulting rooms and an attendant apothecary at all times. The Company of Apothecaries, who had already sworn to 'suitably comply with our just and real intention and désigné of serving the public in affording medicines prescribed by us to such poor at rates answerable to the lowness of their condition', had no intention of giving ground.[22] Bitter battles ensued, erupting into violence on one occasion when a velvet-coated physician and his friends entered the dispensary and attacked the two apothecaries' apprentices in their blue aprons.

The founding of the London Dispensary sets out the separation between the doctor and the maker of medicines, and is a perfect example of the struggle between the medical profession and drug manufacturers. It's also the moment that the quality of medication was brought into the public realm, rather than remaining solely a matter of commerce.

Apothecaries' shops first became sophisticated retail outlets in

Italy, France and Holland, with display and attractive packaging part of the shopping experience. Of the different kinds of retailers operating in London in the late 1600s, apothecaries tied up nearly 40 per cent of their capital in their shop fixtures and fittings. Although there would have been significant investment in manufacturing equipment such as stills, it indicates that a large amount of money was spent on display. The shop of John Arnold, London apothecary, had an inventory of 117 glasses, 295 gallipots and jars, which we associate with old apothecaries' shops today, as well as 183 boxes and barrels.[23] The interior was a carefully balanced blend of form and function, usually spread over two rooms, so that more expensive or dangerous items could be stored at the back, and also allowing for privacy should the need arise. Apothecary shops became synonymous with exoticism, some showing stuffed alligators or snakes, or strange creatures in jars. In April and June of 1633, London apothecary Thomas Johnson displayed in his window the first bananas known to have reached England. These shops were designed to entice the customer and all of this was a stage set that physicians such as Sydenham and Dover were familiar with. Dover abhorred corrupt apothecaries, particularly those who operated freely without obtaining prescriptions from a doctor. The relationship between the two professions was a finely balanced one. Clearly, Sydenham and Malthus worked closely together, but it was Malthus who would have physically made laudanum in the Pestle & Mortar on Pall Mall. Yet, physicians felt on the whole that they were more qualified than apothecaries, and that no apothecary should dispense without prescription. It was an ongoing and often fraught debate.

Meanwhile, Dover had made enough money to take a trip to the West Indies in 1702. In 1708, he decided to invest significantly in a pair of ships, the *Duke* and *Duchess* out of Bristol, to sail around the world, and set off late the following year. It was a remarkable journey. On 1 February 1710, they were off the coast of Chile near the supposedly uninhabited Juan Fernández Islands, when a light was sighted on one of them, Más a Tierra (Closer to Land). Dover led a landing party to investigate, and there found Alexander Selkirk, Scottish privateer, who had been cast away on the island some four years before with only a musket, hatchet, knife, cooking pot, a Bible and his clothes. Selkirk was later one of the inspirations for Daniel Defoe's *Robinson Crusoe*. Selkirk accompanied the ships back to England.

Later, off the coast of Ecuador, the expedition picked up plague after a battle with the locals, and this was a decisive moment for Dover. As head of the medical services on board, he treated 180 sailors with methods he had learned from Sydenham, and lost no more than thirteen. The surgeons on board 'made heavy complaint' to Dover about the lack of medicine for such an amount of sick men, although Dover had been sure that the ships were well provisioned when they set out.[24] Returning to England in 1711, Dover had doubled his original investment, and had enough money to finally live a more leisured life.

Sydenham's laudanum recipe had been disseminated across Europe and America, and new versions of it were already being invented. A Leiden-based chemist, Jakob Le Mort, produced his own version of laudanum. It was significantly less powerful, and contained honey, liquorice, aniseed, camphor, salt of tartar and flowers of Benjamin, as well as opium. It appeared in London in 1721 listings as an *Elixir asthmaticum*, although it was commonly known as paregoric. It rapidly became one of the staples of the household medicine cabinet, used to treat coughs and asthma – as the official title would suggest – to ease diarrhoea, and to quiet restive or teething children.

In 1729, Dover published his best-known work, *The Ancient*

Physician's Legacy to his Country, to great success. Both a robust home medical manual and an outlandish advertisement for his own services, Dover's book is full of wild inaccuracies in its descriptions of both diseases and cures, but it is a marvellous read and ran to eight editions. Although it has many weaknesses, the *Ancient Physician* is excellent on pharmacology, and dispels some of the myths surrounding drugs of the time, particularly that of 'signatures'. This tradition essentially paired ailments with drugs that either resembled them somehow, or had the same name: liverwort for liver problems, for instance. Dover dismissed these cures as nonsenses, including the ancient alchemical talisman of a bezoar stone, long carried to ward off gall and kidney stones among richer classes, which he refers to as 'that petrified Matter of Disease, cut out of the Paunches, Galls and Bladders of some of the nastiest creatures in being'.[25] He had no time for theriac or mithridate, or any sort of 'such good-for-nothing Compositions'. He did, however, advocate the ingestion of large amounts of mercury for everything from asthma to worms, which brought outrage from the medical community and earned him the name 'Dr Quicksilver'. But most importantly, the *Ancient Physician* introduces the recipe for what would become, along with laudanum and paregoric, one of the most popular medicines of the next two centuries:

Take Opium one Ounce, Salt-Petre and Tartar vitriolated, each four Ounces, Ipocacuana one Ounce, Liquorish one Ounce. Put the Salt-Petre and Tartar into a red-hot Mortar, stirring them with a Spoon till they have done flaming. Then powder them very fine; after that slice in your Opium; grind these to a Powder, and then mix the other Powders with these. Dose from forty to sixty or seventy Grains in a Glass of White-Wine Posset, going to Bed.—Covering up warm, and drinking a Quart or three pints of the Posset-Drink while sweating. In two or three Hours, at farthest, the Patient will be perfectly free of Pain.[26]

Like Sydenham, Dover himself gave away the recipe, but the medicine took his name immediately and Dover's Powder was used as a general panacea until after the Second World War. It was often found in bulk in the medical panniers of captured Italian troops, and wasn't banned in India until 1994. The success of the book, and his piratical adventures at sea, had made Thomas Dover a comfortable man, and he retired to live with his friend Robert Tracy, to whom the *Ancient Physician* was dedicated, before dying in 1742.

The New Culture of Intoxication

'Life is a pill which none of us can bear to swallow without gilding; yet for the poor we delight in stripping it still barer.'[27]

James Boswell

Thomas Dover expired just as Britain was at the height of the Gin Craze. Introduced from Holland after the Restoration of 1660, gin exposed London's drinkers to strong liquor for the first time. Traditionally a nation of beer drinkers, they aspired to drink Continental spirits such as brandy, but that had been banned by King William III in 1689, and an Act of Parliament passed to 'encourage the distilling of brandy and spirits from corn' was passed in 1690.[28] Raw gin could be anything up to 140 per cent proof, and tales of strokes and blindness were not uncommon. And as acceptable gin can be made with bad grain, whereas decent bread cannot, farmers loved the industry and the British government wholeheartedly promoted home-grown distilling, but soon it had a terrible crisis on its hands. London's working population were mostly self-employed casual labourers, including the semi-skilled such as seamstresses and tailors; their careers were feast or famine. Gin became so cheap, and was so intoxicating, that people who had been paid and subsequently indulged were then reduced to a state where they were unable to seek labour in the coming days. A labour force previously reliant on nourishing beer and ale was ruining itself on spirits, as a treatise comparing the two describes, noting the full effects of a gin hangover:

> *His eyeballs, see, in hollow sockets sink,*
> *Bereft of health and sleep by burning drink . . .*
> *His liver even vitrifies his blood,*
> *His guts from Nature's druggery are freed,*
> *And in his bowels salamanders breed*[29]

Added to the sheer availability of gin was the fact that gin shops did not need a licence, so gin could be sold in private establishments, and men and women could drink together, with the consequent loss of inhibitions. In one case, William Bird's maid, Jane Andrews, was left in charge of his Kensington house, but instead went out to a gin shop, got drunk, and invited three of her fellow patrons back to her employer's house, where she 'proposed to the company that they, and she, should go to bed together', which they did.[30] This sort of behaviour threatened the ruling class with a lack of order they could not tolerate, particularly in their own homes, and measures were put in place to curb gin drinking, namely a series of five largely ineffectual Acts of Parliament, passed between 1729 and 1751, as the craze reached its peak.

The Gin Craze is linked to the trend for consumption of opium and all other intoxicants by a number of important factors. Gin itself was not necessarily addictive, and was often actively unpleasant to drink, but it fulfilled a need in the working-class population that had been suppressed by the move from the land to towns and cities, primarily London: namely, the need to celebrate the brief interlude of not being at work. The sheer strength of gin meant that it rendered most drinkers drunk very quickly, and publicly. The public and profligate nature of this binge drinking was what was most troubling to the governing classes of the time. The aristocrats and politicians also drank, but their intake was deemed a private matter. They were torn: were the labouring poor being paid too much, so could therefore afford such drunken abandon, or did the economy benefit through their profligacy?

Contemporary writers discussed and usually lamented the rise of luxury constantly. The goods flooding into Britain from all over the New World, Europe and Asia were no longer the exclusive preserve of the royal court. The new middle classes now enjoyed tea, coffee, silk and ivories, as well as opium, ambergris and other expensive products. Many in the old guard were reminiscent of Pliny the Elder in his diatribes against silk, although there were conflicting voices. Daniel Defoe argued in favour of the national distilling trade, with the notion that domestic consumption was a positive thing. Bernard Mandeville's poem 'The Grumbling Hive: Or, Knaves turn'd Honest', published in 1705 just as gin started to become popular in London, imagined that private vices and the need to consume were what kept society cohesive, despite the complainers. When, inside the hive, 'Honesty fills all their Hearts', many die and the bees become dull and less productive. Mandeville concluded with 'Bare Virtue can't make Nations live, In Splendor'.[31] Many writers realized that the state increasingly depended upon an urban population who could be taxed on their consumption, no matter how poor. The

Gin Craze was the perfect example of this debate, and one of the best-documented early social crises that revolved around working-class intoxication.

The middle-class hand-wringing in the endless tracts on luxury was, of course, as meaningless to the men and women inhabiting the gin shops of Covent Garden as the habits of Jahangir and the alcoholics of the Mughal court. Gin was a way to escape the daily miseries and drudgery of their lives, and soon the collective pursuit of oblivion on London's streets was out of control. The 'meaner, though useful Part of the Nation, as Day-Laborers, Men and Women Servants and Common Soldiers, nay even Children are enticed and seduced to taste, like and approve' railed the pamphlets, as London's working classes were 'frequently seen in our Streets in such a Condition abhorrent to reasonable creatures'.[32]

Charles Davenant, the politician and writer, who had initially argued in favour of the gin industry, realized that gin was, 'a growing fad among the common people and may in time prevail as much as opium with the Turks, to which many people attribute the scarcity of people in the east'.[33] Politicians and economists alike were forever afraid of a fall in population, reducing the workforce and available military manpower, as well as decreasing tax revenues, but the fear of gin taking over and decimating the labouring population was real. Bearing in mind that gin was primarily consumed and produced in London, then the figures are alarming. In England and Wales in 1700, total consumption was around 1.23 million gallons. By 1714, that figure was up to almost 2 million gallons per year; by 1745, 6.4 million and, by 1751, 7.05 million. So by the end of that period, it amounted to a gallon per head of the whole population, per year.[34]

The Irish faction of St-Giles-in-the-Field succumbed rapidly and with shocking consequences such as desertion, child malnutrition and prostitution. There was a corresponding rise in crime, and much of it involved drunken violence and theft. The reality of social unrest and women left destitute and inebriated on the streets mobilized London's new middling classes, as well as the government, to work towards social change. New organizations, such as the Society for the Promotion of Christian Knowledge (SPCK) founded in 1689, the year before the Distilling Act, had risen up to try and take positive action by distributing pamphlets and engaging with the unfortunates. Others, such as the Society for the Reformation of Manners, were less positive, seeking to catch miscreants behaving lewdly in order to have them prosecuted.

By the 1730s, things were in a desperate state in London. One particular case shocked the city and the nation, and galvanized the reformers and the government. Judith Defour worked as a throwster, twisting silk fibres into thread. She had a weakness for gin, and often turned up to work a little worse for wear, but otherwise seemed a normal employee. She had a daughter, Mary, aged a little over two years old, but was no longer in touch with the father and money was scarce. For this reason, and perhaps the drunkenness, Mary had been staying in the parish workhouse. One Sunday, Judith collected her for a visit, already the worse for wear. Whether she knew Mary had been outfitted with a new set of clothes that week or not, was never established. After keeping her daughter out for longer than she should, Judith carried her into the fields behind Brick Lane in the eastern part of London and choked Mary with a piece of linen. She insisted she was aided by a woman named 'Sukey'. Stripping the body, they left it in a ditch and took the clothing to a dealer where they 'sold the Coat and Stay for a Shilling, and the Petticoat and Stockings for a Groat. We parted the Money, and join'd for a Quartern of Gin'.[35] Defour insisted, even in the face of a guilty verdict and a sentence of death, that it was Sukey who had made her kill her daughter. Defour's own mother said in court that 'She never was in her right Mind, but was always roving.'[36] The author Henry Fielding, the Covent Garden magistrate in charge of overseeing so many cases in which intoxication played a part, was convinced that 'the *gin*' alone was to blame for many crimes, 'for the intoxicating draught ... removes all sense of fear and shame, and emboldens them to commit every wicked and desperate enterprise'.[37] Fielding, it may be noted, ridden with gout and dropsy, died of alcoholism in Lisbon in 1754.

The Defour case became notorious, bringing together as it did the societal fears of the age: a woman of loose morals, drunkenness, and a vulnerable and ultimately murdered child. For men to carouse drunkenly in the streets was one thing, and to be expected, but for women to lose themselves to drink was quite another. Infanticide was a constant preoccupation of reformers during the craze, as were the 'diminutive, pygmy ... withered and old' children of gin-drinking women.[38] A man deeply affected by seeing these children in the street, 'exposed, sometimes alive, sometimes dead, and sometimes dying', was Thomas Coram, an abandoned child himself who had led a hard life at sea.[39] Coram spent the 1720s and 30s campaigning for enough money to begin London's Foundling Hospital, hoping to house some of these infants, and was in the end successful, mainly thanks to well-known campaigners such as the Duchess of Somerset and William Hogarth. On the first day of admissions on 25 March 1741, far more women applied than there were places for children, and 'a more moving scene can't well be imagined'.[40]

In contrast to the horrendous damage effected by the Gin Craze, opium and its derivatives kept a low profile in the same decades. By now an accepted medicine, widely available in larger cities, there is little commentary. In an examination of the records of the Old Bailey, opium and laudanum appear as poisons deployed in killings or robbery, but in fewer than a dozen cases in the years of the craze. In two cases the perpetrator was also the user. One regards a robbery committed on the EIC premises, by a former employee and clearly hardened taker of opium, Thomas Abram, who attempted to get away with stealing 1,100 guineas and various property. When questioned as to why he committed the crime, Abram pleaded that he was unsound of mind, and called his doctor and apothecary to testify to the fact. When Dr Cromp was asked how much opium his patient took when he was 'under an Indisposition of the mind', the doctor 'reply'd, more than he would have him or any other Person take, for it might do him an Injury.'[41] The other regards a highway robbery committed 'in a common road near Hackney' by a Richard Montgomery, who after the robbery went with an accomplice for dinner, before pushing up the sash window and 'would have got out at the Window, saying, that he must go and fight the Indians' and after this 'he said he would take some Opium, for he had a Mind to take a Journey to the other World'. Montgomery's lawyer confessed that 'Lunacy had ran in the Blood of the Family ... To corroborate this Mr Collier Sen. (altho' the Prosecutor) was so generous as to confess, that his Wife coming to understand what Family he is of (for Montgomery is a fictitious Name) she knew several of them to be weak in their Intellectuals ... The Jury brought in their Verdict that he was Non compos mentis.'[42]

Thus, opiates accounted for an insignificant proportion of the cases presented to the Old Bailey, rather than the 1.5 per cent of all cases involving 'drunkenness' in the same years. The Gin Craze reached a peak in 1751, when William Hogarth issued his famous *Beer Street* and *Gin Lane* prints, showing the contrast between a happy state of consumption amongst the clean and robust citizens of the former and the ruined hags and inebriates of the latter. The

Gin Act of the same year raised prices sufficiently to curtail demand, and attempted to eliminate small drinking shops. But consumption had reached so high a level that it was unlikely that this was sufficient in itself. A combination of changes in society, as well as the influence of reformers, contributed to the end of what was a calamitous localized episode of alcoholism. Ultimately, the trigger for the Gin Craze is obvious, with the passing of the 1689 Act, but reasons for the end of it are unclear. These bouts of collective addiction have struck societies across the world periodically, but, like plague, they eventually lessen and then abate for reasons that remain essentially unknown. The feverish 'itch of gambling' seen amongst the British aristocracy of the late eighteenth century is an example in microcosm.

From the middle of the seventeenth century onwards, there had been attempts, in poetry and sermons, to vocalize what it was to be dependent upon a substance, namely alcohol, and to understand addiction. It was, however, the Gin Craze that was the very beginning of a willingness across society to understand what lay at the heart of alcoholism, and thus all addictions. From Henry Fielding, who believed firmly that it was, as often as not, the drink and not the drinker who was guilty of the crime, to certain members of the government, to campaigning aristocrats and artists, there was a movement towards addressing the needs of those brought to the most desperate of circumstances by what was still termed 'intoxication'.

From The Anatomy of Melancholy to the new Empiricism: Opium Under the Eighteenth-Century Microscope

The years of the Gin Craze saw a change not only in the attitude to intoxication, but to sensibility in general. What, in the seventeenth century, had been regarded as pertaining to the physical senses was increasingly coming to mean a sensitivity to the world at large. Robert Burton (1577–1640) was an Oxford scholar who wrote the first work to address problems with mental health directly, in 1621. *The Anatomy of Melancholy, What it is: With all the Kinds, Causes, Symptomes, Prognostickes, and Several Cures of it* was revelatory in its time, and influential for the following century and a half. Burton wrote from a personal perspective (albeit under a pseudonym), 'I write of melancholy, by being busy to avoid melancholy', and in his view there was, 'no greater cause of melancholy than idleness'.[43] The work is wide-ranging, and combines a medical textbook with a philosophical treatise, touching on many aspects of what are now primary concerns of modern mental health. His writing on insomnia and its attendant 'continuall cares, fears, sorrows' struck a chord and his words are referenced throughout the coming years by many other writers. He insists it must be 'speedily helped, and sleep by all means procured, which sometimes is a sufficient remedy of itself, without any other Physick'. For this he recommends the basics of 'Poppy', as well as 'mandrake, henbane and hempseed' or more complicated medicines he refers to as 'opiats'. What follows are extensive instructions on how to take these concoctions, what foods to eat, even how to lie in bed, in a fashion that 'may procure sleep to the most melancholy man in the world'.[44]

Burton's book is long-winded and repetitive, but there are enough sharply drawn observations on the state of what is now known as clinical depression for it to have been the most influential work on mental health for readers and writers in the next two centuries. It's also apparent from the complicated recipes for his cures that, even by the time he was writing, many people were in a state of almost constant self-medication, whether it be the sleepless rural poor with their boiled hempseed posset, or the gentleman in his chambers applying leeches and opium behind his ears. The direct link between mental health, mental distress and opiate use is implicit in Burton's work, and *The Anatomy of Melancholy* became a standard text for such gentlemen in the eighteenth century, as the Enlightenment began. Samuel Johnson (1709–1784), one of the most gifted Englishmen of his time – and a man who struggled throughout his life with depression, as well as alcoholism – said it 'was the only book that ever took him out of bed two hours sooner than he wished to rise'.[45]

By the time Johnson was reading Burton, Europe had changed significantly. Borders had realigned. The Ottoman and Mughal empires were on the wane, and the Safavids were finished. Constant and inconclusive wars had exhausted all their resources, and devastated the borderlands. European trade with Iran, Egypt and Syria dwindled away, but increased significantly with Istanbul and the Balkans. Although the white Egyptian Theban opium remained the pinnacle, Turkish opium, rather than Persian, became Britain's main supply, imported in 'flat pieces or cakes; covered with leaves, [in] which are frequently small capsules of [dockweed]. It has a peculiar, heavy, strong odour, and a bitter, nauseous taste, attended with some acrimony when long-chewed. Its colour is reddish-brown or fawn-like.'[46]

This Turkish opium, and even basics such as China tea and coffee from Yemen, were freely available and the new way of life for many. By the middle of the century, not only had consumption become more sophisticated, intellectual life had assumed a new importance. Philosophers such as Voltaire and Jean-Jacques Rousseau were writing works on tolerance and citizenship that were widely disseminated. Science had moved firmly towards empirical rationalism. And in 1753 the exceptional Swedish botanist Carl Linnaeus classified the opium poppy into the genus and species *Papaver somniferum*, and counted the seeds in one head with a pin to find over 32,000. The classification system Linnaeus devised, now known as binomial nomenclature, revolutionized natural science in the latter part of the century and forced scientists across all disciplines to organize themselves on a similar model, far superior to the personal and idiosyncratic methods used before.

Opium, through the old manuals, apothecary shops, and increasingly, through laudanum, paregoric and Dover's powder, had found itself a place in almost every home. The government preoccupation with distilled spirits and the disaster of the Gin Craze meant that few were looking at the faithful medicinal standby. Then, in an age of publishing and pamphleteering, a few dissenting voices began to emerge, and over the course of the eighteenth century a series of works on opium appeared that demonstrated changing attitudes to the drug amongst the medical community. Many of these were by men working or educated at Edinburgh University, which produced some of the foremost medical minds in the world in the latter part of the century.

First, though, Welsh doctor John Jones wrote a tract on *The Mysteries of Opium Reveal'd* (1700). His observations on the effects of opium were clear and accurate, and also show how far poppy cultivation had spread: his preference was for Egyptian opium owing to its proximity to the equator, reasoning that it is stronger from there because of the heat, and better than if it is 'made' in England or Germany. Even that made 'in the Languedoc, which borders upon the Mediterranean' was stronger.[47] His notes on the effects of long-term use, all the symptoms 'observable in old Drunkards', show the dangers of opiate abuse but the tone is without judgement, and he views opium overall in a positive light. His observations on the operation of opium on the senses are some of the first to include the feeling of transportation, a dreamlike removal from the ordinary world that shows an intimate familiarity with the mental effects of the drug: 'thus the *Sound* of a Pin's Head, falling into a Brass Cauldron, is heard at some distance', like '*Guns, Bells* &c., are better and farther heard along hollow *Valleys*, than upon *Plains*'.[48]

The book ends, somewhat bizarrely, with a final chapter on the external uses of opium, which concludes with the terse advice that it can 'excite to Venery by its titillating Volatile Salt, if applied to the Perineum', followed by a prayer dedicated to William Harvey's discovery of the circulatory system.[49]

In contrast to the useful but eccentric advice of writers such as Jones, after the Gin Craze, texts begin to appear warning of the dangers of opium. In 1742, the year of Dover's death, Charles Alston, a professor of botany and materia medica in Edinburgh, produced a paper, *A Dissertation on Opium*, the first pharmacological study of opium, some of it conducted on poppies he grew himself. He was convinced that opium worked on the nerves, not by 'rarefying' the blood, although he wouldn't be proved right for another century.

George Young (1692–1757), a surgeon and doctor also working in Edinburgh, published in 1753 a treatise on opiates in which he warned, 'Everybody knows a large dose of laudanum will kill, so need not be cautioned on that head; but there are few who consider it a slow poison, though it certainly is so.'[50] Young, strangely, was against giving opiates in cases of extreme pain, such as kidney stones, for which it is doubtful his patients thanked him, but he wrote sensibly on the need to moderate opiate intake, and tested extensively on himself. His work with pregnant women and children was also the clearest to date. On morning sickness, he dismissed the idea of humours and attributed it instead to 'some change in the uterus, which we cannot explain: yet it is a change which, by sympathy, seems to affect the whole nervous system'.[51] He recommended the use of laudanum in childbirth, although only enough to alleviate pain and not to suppress the mother. For weaning children, he recommended it in small doses, and not as an antidote to being 'crammed every day by their fond mothers with a variety of jellies, sweet-meats and preserves'.[52]

A decade later, in 1763, John Awsiter, apothecary to Greenwich Hospital in south-east London, published a small book on 'the Effects of Opium considered as a Poison'. Opium as a poison was clearly nothing new: from ancient times to the records of the Old Bailey, people had used opium and subsequently laudanum to either drug or poison their victims, but Awsiter's first line declares, 'Gentlemen, I was Induced to Write this Essay from a Desire of throwing a Light upon a Subject, hitherto but triflingly, and at best, obscurely treated.'[53]

The apothecary was in no doubt that opium was 'first intro-duced to dissipate Anxieties, Pains and Perturbations of the Mind, which appears not unlike the Effects of Intoxicating Drinks, so requested in *Europe*'. He asserts that opium is not in 'common use' in England, but that nor should it be, for famil-iarity with the drug would remove 'the Necessary Fear and Caution, which should prevent their experiencing the extensive power of this Drug; for there are many Properties in it, if uni-versally known, that would habituate the Use, and make it more in request with us that with the Turks themselves, the Result of which Knowledge must prove a general Misfortune'.[54] However, he then goes on to describe the successful treatment of enough overdoses to indicate that opiate abuse was rather more wide-spread than he originally indicated, and includes purges, emetics, and keeping the patient awake and mobile. After treating an eighteen-month-old girl for an overdose, Awsiter also warns against nurseries whose practice it is to give their charges syrup of poppy such as 'Godfrey's Cordial, which is a Composition very binding, has Opium in it, and was never designed by the Author for such Purposes'.[55] Godfrey's Cordial became one of the most popular proprietary medicines in America by the end of the eighteenth century and was in use worldwide until the 1970s.

Awsiter's modest book of cautionary tales reveals the extent of knowledge about opiate overdose amongst London's medical professionals; until recently, the immediate treatment for overdose was little different. The book is valuable, though, for its practical knowledge, clearly acquired by personal experience and expressed in a useful and thorough fashion. This spirit of empiricism pervaded the latter part of the eighteenth century as the Enlightenment progressed and intellectual horizons broadened.

John Leigh (1755–96) was an American doctor from Virginia working in Edinburgh when, in 1785, he produced a groundbreaking paper on opium, which he dedicated to George Washington. It won Edinburgh University's Harveian Prize and was published to acclaim the following year. 'No writer,' he says of opium's obscure origins, 'has yet offered to the world any satisfactory account of the manner in which this valuable remedy, or its virtues, were first discovered; hence the imaginations of many have been busily set to work, and a variety of fruitless conjectures brought forth to fill up this historical charm.'[56] Of his many experiments – upon volunteers, animals and himself – he made minute observations under early laboratory conditions, often using the 'common crude opium of the shops' of Edinburgh, estimated to be only one third as strong as that available from the London Dispensary, which Leigh preferred for all his recipes. In one experiment, he extracted opium 'essential oil' and 'prevailed' upon a healthy man to take fifteen drops of it, 'with some difficulty', but it 'brought on such a vomiting as deterred me from making further experiments of this nature'.[57] This did not deter him, however, from other experiments, such as the time he 'threw a quantity of my strong solution into the rectum of a rabbit', and 'into the vagina' of a dog, and dosed young teenagers to test their tolerance. He does at least admit that he designed these experiments to be 'free from artificial gloss'.[58]

Edinburgh's influence on European medicine during this time was remarkable, although some of it somewhat less fact-based than Leigh's empiricism. A contemporary of Leigh's, Dr John Brown, devised the Brunonian System of health, based on stimuli: all disease was caused by over- or under-stimulation. Emetics and purges were needed for those in an excited state, and opium and hearty meals for those in a state of lethargy. Verging on outright quackery, the Brunonian System was hugely popular in Germany and Italy, and proved influential for a few decades until it was finally discredited.

Samuel Crumpe, an Irish physician working in Limerick who had studied with Leigh in Edinburgh, was rather more sensible in his outlook. In his 1793 work *An Inquiry into the Nature and Properties of Opium*, he begins 'It appears rather singular, that almost every circumstance relating to this remarkable medicine has been the subject of dispute ... Late experience, however, seems to have so far ascertained the manner of its production and preparation, as to remove every difference on these points.'[59] This was broadly true, and not least because of the efforts of men like Crumpe, who injected an opiate solution into his skin, eye and penis, and also ground some to powder so he could snort it. His overall observations of this were 'heat and pain', followed by numbness, and he concluded that opium was of no use in the treatment of gonorrhea. Crumpe's calm descriptions of scraping the skin from his wrist, examining his eyes and urethra, and his tendency to sneeze after inhaling are admirable in their restraint, as, unfortunately, is his description of 'laying bare the thorax of a dog which had just been hanged' so that he might apply opium 'milk' directly to the pericardium of its heart. It revived the heart 'for about a minute'. He conducted further experiments on dogs, rabbits and frogs, and gives comprehensive descriptions of not only withdrawal symptoms, but how to treat diseases from smallpox to rheumatism with opiates, and relates how he treated a woman during a miscarriage. On 'Mania', he observes, 'I fear our knowledge of the pathology of this disease is so limited, that the practice must be, for the most part, empirical.'[60]

Both talented writers and scientists, Leigh's and Crumpe's works on opiates are the most accurate and useful of any that had gone before. Leigh returned to America in 1786, married and became a notable if not distinguished manager of a lottery, before dying at forty. Crumpe died suddenly aged twenty-nine, having won the prize of the Royal Irish Academy for his work on employment and the economy in Ireland. These significant losses to the scientific community were no doubt much to the relief of Edinburgh's and Limerick's dogs, rabbits and frogs.

'This odious disease': Early Addiction Theories in America and Britain

The close similarities, if not collaboration, between American and British physicians so soon after the American War of Independence may seem surprising, but it was far from unusual, and was particularly important in the early study of addiction. A large, self-improving middle class burgeoned in both countries in the 1740s and 50s, and many educated families had members on both sides of the Atlantic, with intertwined business interests and close personal ties. Debates on the American War in London's inns and taverns had more often than not voted in favour of immediate peace, even if the colony was lost as a result. Exchange of information and commercial goods was by this stage well established, and many British businesses had an outpost on the East Coast of America, or had frequent contact with them. Many early American newspapers carry advertisements for stock arriving from their London shop, or purchased from London. In the *Boston News-Letter* of 26 November 1761, Charles Russell of Charleston advertised that 'At his Shop at the Sign of GALEN'S HEAD opposite the Three Cranes and near the FERRY', there were to be had all manner of 'the latest Drugs, and Medicines, Chymical and Galenicals' from London, including Bateman's and Sloughton's Drops, Lockyer's, Hoopers and Anderson's Pills, British Oyl and Daffy's Elixir.[61] These drugs were by this time known as patent medicines, and of wildly varying quality. Bateman's Pectoral Drops were stock paregoric, and there was no Dr Bateman; Lockyer's Pills were alleged to contain sunbeams, marketed by Lionel Lockyer, a quack in Southwark.

Americans were not only fans of prepared patent medicines, they also took opium in simpler forms. French-born J. Hector St John de Crèvecœur travelled the East Coast and wrote a memoir titled *Letters from an American Farmer*, exploring what was then life on the frontiers and the American tenets of independence and self-reliance. Of Nantucket island, he wrote, 'A single custom prevails here among the women at which I was greatly surprised and really am at a loss how to account for . . . They have adopted these many years the Asiatic custom of taking a dose of opium every morning, and so deep-rooted is it that they would be at a loss how to live without this indulgence.'[62]

As well as patent medicines and opium, early Americans were drinkers on a similar scale to their British counterparts of one hundred years before: rum from the West Indies was a popular strong drink, but small beer and cider were the most popular, taken at almost every meal. As pioneers moved to the Corn Belt their success at farming meant that, like the European grain gluts that contributed to the Gin Craze, Midwestern Americans began to make whiskey from their crop surplus, and ship it back east. From the late 1770s, there was a marked rise in the consumption of spirits, and the attendant addiction. East Coast clergy were the first to write on this alarming phenomenon, including the abolitionist and Quaker Anthony Benezet (1713–85), who in 1774 wrote *The Mighty Destroyer Displayed*, about the rising tide of alcohol abuse in Pennsylvania, where 'Drops beget drams, and drams beget more drams, until they come to be without weight and without measure.'[63]

Benezet's student and friend Benjamin Rush, a Founding Father of America, was also concerned about what he thought of as a rising tide of not only intoxication, but disease. Rush's *Inquiry into the Effects of Ardent Spirits on the Human Mind and Body* of 1784 is a landmark work in the understanding of alcoholism, and was the beginning of the disease theory: 'This odious disease (for by that name it should be called) . . .'[64] Rush proposed that this disease should be properly treated by physicians, in the correct environment. The gravity of the work is belied in the opening pages, displaying a table of his own devising correlating certain drinks to the result in temperament, appearance, actions and outcomes. Small beer, for instance, results in 'Serenity' and cider in 'Cheerfulness', but rum in 'Peevishness', brandy, 'Fighting and Horse Racing' and gin, 'Perjury'. Should the latter be taken morning and evening for a sustained period, the outcome can only be 'Burglary' and 'Death'.[65]

Four years later, on 4 July 1788, Rush led 17,000 citizens on an Independence Day march, at the end of which they celebrated with beer and cider, but no distilled spirits. In a sad irony, Rush and Benezet watched their friend, Reverend Nisbet – who had brought his family to America from Montrose in Scotland – lose his son Tom to the most desperate alcoholism. After a series of misadventures involving debt and an aborted career at sea, Tom had walked away from a friend in New York 'without a word', drunk, confused, and injured, and trekked towards home for weeks, before taking a canoe trip down the massive Susquehanna River at the beginning of winter. Arriving home in an appalling state, he was eventually confined in Pennsylvania Hospital.[66] The strain killed his father in 1804, and Tom followed him to the grave a few months later, insane, unrecognizable and still in Pennsylvania Hospital. Rush continued to campaign against distilled spirits, and went on to devise a 'Plan for an Asylum for Drunkards to be called a Sober House' in 1810, the first American to suggest such special care.

By the time Rush devised his plan for the Sober House, his pamphlets were selling in their thousands. In England, in the year Tom Nisbet and his long-suffering father died, Thomas Trotter, recently retired physician to the Fleet Prison, published *An Essay, Medical, Philosophical and Chemical, on Drunkenness, and its Effects on the Human Body*.

Unlike almost all those who had gone before him, Trotter studied inebriation alone, divorced from religion or morality. His subject was 'the drunkard, exposed in the street and highway, stretched in the kennel ... allowed to perish, without pity and without assistance; as if his crime were inexpiable, and his body infectious to the touch'. This level of intoxication, he averred, was classless, and 'might be seen in all ranks and stations of life'. Trotter sets out his stall clearly from the start: 'In medical language, I consider drunkenness, strictly speaking, to be a disease.' The prison doctor is also convinced of the similar nature of dependence upon alcohol to that of cannabis and opium. 'The effects of opium,' he writes, are 'nearly alike to those of ardent spirit' and it 'is well known that many of our fair countrywomen carry laudanum about with them, and take it frequently when under low spirits'.[67]

Trotter's *Essay* is a work of great humanity, and although it was not the first to couch persistent drunkenness as a disease, it was the first to treat it without judgement and to compare it to the abuse of other substances. It was republished extensively in America, by that time firmly in the grip of whiskey fever, and inspired temperance preachers and physicians alike in the promotion of what would be known from this point forwards as Sobriety.

A Different Form of Experimentation: The Romantics

In a new age of empiricism and scientific thought, one of the greatest literary movements in Europe, Romanticism, flowered. Nostalgic, rebellious, intellectual and daring, the Romantic movement was a reaction to endless wars, radical changes in the pace of life and the relentless pace of invention and discovery in the latter part of the eighteenth century.

It was perhaps inevitable, with his theories of maintaining 'excitability' and experiencing stimuli, that the member of the Edinburgh school of doctors who ultimately influenced the main members of the Romantic movement was the erratic, self-medicating John Brown. Brown's pupil and acolyte Thomas Beddoes (1760–1808), himself a controversial figure who introduced the notion of hypochondria in his essay *Hygëia: or essays moral and medical, on the causes affecting the personal state of our middling and affluent classes* in 1802, counted the prominent

Romantic figures Thomas De Quincey, Samuel Taylor Coleridge and Tom Wedgwood among his friends and patients. All were opium addicts. Moreover, all the major Romantic poets except William Wordsworth are known to have experimented with or habitually taken opiates, namely, laudanum.

Laudanum and paregoric were by this time endemic in Britain, taken by people of all classes and incomes. The greatest consumers of opiates were those in the poor industrial county of Lancashire, and the poor rural counties of Lincolnshire, Cambridgeshire and Norfolk. In Lancashire, the predominant users were mothers managing long working hours with large families; in the Fenland counties, men used it to ward off the 'severe ague' associated with working in cold and wet conditions, and to allay the boredom of hours in the fields. In Manchester, where cotton-spinning predominated, 'on a Saturday afternoon, the counters of the druggists were strewed with pills of one, two or three grains, in preparation for the known demand of the evening'.[68] In the east of England, from the Wash south to Cambridge, demand for laudanum was huge, and it was known as 'opic' or 'elevation'. The working people of the fens had traditionally cultivated white poppies to make poppy-head tea, imbibed to ward off the chills of the marsh and to settle children's stomachs, but increasingly they were turning to shop-bought patent products. For the inhabitants of these poor communities, both urban and rural, laudanum was cheaper than alcohol, could be used by the whole family and bore little social stigma.

For the Romantic poets, removed from these mundane working lives, laudanum was a different means of elevation. Or at least so they believed initially. De Quincey, Coleridge and Wedgwood all began misusing laudanum in their teenage years, and their lifelong addictions display all the hallmarks of opiate abuse throughout the past two centuries.

Samuel Taylor Coleridge (1772–1834) began using laudanum at nineteen, although his dependency took almost another decade to become problematic. In 1797 he composed his three greatest poems, *The Rime of the Ancient Mariner*, 'Kubla Khan' and *Christabel*. 'Kubla Khan' is famously the result of an opium-inspired dream. Coleridge related how he had 'retired to a lonely farm house between Porlock and Linton, on the Exmoor confines of Somerset and Devonshire' where he had been prescribed an anodyne for a 'slight indisposition'. Sitting down to read, he chose *Purchas*, with its tales of the Mughal Empire and the magic of the East. He fell asleep reading the sentence, inspired by Marco Polo's description of Xanadu, 'Here the Khan Kubla commanded a palace to be built, and a stately garden thereunto: and thus ten miles of fertile ground were inclosed with a wall'. After a three-hour opiate vision, Coleridge woke and wrote down all he remembered, before he was interrupted by a person from Porlock. On returning to his desk, the vision had dissipated 'like the images on the surface of a stream into which a stone had been cast'.[69] But before the rude interruption, the immortal opening lines were already on paper.

> *In Xanadu did Kubla Khan*
> *A stately pleasure-dome decree:*
> *Where Alph, the sacred river, ran*
> *Through caverns measureless to man*
> *Down to a sunless sea.*
> *So twice five miles of fertile ground*
> *With walls and towers were girdled round:*
> *And there were gardens bright with sinuous rills,*
> *Where blossomed many an incense-bearing tree;*
> *And here were forests ancient as the hills,*
> *Enfolding sunny spots of greenery.*

From this point on, Coleridge was a dedicated user of laudanum, although he would never again be as productive as he was in 1797. In his abuse of laudanum, he was joined by his great friend Tom Wedgwood, son of Josiah. The Wedgwood family supported Coleridge at a time when he was particularly impoverished, and the friendship between Tom and the poet remained a constant. Delicate and sensitive, Wedgwood passed most of his life in ill health and experimented with various drugs to cure himself. He was charming, if quiet and often despondent, and suffered long bouts of depression. His experimentations with silver nitrate and a camera obscura succeeded in producing images that were the first photographs. Unfortunately, they were sensitive to light and faded as fast as their creator. Tom did, however, also have time to experiment with a lot of drugs, something he and Coleridge obviously enjoyed together, as Coleridge's words suggest: 'We will have a fair trial of Bang. Do bring down some of the Hyoscyamine pills, and I will give a fair trial of Opium, Henbane, and Nepenthe. By-the-bye I always considered Homer's account of the Nepenthe as a "Banging" lie.'[70]

At a high point in Coleridge's use of opium, in 1805, Tom Wedgwood's 'poor, broken life' came to an end.[71] Alleged by his family to have passed away from a stroke, descriptions of his miserable death are more redolent of a drug overdose. 'What a day for poor Jos,' wrote his sister-in-law to her own sister, Emma, 'watching him dying for 12 hours.'[72]

There is, ultimately, little wonder the Romantic poets began to turn upon themselves. Robert Southey, another prominent poet, savaged Coleridge's selfishness: 'Every person who had witnessed his habits, knows that for the greater – infinitely the greater part – inclination and indulgence are the motives.'[73]

Yet the Romantic notion of opium persisted. Thomas De Quincey (1785–1859), who first took opiates to treat trigeminal

neuralgia, credited laudanum as the root of his creativity, referring to the 'marvellous agency of opium' the 'true hero of the
tale'.[74] His work of 1821, *Confessions of an English Opium-Eater*,
is central to the Romantic concept of opium as a font of creativity. Throughout his long life, De Quincey used laudanum,
sometimes in mammoth doses; his periods of low usage were
unproductive. Of all the Romantics, De Quincey's affinity for
opiates and their effects was genuine. The visions he experienced,
which he noted were 'chiefly architectural', spent in Italianate
landscapes, are remarkable:

> The sense of space, and in the end, the sense of time, were both
> powerfully affected. Buildings, landscapes, &c. were exhibited
> in proportions so vast as the bodily eye is not fit to receive.
> Space swelled, and was amplified to an extent of unutterable
> infinity. This, however, did not disturb me so much as the vast
> expansion of time; I sometimes seemed to have lived for 70 or
> 100 years in one night; nay, sometimes had feelings represen-
> tative of a millennium passed in that time, or however, of a
> duration far beyond the limits of any human experience.[75]

It was not all creative bliss, however. In a bizarre encounter in
1816, recounted in his *Confessions*, he was living in Dove Cottage,
Grasmere, in the English Lake District, when a 'Malay' knocked
on the door. De Quincey's maid fled, leaving her master to speak
to the man. In a show of hospitality, De Quincey offered the
man enough opium to 'kill three dragoons and their horses' and
watched as the man ate the whole, and left. De Quincey struggled with the encounter for a long time, wondering if he had
overdosed the man, but 'I never heard of any Malay being found
dead.'[76] Despite a telling lack of evidence of the Malay's existence at all, De Quincey continued to suffer with anxiety over the

episode. Unlike Coleridge, whose readings of tales of the East were an inspiration, for De Quincey, they were the stuff of nightmare:

> The Malay has been a fearful enemy for months. Every night, through his means, I have been transported into Asiatic scenery . . . in China or Hindustan . . . I was stared at, grinned at, chattered at by monkeys, by parquets, by cockatoos. I ran into pagodas, and was fixed for centuries at the summit, or in secret rooms; I was the idol; I was the priest; I was the worshipped; I was the sacrificed . . . Thousands of years I lived and was buried in stone coffins, with mummies and sphinxes, in narrow chambers at the heart of eternal pyramids.[77]

From his late teenage years, De Quincey lived entirely through the spectrum of opiates. He neither wanted nor really attempted to cease using them. He married and had a family, although their existence was precarious. He believed opium accentuated dominant features of the personality, and 'If a man "whose talk is of oxen" should become an opium-eater, the probability is that (if he is not too dull to dream at all) he will dream about oxen.'[78] Yet for all his dreams of higher plains, he was also the man who, when called upon one day by his friend John Wilson, was wearing a 'Sort of grey watchman's coat, evidently made for a man four times his size, and bought probably at a pawnbroker's shop'. Halfway through a rant on transcendentalism, the coat fell open to reveal a naked De Quincey beneath. 'You may see I am not dressed,' Thomas observed soberly. 'I did see it,' replied Wilson. De Quincey wrapped the coat back 'round him and went on as before'.[79]

Coleridge died in 1834, an unhappy addict confined to his doctor's house in Highgate. Thomas Carlyle, the Victorian philosopher, visited him, hoping to discuss transcendentalism, but soon grew bored, for 'To sit as a passive bucket and be pumped into, whether you consent or not, can in the long-run be exhilarating to no creature.'[80] De Quincey lived to the age of seventy-four, managing short periods of abstinence, and died in Edinburgh, ending a life riven by disputes, nightmares, debt and drug dependence.

In the Arms of Morpheus: Friederich Wilhelm Sertürner

By 1800, European chemists had been advancing the causes of the natural sciences into various different modern disciplines. Organic analysis was a particular speciality for British, French and German chemists, as they sought to find out how various drugs work in the way that they do. The medical profession was becoming ever more structured, and it and the general public were calling for more specific and higher-quality medicines.

In 1804 – as De Quincey began his career in laudanum, Coleridge reached a high in consumption, and Tom Wedgwood went into terminal decline – the history of opium took another huge stride forward. Romanticism and *Naturphilosophie* developed in tandem at the beginning of the nineteenth century and played an important role in scientific, as well as literary, life. Friedrich Wilhelm Adam Sertürner, a twenty-year-old German pharmacist on the outskirts of what is now Paderborn, isolated meconic acid from opium latex, which he identified as the sleeping agent. The following year, and the year after that, his discoveries were published in a publication for practising apothecaries, Johann Trommsdorff's *Journal der Pharmacie*. The result was, at the time, a damp squib. The field of organic chemistry was struggling to find the same sense of order that had prevailed in inorganic chemistry and botany and Sertürner was left to continue his experiments, but his work was disrupted by Napoleon's invasion and he had to move to another pharmacy in Einbeck. At the same time, the Parisian chemist Armand Séguin was also working on opium latex, attempting to isolate the active ingredients. Despite conducting extensive experiments, many chemists and pharmacists did not really know what they were looking at, but in 1804, he reported to the Paris Institut that he had obtained from opium a plant acid and a white, crystalline substance that dissolved in alcohol and turned syrup of violets slightly green. The syrup of violets test was used to identify alkali substances. In the same year, French industrialist Charles Derosne had also obtained the white crystalline substance, but he did not understand its alkaloid nature. He called it a salt because 'I do not know the proper name to assign to it.'[81] In 1811, Sertürner published again on the substance he had discovered, and agreed with Derosne that it was salifiable, or capable of forming a salt.

In 1817, Sertürner published in the *Annalen der Physik* that he had identified the active substance *Morphium* from opium latex.[82] He had tested the substance on himself and three volunteers in the laboratory, and within forty-five minutes had almost poisoned all of them. Only the downing of vinegar as an emetic prevented the experiment going badly wrong. But still, Sertürner was now sure he had found the active sleeping agent in opium.

French chemist Joseph Louis Gay-Lussac worked with pharmaceutical chemist Pierre Robiquet on Sertürner's findings, and declared it the first discovery of an organic base. Sertürner had identified the alkaloid that was morphine. Before 1810, alkaloids were unknown, and in less than fifty years almost eighty had been documented. His work had an almost instant and far-reaching effect, allowing others to rapidly identify such

compounds as quinine and strychnine, as well as the other alkaloids present in opium base.

European commercial competition was by this time fierce, and
publications were translated quickly and widely disseminated. In
1821 Thomas Morson, a London apothecary, was manufacturing morphine, and following a decade of research and testing,
German pharmacy H. E. Merck, having long outgrown the
Engel-Apotheke, began to refine and distribute it in bulk, featuring it in their 1827 brochure of all known alkaloids. It was
immediately in demand.

Sertürner, meanwhile, struggled again at the end of the Napoleonic Wars and had to move to Hamelin. Despite his discovery,
and his valuable observations on the Asiatic cholera outbreak in
Germany in the early 1830s, he died in obscurity in 1841 and was
buried back in Einbeck.

Morphine heralded a new era in drug manufacture and consumption. A new, clean chemical product, fitting for the age, it
produced miraculous results instantly, and appeared to have no
side effects. People previously crippled by pain got up and
walked from their doctor's office. Named for a god, it is also a
demon, and by the 1840s, Western doctors realized there was
a dreadful problem with this wondrous new cure. Sertürner, in
the name of science and a good night's sleep, had unwittingly
unleashed a monster, just as, on the other side of the world, the
British Empire was engineering one.

Chapter Five

THE CHINA CRISIS

The Indian News and Chronicle of Eastern Affaires

Although Britain and America continued to obtain their opium mainly from Turkey, Iran and sometimes Egypt and the Levant, as well as the new small-scale home-grown attempts at cultivation, on the other side of the world, an entirely different supply chain had been constructed. After the Battle of Plassey in 1757, the East India Company had consolidated its grip on trade at each of its factories, and finally rid itself of the challenge from the French East India Company in 1763. Government-authorized rogues such as Robert Clive (1725–74), better known as Clive of India, had made massive gains for the British Crown, snatching huge swathes of the country to establish British dominance in Bengal. Clive was an opium addict his entire adult life, having first taken it during a nervous breakdown as a young man, and it is likely he died of an opium overdose at his grand house in Berkeley Square in 1774. During his career, the EIC had changed radically from a band of merchant adventurers into a mighty bureaucratic and military machine that governed millions of people. As it grew, the EIC recruited Indians into the ranks, from all castes, although the British-trained officers who arrived from the company's own military academy outranked any native soldier.

Initially focussed on the acquisition of land and trading rights, the EIC had become a quasi-governmental force in a land riven by the infighting of the local rulers and the decline of the Mughal Empire. Once it had consolidated its interests, it looked to its global concerns to facilitate international trade, and by the late eighteenth century, it had a clear solution: tea.

The British opium trade with China resulted largely from the domestic demand for tea. From the modest imports of the 1660s, when Samuel Pepys had first tried the 'China drink', a century later, Britons had become insatiable consumers of tea. Tea exports from Canton had more than quadrupled, with the EIC importing 25.5 million pounds between 1785 and 1787.[1] So huge was the appetite for the drink that it, like gin, had become a political issue, with commentators writing on tea's ever-growing place in the economy.

Jonas Hanway (1712–86), a governor of the Foundling Hospital and founder of the Marine Society, who had opinions on everything (as evidenced by his seventy-four privately published pamphlets), thought tea deleterious to the constitution both of the individual and the economy. His publication of *An Essay on Tea, Considered as Pernicious to Health, Obstructing Industry and Impoverishing the Nation; also an Account of its Growth, and great Consumption in these Kingdoms* in 1756, attacked tea from every possible angle. Not only was it a luxury that working people should avoid, along with gin, it was damaging to health. On a broader level, it caused hard currency to leave the British Isles to pay for it. Hanway shunned it as a fashionable nonsense and wholeheartedly recommended abstinence, citing 'parsimony as the best remedy against augmenting the public debt', which was swelling as the British government took further loans from the increasingly wealthy EIC in return for allowing it to continue trading.[2]

Dr Samuel Johnson, who after giving up brandy had become 'a hardened and shameless tea-drinker, who has, for twenty years, diluted his meals with only the infusion of this fascinating plant', wrote a rebuttal in the *Literary Magazine*, arguing that tea was beneficial to health.[3] To Hanway's impassioned plea that 'If a quarter the sum, now spent in tea, were laid out, annually, in plantations, in making public gardens, in paving and widening streets, in making roads, in rendering rivers navigable, erecting palaces, building bridges . . . should we not be gainers, and provide more for health, pleasure, and long life, compared with the consequences of the tea-trade?'[4] Johnson agreed that 'Our riches would be much better employed to these purposes; but,' he objected pragmatically, 'let us first resolve to save our money, and we shall, afterwards, very easily find ways to spend it.'[5]

Hanway was also convinced that while Britain imported 3 million pounds of tea annually, at least 2 million was brought in by smuggling, and where previously it had come in via the Orkneys, much of the trade had now been displaced by the Seven Years War (1754–63) to the Isle of Man, Devon and Cornwall. The only way to estimate the value of the Free Trade at any given time is as a multiple of what is impounded. The EIC held the monopoly on the legal trade of tea into Britain, and after 1724, it was stored in bonded warehouses until duty had been paid. For Devonian and Cornish smugglers, tea was available at the same time for between sixpence and one shilling a pound in France, and when landed at home, it was worth up to seven times as much.[6] Along the peninsula, the main industry was smuggling, owing partly to the decline of tin mining after 1700. Tea, like tobacco, was the perfect commodity to smuggle: unlike brandy, it wasn't heavy and was less prone to spoiling than silk, another contraband favourite.

Smuggling is, by nature, an opportunist activity, and almost everyone at sea engaged in it. The ships of the West and East India Companies often hovered outside Falmouth or in the Channel so that crews could sell what they had acquired privately on their journeys. In 1763, three EIC ships there were said to have offloaded £20,000 of contraband into the local smuggling population, at a time when Cornish wages struggled to reach £20 a year per working man.[7] Offloading in this fashion became so rife that the government began to pilot ships up the Channel and the Thames to stop it happening, reinforcing this after 1718 with a series of Hovering Acts. Yet it was impossible to stop the rife free trading that went on between Britain and the Continent from the south coast. Large, nimble ships began to appear with improved rigging and shallow drafts for entering smaller harbours, capable of carrying up to 10,000 gallons of spirits or twelve tons of tea, indicating the sheer scale of trade. What part, if any significant one, opium played in the British smuggling trade of the eighteenth century is impossible to say, although exhibits in Liverpool's National Border Force Museum indicate opium was indeed smuggled. However, tea and spirits were the mainstay of the British smuggling trade, and demand was only growing. It was also growing in America, and British Americans relied heavily on the Dutch for cheap, coarse tea, rather than pay the tax on expensive tea from Britain. The refusal of Americans to pay the duty for 'British' tea of course culminated in the Boston Tea Party of 1773, when the protestors, the Sons of Liberty, tipped 342 chests of tea from EIC ships into Boston harbour.

The Commutation Act of 1784 attempted to regulate the EIC's monopoly, and also the tea trade between China and Britain. This resulted in the company buying up most of the available stocks of Canton and also from the Continent, which helped reduce smuggling. But it also had the effect of driving up the price of tea in Canton, and thus in Britain. It did not slow down demand, though, but seemed rather to have the opposite effect. From 1783 to 1792, Canton exported 285 million pounds of tea, which was over 100 million more than the previous decade, with nearly 60 per cent of that arriving in London through the EIC, in which time the company made £5 million profit from its monopoly on the trade.[8] Favourite black varieties were bohea, congou and souchong, and singlo and hyson in green. Many Chinese tea dealers were unable to meet the demand, and tales of trunks packed with rubbish instead of tea, or poor quality, adulterated product were soon rife. Still, demand throughout Britain grew, and by the end of the century it was a staple in every grocer in the land. The British were, by far, the biggest consumers in the West, and the trade was of immense value to the economy.

Attempts were made to cultivate Chinese tea in British India, to supply the demand. Indians already drank tea, as the German writer John Mandelslo had remarked on his visit there in the 1630s, but it wasn't until 1780 that Governor General Warren Hastings acquired tea plants for Bhutan and Bengal. In 1788 the naturalist Joseph Banks corresponded with the Botanical Gardens of Calcutta to try and establish a crop there. The EIC naturally opposed anything that might compromise their hold in the Chinese tea market, but others could see the potential for an Indian tea industry to rival that of China, although it was not until the 1830s that an organized effort was made to create it.

In this period, a complex culture evolved around the preparation and consumption of tea: the heating of the cup, the addition of milk and sugar, and when it should be consumed. Anna, Duchess of Bedford (1788–1861), is credited with introducing the ritual of afternoon tea, to be taken between 4 and 4.30, and not lasting more than one hour. The addition of West

Indian sugar was, in itself, a complex political and social subject. Abolitionists refused sugar pointedly, and poet William Cowper even wrote a colourful storybook for children on the human evils of sugar, entitled *The Negro's Complaint*. Yet soon, tea was the staple of both polite society and the working people.

The struggle was to keep this market afloat on a complicated system of credits, cash payments and the EIC working 'in hand' across thousands of miles of ocean. Currency had always been in relatively short supply in Britain, so continuing to export the massive amounts of bullion required to exchange for such a quantity of tea was soon not even an option. And as British goods were of no interest in China, the shortfall had to be met somehow. British India, rapidly on the rise, did however have goods to trade. Indian cotton and opium were both in high demand in China, and so in Canton the EIC established an equitable trade exchange. It was the beginning of a trade exchange that had disastrous results for China.

The Seven Years War saw Britain ally itself with Prussia and Portugal against France and Austria, and later, Spain. In Europe, it was a tedious, slow-moving land war, but in the colonies things happened much more rapidly and there were fortunes to be seized. At the beginning of the war, the old European powers were still making a play for the new worlds across the seas, but by the end of it, Britain dominated the eastern seaboard of North America, India and the Caribbean. Young men such as Robert Clive had followed in the footsteps of the first clerks, and used the EIC's mandate to make war in the name of trade to their own and Britain's advantage.

Robert Clive was, by any measure, an extraordinary man. Born in 1725 into the Shropshire gentry, he had shown his colours early, when his uncle declared, 'I am satisfied that his fighting (to which he is out of measure addicted) gives his temper a

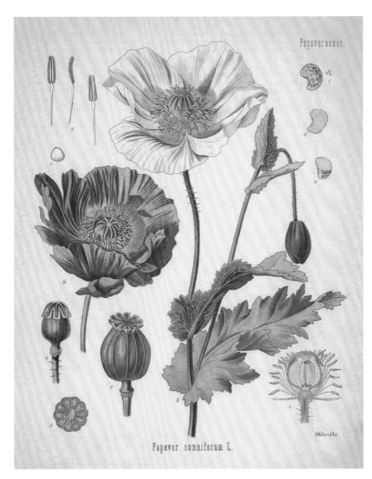

Papaver somniferum: a white opium poppy (*Stedman's Shorter Medical Dictionary*, 1942).

Scarified opium poppy heads during the harvest in Kandahar, Afghanistan, May 2002.

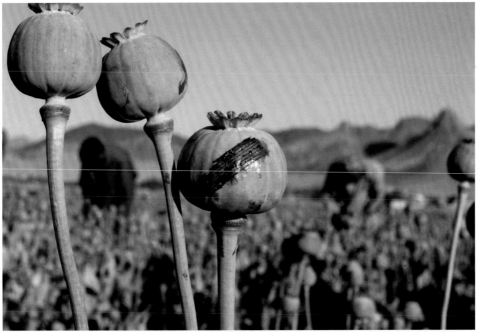

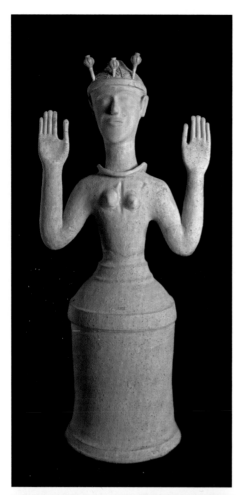

The terracotta figurine of
the Poppy Goddess, divinity
of sleep or death. From the
sanctuary of Gazi, Crete.
1350 BC.

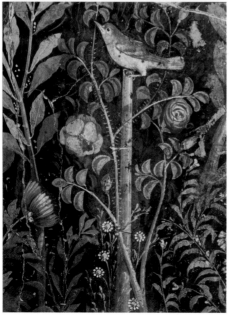

Fresco detail from the garden
room of the House of the
Golden Bracelet, Pompeii,
depicting opium poppies growing
with roses on an ornamental frame.

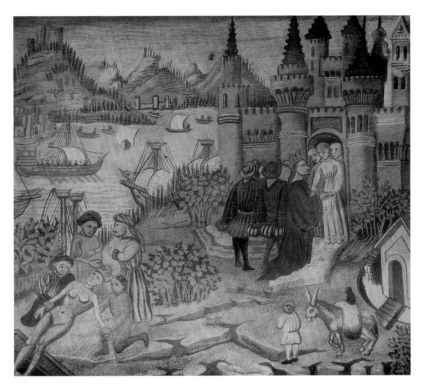

The medical school at Salerno, showing the arrival of Robert, Duke of Normandy, seeking treatment for wounds sustained during the First Crusade, 1099.

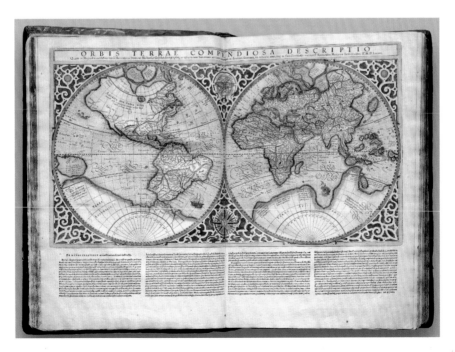

The Mercator projection, as published by Gerardus Mercator in Duisburg, 1596.

Thomas Sydenham, who created the first commercially successful and widely available preparation of laudanum.

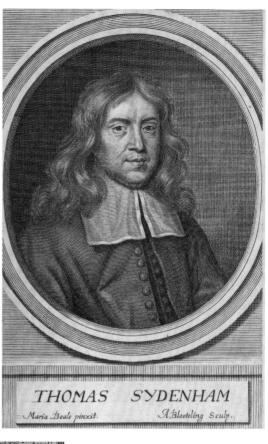

THOMAS SYDENHAM

Maria Beale pinxit. *A. Blooteling Sculp.*

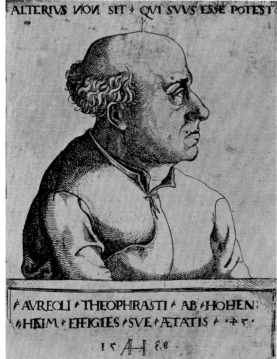

ALTERIVS NON SIT ⊹ QVI SVVS ESSE POTEST

⊹AVREOLI ⊹THEOPHRASTI ⊹ AB ⊹HOHEN⋮ ⊹HEIM ⊹ EFFIGIES ⊹SVE ⊹AETATIS ⊹ ⊹ ⊹·

I ⊹ AH ε.ε

Left Paracelsus, who mixed exotic ingredients such as musk and ambergris to create the mysterious preparation 'laudanum'.

OPPOSITE PAGE

Top The Engel-Apotheke of Friedrich Jacob Merck, Darmstadt, shown here *c.*1790.

Bottom Robert Clive, 1st Baron Clive of Plassey. He was a long-term user of laudanum and died in his home in Berkeley Square, London, after an overdose.

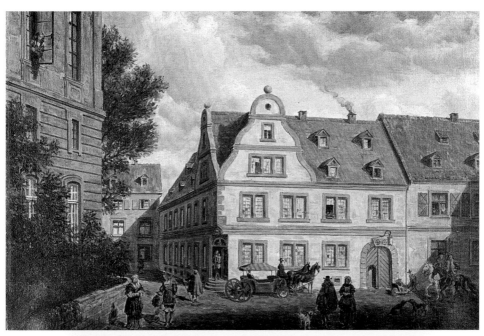

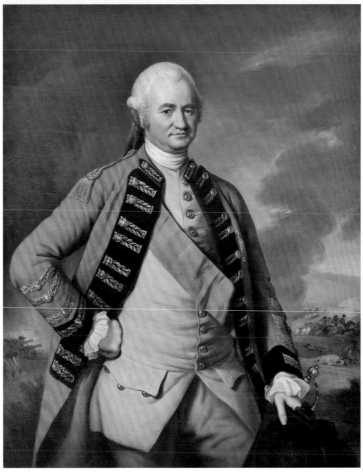

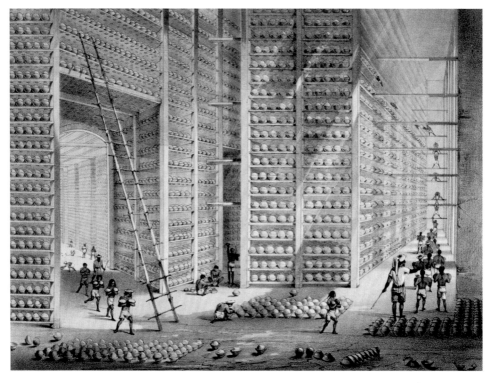

'The Stacking Room' of the British East India Company's
opium factory, Patna, India, *c.*1820.

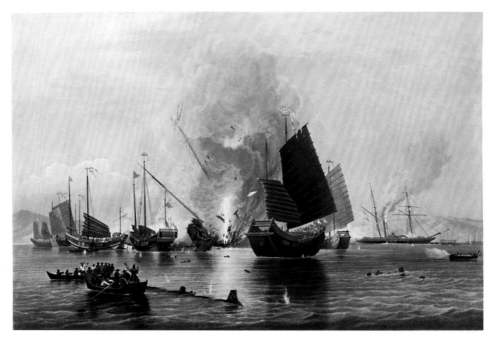

The British East India Company's iron steam ship *Nemesis*, with boats from the *Sulphur*,
Larne, and *Starling*, destroying Chinese war junks in January 1841, by E. Duncan, 1843.

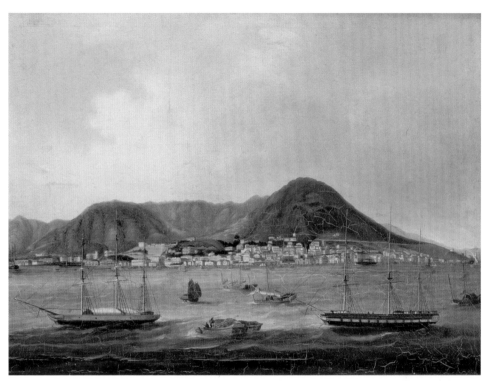

Hong Kong, *c.*1850, depicting the early settlement and the harbour.

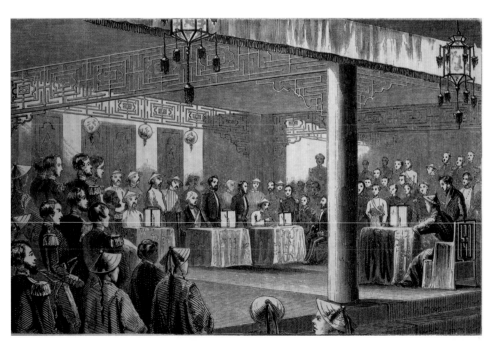

Signing of the Treaty of Tientsin, 1858.

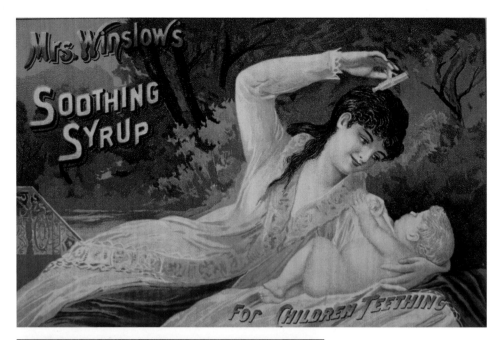

Mrs Winslow's Soothing
Syrup, trade card, 1887.

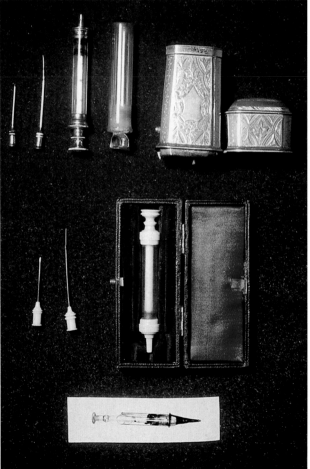

Two examples of
Alexander Wood's
hypodermic syringe,
the first in a chased silver
case with glass barrel and
silver fittings; the second
in a leatherette case,
with glass barrel and ivory
fittings. Latter part of
the nineteenth century.

fierceness and imperiousness, that he flies out upon every trifling occasion: for this reason I do what I can to suppress the hero, that I may forward the more valuable qualities of meekness, benevolence, and patience.'[9] Suffice to say, his uncle failed: Clive was a tearaway who ran protection rackets in the local market town and once climbed the church steeple, to the alarm of onlookers. Unsurprisingly, his father shipped him off to Madras as an EIC clerk, aged eighteen. Clive was part of a British contingent who went out as clerks and became co-opted into the military mentality of the EIC as it expanded across India. In Madras, he worked in the factories, but became depressed and isolated in his new circumstances, trying and failing to commit suicide twice. In 1746, when fighting broke out between the British and French forces in India once more, Clive gave up his desk job and became a soldier. Few can claim to have changed history with a single decision. Robert Clive is one.

The Mughal Empire was a spent force by the time Clive arrived in Madras. They had not sustained the glory of their earlier rulers, and their lack of infrastructure had ultimately left them weak and vulnerable. Harried by independent leaders, the nawabs, and Hindu warrior tribes such as the Marathas, they had lost Delhi in 1739, a terrible blow to their power. Britain and France, seeing their chance to take power, were soon engaged in the Second Carnatic War, beginning in 1748, giving Clive his opportunity to shine. But a health breakdown occurred, allegedly from gallstones, and in 1750, he was sent to Bengal to recover as the war continued without him. There he became a regular opium user, something that would continue for the rest of his life.

Then, in 1751, Clive achieved a feat of arms that changed the balance of imperial power in Britain's favour for almost two centuries. The Siege of Arcot, outside Madras, fought against

Chanda Sahib, the nawab of the Carnatic who was assisted by the French, saw the British troops of the EIC who were holding the small city facing numbers that have been estimated to have been as high as fifty to one. Embattled by the nawab's men, the French, and fighting elephants in armour, Clive took charge and rallied the artillery. After an ugly battle, lasting only an hour, it was over. The reputation of the English forces was assured, and Clive's career was transformed.

After Calcutta was captured by the Bengali army in 1756, the infamous Black Hole incident, in which 123 out of 146 British, Anglo-Indian and Indian prisoners died, created anti-Indian feeling. At the Battle of Plassey, Clive, by this time a colonel, was given the opportunity to be successful once more. Having bribed various members of the nawab of Bengal's army to opt out of fighting, Colonel Clive engaged some 50,000 soldiers and a brigade of war elephants with only 3,000 men, and won. Critics remain sharply divided on just how competent Clive was as a military commander, but nevertheless it was an act of theatre, a political coup, and a victory on an enormous scale, and one that allowed Britain to establish its dominance in India, rapidly pushing out the French and Dutch.

In 1762, Clive was created Baron Clive of Plassey and knighted in 1764. He reaped vast wealth in diamonds, emeralds and gemstones, and Britain now controlled the most productive opium-growing areas of India. Nabobs, as they were known, such as Robert Clive had no real interest in staying in India and establishing a new infrastructure. In the Caribbean, land was key, and people arrived with a view to becoming planters, but in India the British speculated in diamonds and other precious stones. After Plassey, Clive had walked amongst 'heaps of gold and silver' as the treasury of the Bengal and the Mughal princes 'was thrown open to him', free to help himself to whatever he pleased.[10] He used some of this new wealth to transact EIC business and for bribing the local nawabs, but he and others also grabbed great swathes of it for themselves. The British nabobs of this period in India were little more than looters, and even lowly clerks were sending diamonds home to their loved ones. By the 1760s, Clive held huge sway with the EIC, and thus with the British government itself, his father acting as a go-between. Sarcastic man of letters Horace Walpole noted 'General Clive's father has been with Mr Pitt, to notify, that if the government will send his son £400,000 and a certain number of ships, the heaven-born general knows of a part of India where such treasures are buried that he will engage to send over enough to pay the national debt.'[11]

The sheer amounts of money involved in the two decades from Plassey onwards were gargantuan, so much so that, in 1772, Parliament opened an inquiry into Clive and the EIC's actions in India. When questioned on the money he had received in India, Clive famously replied, 'Mr Chairman, I stand astonished at my own moderation.'[12] In the end, the wealth counted for little: Clive became increasingly ill and depressed at the vicious attacks on his character in the British press, and ever more dependent upon laudanum. The general feeling was against the nabobs and their diamonds, and people worried not only about corruption in India, but also how this new wealth might affect national policy if used to corrupt effect at home. All of this put paid to Clive's political aspirations. On 22 November 1774, he was playing cards at his house in Berkeley Square when he excused himself from the party and went to his study. There, he took a substantial dose of laudanum, and is alleged to have opened his own throat with a penknife, although there was no inquest. The papers, so unforgiving of his actions in India for over a decade, were suddenly silent, and the body was interred in a church in Shropshire, near his birthplace. His tombstone bears only the indisputable legend: Clive, Primus in India.

The British Opium Smugglers

Clive's efforts in India had not only lined his own pockets, but placed Britain in control of the major opium-growing regions of Patna, Benares, Behar and Malwa. Production also went on in various independent states, and was either for purchase or domestic consumption outside British control.

As in many of the world's opium-growing regions, poppy agriculture is not a matter of a straightforward exchange with a farmer, and this was also true in India. The caste system and entrenched hierarchies meant that the farmer was at the very bottom of the production line and earning very little, as a series of middlemen – in India's case, higher-caste landowners – took their profit along the line. In theory, the farmer himself delivered the opium crop to the EIC or 'government' agents, but this was rarely the case, and opium farmers ran their own smuggling sidelines, something the company rapidly became used to.

The appetite for opium inside India was high, although not comparable to China's voracious demand. Opium smoking, and more usually eating, was a common pastime of male workers, who would smoke *madakwala* in a hookah, or *chandu* in a *nigali*, like a rough cigarette with paan. The common sight of smokers at an Indian opium 'shop', rather than the Chinese den, is described in an early British trade monograph on northern India. These shops were taxed by the government, although many ran illicit operations on the side, buying their opium direct from the farmers. As in China, Indian opium smoking was a highly social event. 'Visit the famous madak shop at Pulgaman at about 8 pm and you will see a small square shop . . . On the opposite side of the street you will see a long shed where other smokers are gathered. They sit in a long line with their backs to the wall and their knees drawn up to their chests . . . the whole forming a medley group of harmless irrationality and helpless intoxication'.[13]

The preparation of both *madak* and *chandu* in India was a long and tedious process, involving drying out the latex, powdering it, evaporation and adulteration, but it rendered a product that was more than twice as strong as crude opium, and had the added advantage that what was left in the hookah bowl could be scraped out and made into pills 'and swallowed by those whose poverty prevents them from smoking the chandoo itself'.[14]

It is likely that women took opium less conspicuously, and it was also associated in India, as in Persia, with female suicide. John Mandelslo, the German writer who travelled in India, witnessed at Cambay the Hindu tradition of *sati*, in which the widow immolates herself on the funeral pyre of her husband. Mandelslo, watching from horseback, was particularly touched when the young woman came and threw him one of her bangles, and 'she came up to the place with so much self-control and cheerfulness [he] was much inclined to believe she had dulled her senses with a dose of opium'. Mandelslo caught the bangle and kept it, 'in remembrance of so extraordinary an action'.[15]

In late-eighteenth-century Bengal, opium for the domestic and export markets was prepared in vast government factories at Patna and Benares, overseen by the EIC, where it was carefully inspected, prepared and packaged on an industrial scale. Large balls were formed in iron moulds, and these balls then coated in opium paste and rolled in poppy leaves. This created a hard outer casing that would survive shipment, and a softer latex interior. The balls were then packed into mango-wood chests, forty to a chest, and the chest sealed and weighed to ensure that the contents weighed 116 pounds. Then, they were transferred to the government warehouse in Calcutta, and auctioned off at one of four sales per year. These auctions, although real enough, were part of what was essentially an elaborate ruse, all linking back to the British demand for Chinese tea.

The rising Chinese demand for opium finally meant that the British had a core product to trade against tea. There was one problem: by the late eighteenth century, opium had been banned in China. This prohibition had little effect on the escalating consumption, but it did mean that the EIC had to come up with a way to get opium into Canton without sailing in there under their own flag. The Calcutta auctions were the answer. Sanctioned British merchant ships, and selected others, bought the opium and exported it to Canton, either sailing in brazenly or distributing their shipments to local Chinese merchant ships, often through Macau. The Chinese government, whilst vocal about the evils of opium, was slow to react against the powerful *hong* merchant faction in Canton, who had no scruples about bringing in such cargo to weigh the British balance of payments for the tea they so desired. Business was, after all, business.

It took less than twenty years for the trade to become a substantial part of the income of the British Empire, and the EIC was swift to ensure it had a monopoly, firmly establishing it between 1773 and 1797. This, however, was not without its problems, for the British Parliament, as much as the revenue was welcomed, had long been suspicious of the actions of EIC agents. The arrival of the nabobs back in London in the 1760s had stirred up a deep distrust of the company amongst London's political classes, and the government continually attempted to regulate the EIC's operations through a series of Acts and the appointment of overseers. To no avail. Out in British India, so far from the control of London, there were stupendous and fast fortunes to be made, and those who were making them were an increasingly independent breed whose loyalty was to themselves first, the company second, and Britain somewhere down the line. There was also the fact that the EIC was still in debt from the wars that had brought its agents such fortunes, and from maintaining what was essentially a whole new infrastructure in its Indian holdings. The money had to come from somewhere, and as the tea and opium trade took off in the last thirty years of the eighteenth century, it was obvious where that money would come from.

By the late 1760s, the company was increasingly using opium to fund the British tea habit, which meant that more high-quality land, formerly used to grow valuable indigo and sugar, was given over to opium poppies between November and March. Less and less land was available for basic food crops. The company was also taxing the land under its control, and the prices were rising, leaving people unable to buy in the food they needed in times of shortage. This had a disastrous effect when in 1768 and 1769 there were poor grain harvests. Coupled with the tax-induced poverty, people began to starve. The company, under the control of Warren Hastings, the first British governor general of India, continued to collect taxes, sometimes using violent means. Hastings later recorded that by his estimate one third of the population had died, thought today to be in excess of 10 million people. The EIC was not responsible for the Great Bengal Famine of 1770, but the actions of its agents and over-seers no doubt exacerbated what was already a catastrophic situation.

Just three years later, Britain and the EIC had established their dominance over the opium trade, and it did so with aggression. After the famine, a bandit culture arose in the now sparsely populated rural areas, which the company had to quell to prevent opium simply leaking away in the night. And the Bengal bandits were not the only smugglers, as privateers continued to purchase low-grade opium from Malwa and run it to China through Bombay. The company became increasingly indignant about this practice, as the Malwa producers, whose opium had traditionally gone to the Indonesian market, were now in direct competition with the company. The Portuguese enclave on the southern Indian west coast were taking more and more trade away, and Lord Wellesley, governor general of India by 1804, called for its 'complete annihilation'.[16]

In China, Britain and the EIC had tried to take the diplomatic route in 1793 by sending George Macartney, 1st Earl Macartney (1737–1806), to Beijing as the British envoy to China, to negotiate the establishment of a permanent British embassy there, as well as other numerous trading concessions, such as an island for British use off the south China coast. The Qianlong Emperor met with the delegation, and accepted the gifts given to the court with polite neutrality, later saying that they were things only fit to amuse a child. The delegation were sent from pillar to post, and told exactly when they would leave the court, having achieved none of their objectives. The Macartney mission was a failure, markedly because the Chinese court and emperor, secure in Beijing, had no interest in making concessions to foreign barbarians, while Macartney and his delegation had severely underestimated the social and cultural differences between the two nations. With hindsight, the mission was a real and unfortunate lost opportunity to establish meaningful ties between China and Britain, but at the time, it only seemed more like a complete humiliation for Macartney himself, who had been sent across the seas on a goose chase somewhat arrogantly termed British diplomacy.

By now there was another player in the game, one that would be a continual thorn in the British side: America. Opportunistic and resourceful, one American merchant ship arrived in the East Indies in the 1790s having sailed there using only a Mercator projection and a school atlas. After 1800, these American merchants were playing a significant role in trafficking opium throughout the South China Sea. Coming out of Baltimore and Philadelphia, these ships went not to India but to Smyrna (now Izmir) on the Aegean coast, often putting in at Batavia before they finished up in China. In opium, American merchants had found something that seemingly had an endless demand. Cash poor, they had to involve themselves in constant rounds of commodities such as sealskin, sandalwood and ginseng to generate the money they needed to keep buying, but sending Turkish opium to China was different, and much simpler. By the early nineteenth century, Perkins & Co. was established in Smyrna to facilitate the trade, and had the strongest ties with Boston. By 1807, the Select Committee of the EIC in Canton was becoming increasingly irritated by the American presence. By the War of 1812, Americans were determined to press their rights to trade across the oceans, and the number of American ships in the South China Sea increased significantly. The EIC was not amused, but there was little it could do, as the Americans operated as sole traders and were too piecemeal to prosecute. This changed with the *Emily* incident in the autumn of 1821.

The American ship *Emily* had arrived in Canton in May 1821 to sell a Turkish opium cargo. She lay at anchor near Whampoa for four months, selling carefully and slowly to maintain the price for their premium product. On 23 September, a seaman argued with a local woman in a boat, and then hurled a jar at her. It struck her in the head and, falling overboard, she drowned. The British consul resident in Canton attempted to persuade the captain to bribe the grieving family, but he refused. The Chinese authorities demanded the seaman be presented for trial. Captain Cowpland again refused, and rallied a committee of American merchants to negotiate with the Chinese. Suddenly, the American faction in Canton were not so piecemeal as they had been. A trial held aboard the *Emily* resulted in deadlock, so the Chinese blockaded all American trade. Stuck in Canton with goods to sell, the Americans gave up the seaman. He was retried and strangled. A man from Canton mysteriously appeared with a ledger totting up what the *Emily* and other ships had managed to sell, and *Emily* was ordered from Canton without further ado.

The British watched all this with alarm. In 1784, the *Lady Hughes* affair had similarly affected the British contingent, when a gunner had fired an honorary salute and accidentally killed a Chinese boatman in a small vessel beneath the gunport. After the gunner was arrested by Chinese authorities and strangled on a murder charge, the British in Canton had applied the Principle of Extraterritoriality, meaning they were a foreign enclave immune from local laws, much to the chagrin of the Chinese. The British were determined to maintain this principle, and from then on there was an increasing accord between the British and Americans in the face of the Chinese authorities in Canton. This, of course, did nothing for American–Chinese relations, but the *Emily* incident was a turning point in the organization of the Western communities of Canton, and one that had far-reaching consequences for China and, ultimately, Hong Kong.

At this time, estimates of the American share of the Canton opium trade are around 10 per cent of the whole, with Britain dominating the market with anywhere between 60 per cent and 80 per cent. The rest was made up of privateering vessels from all over the world. Trade was flourishing, with Chinese demand continually increasing through the nineteenth century, despite yet another call for total prohibition from the emperor and the Qing government in 1799. In 1810, the edict had been reaffirmed, with the emperor declaring, 'Opium has a harm. Opium is a poison, undermining our good customs and morality . . . However, recently the purchasers, eaters, and consumers of opium have become numerous. Deceitful merchants buy and sell it to gain profit.'[7] Beijing was too far from Canton for it to have any effect on the reality of trading there, and whilst relationships between the Chinese merchants and the Western traders were civil at the best of times and often strained, the rising revenue smoothed out many of the conflicts. This was aided by the British and Americans adopting the system of trading out of Lintin Island, located on the eastern side of the delta near Hong Kong island. Owing to the complicated system of bribes, backhanders and the struggle to get paid, Lintin soon seemed like the perfect solution for the Western merchants.

Western ships would stop at Lintin and place their opium into an innocent-looking storeship there, before proceeding upriver with their legal cargoes. Chinese merchants and smugglers would then buy opium tokens at Whampoa or Canton, before sliding down to Lintin to retrieve their goods. The merchants kept their noses clean, removed the need to bribe Chinese officials, and the Chinese traders got the opium. The Americans and the British had taken their business offshore.

The Opium Giants

'As respects Opium I must take all the blame'[18]

The spirit of free trade that pervaded in Canton was rapidly attracting respectable merchants from all over the world who wished to take advantage of the profits to be had there. William Jardine and James Matheson were both from Scotland.

Jardine, born in 1784, graduated from Edinburgh University with a degree in medicine and became a ship's surgeon on an East Indiaman. The Scottish contingent serving aboard East India Company ships was a large one: between 1777 and 1813, 28 per cent of all commanders of East Indiamen were Scots.[19] Soon, Jardine was supplementing his income by bringing back opium from India. In 1819 he set up on his own, determined to trade in opium, and by 1822 had arrived in Canton.

Matheson, born in 1796, was sent as a teenager to Calcutta to work in his uncle's trading company, Mackintosh & Co. After an argument with his uncle when he forgot to deliver a letter to a departing ship, he left for Canton, hoping to improve his fortunes. In Canton, Matheson became a free agent specializing in goods from India, including opium and cotton. Bright, organized and cheerful, he was invited to join one of the principal five Trading Agencies of Canton, Yrissari & Co. He inherited the business on the death of the senior partner, leaving him in a fortunate position. Winding up the business, he was free to go into partnership with the Jardine family in 1827. They operated under the name of Magniac & Co., dealing in India goods, but predominantly opium. William Jardine used his influence, and extraterritoriality, to become the Danish consul, meaning that he was exempt from the EIC's rules.

The company Jardine Matheson was soon prominent in the Canton opium trade. In 1831, it built the opium clipper the *Sylph*, which made the run to Macao in seventeen days and seventeen hours, heralding a new age in competitive shipping times for the drug. It also meant she was relatively safe from piracy, owing to her speed and nimbleness on the water. Clippers were primarily coasting vessels, shallow and relatively small. Their capacity was optimized by carrying a small amount of imported goods along with a large central cargo of opium, which was then to be traded up and down the China coast, thus avoiding what the British viewed as the extortionate fees to be paid in Canton.

By this time, the firm was making tremendous profits. Goods of all kinds were starting to be traded between Canton and Britain, not just tea and opium, but trade in Canton remained precarious, something William Jardine complained about constantly. 'We are in a sad, stupid state,' he said in 1832, regarding the lack of protection afforded to merchants by the British government, although he did acknowledge the role of the Select Committee of the EIC as the only positive power for protecting the goods and rights of the trading houses in the face of shifting Chinese regulations.[20] Then, in 1833, the British Parliament passed the Government of India Act and divested the EIC of all its trading rights and monopolies, rendering it a purely administrative body, active in India. Once *the* opium giant, the East India Company's trading days had come to an end.

This change, however, had not come about because of the competition in Canton, but because of the Industrial Revolution back in Britain. The new industrial towns in the Midlands were turning out cheap cotton goods that had found a ready market in India, and the manufacturers were keen to open up new markets. Tenacious and political, they had lobbied Parliament continuously, and finally the British government caved in. By 1834, the EIC was gone from Whampoa Anchorage and Canton was an open market. In the same year, Jardine Matheson sent the first private shipments of tea to Britain, and rapidly established a successful business sending the finest Chinese teas back across the world, whilst simultaneously shipping opium and cheap British goods back to Canton.

The removal of the EIC's control of the Canton trade did not suddenly open it up in the way that many in Britain had hoped, for the Chinese were still in control, and remained as resistant to foreigners as ever. The British government had also replaced the presence of the EIC with a superintendent to keep the British merchants in order, hardly something Jardine Matheson was in favour of. At this stage there were a dozen British firms trading out of Canton, including Dent & Co. and Jardine Matheson, six Indian companies, and two American firms, Russell & Co. and Perkins & Co. But it was Jardine Matheson which conducted one third of all Canton trade in the run-up to the First Opium War. It flew its own flag, blue with a white cross, based on the flag of its founders' Scottish homeland, and had the most prominent merchant fleet on the water out of Canton, plying clippers which put the huge old teak ships, some of which were over a century old, to shame.

Jardine had earned himself the nickname 'The Iron-headed Old Rat', owing to his business capabilities, and his nonchalance at once being hit over the head with a club by an assailant. No one but him was allowed to sit down in his office, which had only one chair.

Matheson, meanwhile, was in charge of the correspondence for the firm and had developed a straightforward and wry sense of humour, apparent in his letters: 'The *Gazelle* was unnecessarily delayed at Hong Kong in consequence of Captain Crocker's repugnance to receiving opium on the Sabbath. We have every respect for persons entertaining strict religious principles, but we fear that very godly people are not suited for the drug trade. Perhaps it would be better that the Captain should resign.'[21]

By the late 1830s, British merchants were selling an estimated 1,400 tons of opium into China through Canton.[22] Things were not all plain sailing, though: the Chinese authorities and many of the merchants remained resistant, deceitful and keen on extortion when they saw a chance to exact a bribe. This irritated Jardine in particular. In 1835, the attempt to operate the steam clipper the *Jardine* between Canton and Macau was thwarted by the Chinese authorities.

Part of the problem in Canton was the heavy presence amongst the merchants of members of Chinese secret societies. Now known as Triads, they were then referred to as the Heaven and Earth Society, although there were (and are) many different regional names. Society lore holds that in about 1674 in Fukien province a group of Buddhist monks formed a protest movement against the invading Manchus, the barbarians who had invaded from the north in 1644. They were betrayed in the 1760s, and their numbers were reduced from 128 to just five, who called themselves the Heaven and Earth Society, and set out on an evangelizing mission across China to bring together fellow rebels. As with freemasonry, these societies became popular with business communities, who used them to maintain links with their all important home villages, but also to reach out to others in the same trade or industry. The British, already suspicious of the cabalistic and disdainful Chinese merchants, detested the existence of these secret societies, about which they were powerless to act, because they increased the already chronic lack of transparency in Chinese–Western relationships in Canton, and now further up the coast.

The fortunes to be made in Canton by the Chinese *hongs* who managed to secure one of the posts surpassed virtually anything that was known in the private hands of an individual. Many of them were from Fujian, such as Puankhequa (Pan Chencheng), Mowkqua (Lu Guangheng), and Howqua (Wu Bingjian). Puankhequa had come from a poor background and worked as a sailor as far as Manila before returning to Canton and building a fortune of millions of dollars. Howqua (1769–1843) was even more successful, and invested his money with Boston merchant banker John Forbes. He worked alongside Mowkqua as the British and Americans became ever more numerous and forceful, but between them, with their vast fortunes, they felt strong enough to resist the troublesome requests and demands of the barbarian foreigners. However, it was by no means universal that the merchants and the *hongs* did not get on. Most of the trouble was caused by the authorities and civil servants in whose nature it was to be as obstructive as possible to both parties, which caused strife on all sides. Some of the *hongs* regularly called on the merchants, and extended hospitality to them. William Hunter, an American who spent many years in Canton, remembered the scale on which the thirteen *hong* merchants lived: 'Their private residences, of which we visited several, were on a vast scale, comprising curiously laid out gardens, with grottoes and lakes, crossed by carved stone bridges, pathways neatly laid with small stones of various colours forming the designs of birds, or fish, or flowers.'[23]

To the fury of the Chinese government, but the satisfaction of everyone else involved, Lintin Island was thriving. Opium imports into Canton had risen from 2,000 chests in 1800 to 5,000 in 1820, and stood at 20,000 in 1834, leading one statesman to lament that the opium trade was 'a subject of deep regret that the vile dirt of foreign countries should be received in exchange for the money and commodities of the Empire'.[24] Yet it was still to no avail. Opium was simply pouring in. To put into perspective just how much money firms like Jardine Matheson were making, when their old partner Magniac left in 1827, it took almost six years for them to finalize his liquid assets. They had so much business they could barely keep the books in order, but when his last goods were traded in 1833, Jardine wrote to him, 'I have the pleasure to enclose your account current (as of June 30), of 403,035 Spanish dollars.'[25] So when the *Jardine* was thwarted on her supposed trip to Macau in 1835, British and American merchants and the British authorities tried to break free of the Chinese hold over them.

In 1834, when the opium imports hit yet another high with the 20,000 chests, the government sent Lord Napier with two British superintendents for trade with China. It was an attempt to ensure the continuation of the trade that the EIC had overseen, but Napier made the grave mistake of trying to circumvent Chinese bureaucratic etiquette in contacting the viceroy of Canton directly. He was prevented as the viceroy refused to accept the letter, and in a show of rebuttal, closed trade with British merchants. Napier ordered two Royal Navy ships to bombard the forts on the Pearl River Delta and war was only avoided because he fell ill with typhus. The British were ordered to leave Canton for Whampoa or Macau, where Napier died. It had been a complete disaster for all sides, but the need for the British and American merchants to have somewhere independent and safe to trade, operating under the principle of extraterritoriality, was now crystal clear.

In 1836, Jardine Matheson began to propose the founding of a trading colony on Hong Kong island, although this was not the immediate favourite choice of others owing to its rocky geography. Bad feeling escalated between the Chinese author-ities and the increasing number of merchants arriving to do business at Canton and down the coast, but the demand for opium was now snowballing throughout China. Perkins & Co. still dominated the Smyrna route, and Lancelot Dent, who had taken over Dent & Co. in 1831, had made it into a powerful force, with strong ties to prominent Calcutta agency houses. Jardine Matheson was, by this stage, unassailable. Or so it thought.

The Incorruptible Lin Zexu and the First Opium War

The Western merchants had, however, not counted on Lin Zexu (1785–1850), a brilliant Chinese bureaucrat who had been appointed by the court in Beijing to scourge Canton and the coast of the trade in opium. There were now estimated to be around 12 million opium addicts on mainland China, and the demand was such that China's silver reserves were flowing back down the Pearl River at an alarming rate. Lin Zexu arrived in Canton in March 1839 and ordered all trade in opium to be stopped immediately and the stocks surrendered. He wrote a long and eloquent open letter to the young Queen Victoria about the evils of the opium trade, which was printed in Canton, and although the letter itself never reach the queen, it was later reprinted in *The Times*. Lin Zexu entrusted the letter to Captain Warner of the *Thomas Coutts*, who returned it to England, but the Foreign Office refused to accept it when they knew what was in it.

> Your honorable nation takes away the products of our central land, and not only do you thereby obtain food and support for yourselves, but moreover, by re-selling these products to other countries you reap a threefold profit. Now if you would only not sell opium, this threefold profit would be secured to you: how can you possibly consent to forgo it for a drug that is hurtful to men, and an unbridled craving after gain that seems to know no bounds![26]

Initially Lin Zexu attempted to be fair, offering to compensate the British merchants for their stocks in tea and rhubarb, for it was a well-understood fact in China that Englishmen would die of constipation without a regular supply of rhubarb. This was

rejected, Canton was blockaded and the merchants were confined to their homes, some threatened with the deprivation of
food and water. Some of the *hong* were put into prison, and some
including Mowkqua and Howqua were put into chains with
manacles around their necks. Lin Zexu was also in the process
of arresting opium smokers and confiscating and destroying
opium pipes in their tens of thousands.

Captain Charles Elliot was chief superintendent of British
trade in Canton when he wrote to the Foreign Secretary, Vis-
count Palmerston, on 6 April 1839 that although he was 'mindful
of the nature of the trade', the 'wanton violence' shown to the
'Queen's officers and subjects, and all the foreign community in
China' meant that 'There can be neither safety nor honour for
either government until Her Majesty's flag flies on these coasts
in a secure position.'[27] Frantic communications from Elliot to
Palmerston ensued about the increasingly fraught nature of the
events in Canton, and the need for Britain to extend protection
to her subjects. Elliot himself was of the mind that if the
emperor wanted to prevent the import of opium then he was
within his rights, but Britain was also within her rights to protect the lives and property of her subjects.

Lancelot Dent, holding a significant amount of opium, was
ordered to surrender it but only gave over a small proportion.
Lin requested he attend a meeting but Dent refused, aware that
he was in danger of being beheaded as an example to the other
merchants. Elliot ordered the British to Hong Kong island while
he negotiated with Lin. When Elliot arrived, the Union flag was
raised and he read out a petition to the effect that all British
subjects were henceforth under the protection of the government, and that they would be compensated if they handed
over their total opium stocks. By nightfall, the merchants had
handed over their stocks, the equivalent of 20,000 chests, for

destruction. The total Lin Zexu confiscated from the merchants was put at over 1,300 tons, and took, starting on 3 June 1839, 500 men twenty-three days to mix it with salt and lime in pits, where it 'boiled like soup', after which it was sluiced into the sea off Humen Island, at which point Lin wrote a poem apologizing to the gods of the sea for dumping such rubbish.

In May the merchants had received orders to quit China forever, and later that year a flotilla set sail from Canton under Charles Elliot, after the Battle of Kowloon in September, sparked by an incident involving a group of sailors drinking rice liquor who subsequently beat a Chinese villager to death. After the Chinese reacted by stopping all trade in food to the merchant community, Elliot ordered British ships to fire on junks outside Kowloon. The battle was over by nightfall, its only real significance being the death of the villager, and the fact that it marked the beginning of the First Opium War.

Elliot was far from the hero of the hour. His anti-opium sympathies were well known in the British government and the merchant communities, and many suspected that, when he had met Lin Zexu, he had colluded with the Chinese official, or at least taken Lin's worst terms. It also turned out that Elliot hadn't quite negotiated the deal as he had imagined it when he spoke under the Union flag on Hong Kong island. The British government had no interest in paying any compensation, regarding it as the business of the Chinese, since they had destroyed the opium stocks. The merchants, led by William Jardine, began a campaign to sway the government to go to war with China, and in spring 1840 an expeditionary fleet left Britain. William Gladstone, the future prime minister, denounced it 'unjust and iniquitous'; he had tried and failed to cure his sister of an opium addiction.[28]

Over the course of the next year, a series of sea battles comprised the First Opium War. Lin Zexu was dismissed in late

1840 and exiled to Turkestan, deemed by the authorities to have failed, like Elliot, in his task. Back in Britain and America, reaction from the public was mixed. The war had brought to light many facts about the opium trade that ordinary citizens were not aware of, and as pro-trade as both countries were, there was a rising backlash against forcing opium on the Chinese people, particularly from the religious communities who had missionaries stationed there. The *North British Review* published a letter to the same effect: 'No man of any humanity can read without a deep and very painful feeling what has been reported of the grief, the dismay, the indignation of men in authority, and the Emperor, on finding that their utmost efforts to save their people were defeated by the craft and the superior maritime force of the European dealers, and by the venality of their own official persons, on the coast.'[29]

Now, this precise situation had resulted in a war between Britain and China. The British victory in the First Opium War was decisive, mainly due to highly advanced technology in terms of firepower and steamships such as the *Nemesis*, the EIC's first iron warship. The Chinese junks and small ships were no match for the organized might of even a small fleet of the navy, and the Chinese losses were heavy, numbering some 18,000 troops. In contrast, less than seventy British sailors were killed in battle.

The war ended on 29 August 1842 with the Treaty of Nanking, known by the Chinese as the Unequal Treaty, the first of several that play a large part in their history of relations with the West and Britain in particular. Signed at Nanking aboard HMS *Cornwallis*, by both British and Qing representatives, it was ratified by Queen Victoria and the Qing Emperor nine months later. Ultimately, the aim of the treaty was the demise of the Canton System, thereby breaking the hold of both the Cohong and the Chinese bureaucrats over free trade. But the British didn't stop there. In addition, they wanted four more treaty ports, at Amoy, Foochow, Ningpo and Shanghai, where the principle of extra-territoriality would be enforced, and a fixed tariff system for duties and taxes imposed, subject to negotiation. The Qing government would pay 6 million silver dollars for the opium Lin Zexu had destroyed, 3 million for the accounts the *hong* still had open with the exiled British merchants and 12 million for the cost of the war. They would also cede Hong Kong to the British Crown in perpetuity. The treaty was a terrible blow for the Chinese, although they did not fully appreciate the repercussions it would have.

The emperor's views on the British and their trade remained clear, even in defeat: 'It is true I cannot prevent the introduction of the flowing poison; gainseeking and corrupt men will, for profit and sensuality, defeat my wishes; but nothing will induce me to derive a revenue from the vice and misery of my people.'[30]

The young Queen Victoria, however, wrote to her uncle, the King of Belgium, like a spoiled child: 'The Chinese business vexes us much, and Palmerston is deeply mortified at it. All we wanted might have been got, if it had not been for the unaccountably strange conduct of Charles Elliot . . . who completely disobeyed his instructions and tried to get the lowest terms he could . . . Albert is so much amused at my having got the Island of Hong Kong.'[31]

The Making of Hong Kong

'Viewed as a place of trade, I fear Hong-kong will be a failure'[32]

The steep, rocky island of Hong Kong was still only sparsely settled when the British decided to take it for its excellent deep harbour, which the British botanical collector Robert Fortune, collector to the Royal Horticultural Society of London, who came to Hong Kong in 1843, described as 'one of the finest I have ever seen: it is eight or ten miles in length, and irregular in breadth; in some places two, and in other places six miles wide, having excellent anchorage all over it, and perfectly free from hidden dangers'.[33] At its widest point east to west, it measures eleven miles and between two and five north to south. Jardine Matheson was, naturally, the first to purchase plots at East Point, for £565, in the Land Sale held by Charles Elliot on 14 June 1841.[34] Alexander Matheson would later admit somewhat sheepishly to a Select Committee that perhaps the firm had begun building 'to a certain extent' before the sale.[35]

When George Pottinger, first governor of Hong Kong, saw the building works of huge godowns and administrative buildings in 1842, he described it as 'one chaos of immense masses of granite and other rocks, that ... by the application of science and extraordinary labour and by an expenditure of about £100,000, have not only made it available for their vast mercantile concerns, but have rendered it a credit and an ornament to the colony'.[36] Jardine Matheson did not move to Hong Kong until 1844, by which time their site covered 3.5 acres, and by 1845, when the botanist Robert Fortune left China again through Hong Kong, he was impressed with the rate of growth, and that Governor Davis had changed the names of the Chinese towns on the south side, which 'used to be called Little Hong-kong and Chuckehew ... into Stanley and Aberdeen'.[37]

Jardine Matheson was by no means the first business to move to Hong Kong, though, and by the end of 1843 there were twelve substantial British firms operating there, various smaller British merchants and six Indian companies. And by the time Jardine returned the following year, there were around a hundred firms in business, of which half were British and a quarter Indian and Parsee. The Americans Russell & Co. had also moved to the island by then, a company of note for their huge success in opium trading but also for employing Warren Delano Jr, the grandfather of Franklin D. Roosevelt.

Many of the place names are from this early time and reflect the variety of companies on the island. There is, of course, Jardine's Bazaar, but also Jardine's Lookout, a 433-metre high point where a lookout was stationed to spy Jardine Matheson ships approaching. The Jardine firm is inextricably linked to the history, culture and landscape of the island, even down to the soundscape, as outside the East Point premises a cannon known as the Noonday Gun was fired each day. The stories differ as to quite why this happened, but the midday firing became such a part of Hong Kong's daily life that when the cannon was destroyed by the Japanese in the Second World War, the Royal Navy replaced it after the occupation.

One dramatic difference with the merchant's return to Hong Kong was that the ships were now coming under steam power, indifferent to the tides and winds of the South China Sea and the Pearl River Delta. Opium was still by far the most profitable cargo, and it was responsible not only for the British colony on Hong Kong, but the success of the island itself. This success did not come immediately and initially the island was beset by piracy and raiding, as well as malaria, which killed almost a quarter of the British garrison in 1843. They were buried quickly, but soon afterwards the foundations for the new island road meant the coffins were unearthed and the bones disturbed. They were still lying by the side of the road years later, exposed to the 'vulgar gaze'.[38]

For the great British merchant houses, now widely called *hongs* in their own right, and their owners *taipan*, meaning 'great manager', these risks and rough conditions were worth it. They were making full use of the excellent harbour for their trade, although the climate and early conditions left a lot to be desired. In 1844, Robert Montgomery Martin, the colonial treasurer, recommended abandoning the island as unfit for general trading.

This was premature. The sheer power of the *hong* merchants and their opium trade on Hong Kong was acting like a magnet not only for Chinese from the Pearl River Delta and Canton, but for people all over the world, and 'people from all countries, from England to Sydney, flock to the Celestial country, and form a very motley group'.[39]

Hong Kong's vast harbour allowed islanders to diversify into shipping, and new steamship companies created fleets as a business rather than a sideline like Jardine, such as the Apcar Line, founded in 1819 and operating out of Calcutta to bring opium to southern China, and the Peninsular and Oriental Steam Navigation Company (still operating as P&O), which went into the Bengal opium business in 1847 with the modest aim of monopolizing all opium routes east of Suez. These steamships soon became a regular sight off the coast of the island.

The rapid colonization of Hong Kong, which brought not only permanent settlers and families but ships' crews and other visitors like Fortune, did not, as might be thought, displace the local population. If anything, relationships between the different nationalities, including the Indian traders as well as the indigenous people, seemed peaceable. Chinese peace officers with the same duties and rights as constables were drafted in 1844, on the principle that no one outside a Chinese community would have any success in governing it.

A considerable number of the Hong Kong population had

been collaborators during the First Opium War, perhaps because they already had strong trading ties with the foreign merchants who called on the island, which had benefitted them more than the Canton System located ninety miles up the river. Unsurprisingly, some of the most enthusiastic of these collaborators were the Tanka water-people. Some of these men emerged as the most important local liaisons on the island for the new settlers, becoming wealthy and popular in their own right. One such was Loo Aqui, who had provisioned the Royal Navy during the war, for which he was rewarded with a large plot of land in the island's Lower Bazaar, making him a rich man. In later life he was widely suspected of heavy involvement with the Triads, police corruption and even piracy, but he was also known in the community for assisting those who were 'distressed, in debt, or discontented'.[40] Another was Kwok Acheong, who joined the Peninsular and Oriental Steam Navigation Company as a young man, and later began his own line of steamships. By 1876, he was the third largest taxpayer in the colony, and the steamship industry was an integral part of the trading there. The building of the Man Mo Temple in 1847 on the island's Hollywood Road was an important moment for the Chinese islanders. Still standing today, it became Hong Kong's focal point for Chinese people of all backgrounds.

The Chinese population on Hong Kong grew rapidly, from 7,500 in 1841 to 22,800 in 1847 and 85,300 in 1859.[41] This was a rare source of tension between the colonists and the Chinese, particularly regarding Chinese living conditions in some parts of the island, and also burial customs, or the distinct lack of them. The poorer Chinese had a custom of laying people near death in a final resting place and leaving them without care. Sometimes they were laid out next to those already dead. This created a public scandal in 1869 and led to the creation of the Tung Wah

Hospital, still in operation. Later, the colony made the hospital embrace Western medicine when the death rate amongst the Chinese population through disease remained significantly higher than that of the colonists.

Many of these Chinese came as builders, constructing in less than two years from 1841 housing for more than 15,000 people and also a magistrate's court, a gaol and a post office, as well as the myriad governmental administrative offices needed to deal with the amount of business the huge firms like Jardine Matheson were conducting. With them grew the Nam Pak Hong trade, a sort of southern Asian entrepôt including everything from rice to pearls to silk and herbal medicines. The Nam Pak Hong trade caused a huge rise in the number of junks arriving in Hong Kong, and the junk trade rose from 80,000 tons in 1847 to 1.35 million tons exactly two decades later, and created fifty-three junk yards on Hong Kong by the late 1850s.[42] The thriving Chinese population hugely outnumbered the colonists, and the shopping and food culture reflected this. They were also the largest ratepayers, as many had invested in land.

Service culture and industry – embodied in men such as Loo Aqui and Kwok Acheong, and the Nam Pak Hong trade – were particularly important for Hong Kong from the start, with the whole island dependent on trade and foreigners arriving. One thing that was becoming increasingly important on the island was credit, and to that end the Hongkong and Shanghai Banking Corporation was established there in 1865. Initially it was started to offer credit to the local steamship businesses that were springing up over the island, or to small industry in the interior, but soon it was working with London's Westminster Bank and was in the very rare position of being a colonial bank able to play off local silver against British sterling. It was able to provide credit in the sorts of numbers the burgeoning industries such as shipping needed, and provide the steady, trustworthy banking system so helpful to the opium trade.

The success of HSBC, now the largest bank operating in the world today, proves the pivotal importance of Hong Kong's location. It may have been rocky, steep, impossibly humid, disease-ridden and prone to typhoons, but this 'wild and uncouth state' had opium, and on that one commodity, it rapidly built one of the world's great trading centres.[43]

The Second Opium War/The Arrow War

For the British, the Second Opium War, lasting from 1856 to 1860, was a conflict distinct from the first; for the Chinese, the Arrow War was simply another insult in a long line of barbaric behaviour towards the Celestial Empire.

In October 1856, a British ship, the *Arrow*, was captured by pirates then resold by the Chinese government at Canton. It was flying the British flag when Chinese marines boarded it, pulled down the flag and carried off the crew, much to the outrage of the captain, Thomas Kennedy, who was aboard at the time. The Chinese had contravened the principle of extraterritoriality once again, and the British consul in Canton contacted the viceroy Ye Mingchen directly, now permitted after the Treaty of Nanking, and demanded the release of the crew and an apology for the insult to the British flag. The viceroy released only part of the crew, and no apology was forthcoming. British ships fired heavily on Canton, and on 29 October entered the city, where the US consul James Keenan, somewhat unwisely, chose to fly the American flag from the viceroy's residence.

Somewhat unsurprisingly, negotiations were a stalemate, and the British continued to bombard Canton periodically until

January 1857, when they returned to Hong Kong. The British government, preoccupied with an upcoming general election, was less than sympathetic to the problems in the Pearl River Delta and not interested at all when the Indian Mutiny rose up in May. However, when a French missionary was executed in mainland China, the French envoy, Baron Jean-Baptiste Louis Gros, lobbied for action and the British and French joined forces to take Canton, which they did in late 1857. Ultimately, Britain and France occupied the city for almost four years. America and Russia, despite the British requests for help, remained neutral.

In December 1857, Britain and France threatened the viceroy with a total bombardment of Canton if the crew of the *Arrow* were not released within twenty-four hours. And they still wanted their apology. They received the former, but not the latter, yet were victorious in what became popularly known as the Arrow Incident.

Back in Britain, opinion on what had happened was divided, and was a frequent subject of parliamentary debate. Richard Cobden, the MP for the West Riding of Yorkshire, recorded his opinion: 'the papers which have been laid on the table fail to establish satisfactory grounds for the violent measures resorted to at Canton in the late affair of the *Arrow*'.[44] The House of Commons passed a resolution against the war, with a majority of just fourteen. The Arrow Incident was a controversial issue in the general election, but the pro-war faction were returned to power.

In June 1858, the British government, now allied against China with America, France and Russia, proposed the Treaties of Tientsin, which would essentially open up China to free trade with the rest of the world. Over two years ensued of battles and diplomatic incidents involving captures of British officers and grisly torture. Southern Chinese 'coolies' fought with the British and French forces, engaging their enemies with sharpened bamboo. The Qing government, meanwhile, was also under huge pressure from the Taiping Rebellion in south-eastern China, where a group of rebels were declaring their freedom to practise their own form of Christianity. For the Qing administration, it was an utter disaster.

Karl Marx, at that time the European correspondent for the *New York Daily Tribune*, wrote a piece called 'Trade or Opium' in which he said Tientsin had 'succeeded in stimulating the opium trade at the expense of legitimate commerce'.[45]

On 6 October 1860, Anglo-French forces entered, looted and burned the splendid Old Summer Palace of Peking. The British also proposed to burn the Forbidden City, but their allies discouraged it, believing it might jeopardize the signing of the treaties. On 18 October, at the Convention of Peking, the emperor's brother, Prince Gong, ratified the Treaties of Tientsin. They had been somewhat modified, and the result for the Chinese was catastrophic. Not only did they have to pay 8 million taels of silver (the equivalent of 400 tons) in compensation to the British and French, they had to open up Tientsin, cede Kowloon to the British, grant freedom of religion, and the right for missionaries to preach in China; the 'coolie trade' in which indentured Chinese servants were carried to America was to be permitted. And finally, the opium trade was to be fully legalized in China. It was the worst outcome they could have hoped for. Then, a fortnight later, the Russians forced what was left of the Qing government to sign a further codicil regarding coastal rights, which allowed them to found Vladivostok in the same year.

Britain and its allies had achieved their aim of forcing China's hand once and for all in terms of free trade. America, desperate for cheap labour after its own civil war, had a new, legalized slave army, and Britain added Kowloon to her rapidly expanding Hong Kong territory. Christianity was pushed onto a people who had survived and flourished without it for thousands of years. But most important of all, the trade in tea and opium would continue, now unchecked and completely legal. There would be no way to check the ravening demand for opium in mainland China, and supply would be unbridled. The Chinese regard this crushing compromise as both the birth of modern China and their most humiliating defeat at the hands of the West.

Ye Mingchen, the viceroy who made what turned out to be such a grave error in Canton, was exiled to Calcutta, where he starved himself to death.

China's Opium Missionaries

'Go ye into all the world and preach the gospel to every creature'[46]

As Chinese coolie labour flooded out of southern China, both opium and Christian missionaries flooded into what had been a closed country. While the early Roman Catholic missions, aside from the Jesuits, had largely met with failure, it was now predominantly American Evangelical Protestants who wished to go and preach to the Chinese people.

There had already been Protestant missionaries in China, notably the Briton Robert Morrison (1782–1834), who arrived there in 1807 on behalf of the London Missionary Society, and in defiance of the EIC's total ban on British missionary activity anywhere in their mandate. To circumvent this, Morrison pretended to be an American.[47] Canton's missionaries throughout the nineteenth century used print to try and spread the word of God. Morrison, who produced a Chinese translation of the Bible as well as a book on Chinese grammar aimed at the English and American markets, was determined to foster a better cultural understanding between East and West. He also founded the Anglo-Chinese College at Malacca.

Both he and his notional successor in Canton, the American Evangelist E. C. Bridgman, were gravely concerned with the effect of opium upon the population. Bridgman, who immersed himself in the Chinese language well enough to write fluent letters to the emperor upon the subject, was particularly keen to see the trade abolished. The *Chinese Repository* was a periodical that ran in Canton between 1832 and 1851, with the aim of informing missionaries working in Asia about the history of China, cultural differences and current events. Bridgman was a keen contributor and in 1836–7 published seventeen articles on the history and state of the opium trade.

The First Opium War was, for many missionaries, a time of hope that the trade had 'received its death blow'. Bridgman wrote back to the American government in 1839, during the Lin Zexu period in Canton, that 'Our little community has been held these two months constantly in painful-fearful suspense. England, India – and Christendom – must now awake to the evils of this "hurtful thing".'[48] Bridgman had a good relationship with Lin, and it was Bridgman who printed Lin's letter to Queen Victoria in the *Chinese Repository* and distributed it in Canton. The new importance of printed propaganda in the Canton trade was mobilizing not only the missionaries, but also the merchants, who printed their own magazines. Jardine Matheson bought at least one printing press, and the Qing government, used to having absolute control of what was publicly circulated, was unable to stop the flood of new pamphlets and periodicals debating Canton and the opium trade.

With the outbreak of the war, Bridgman and his compatriots, now well established in Canton and immersed in the culture of the factories, felt they could be more vocal about the evils of the opium trade. But they still had one significant problem: Jardine Matheson and Dent, in the spirit of Christian fellowship in the face of the Chinese, or for public relations reasons, were generous contributors to the various missionary projects. Such a detail moderated Bridgman's language, but did not stop him speaking out about the trade in print. The only problem with the missionary press in Canton was that the matter was given over to the merchant-missionary debate about the opium trade, rather than the realities of the situation. Whilst the missionaries were no doubt doing good work on the ground, their printed debates made the subject a theoretical and theological one. However, their published works, when exported back to America, where people had never seen an opium den, but were filled with evangelical faith, had a powerful effect on public opinion.

The American Board of Commissioners for Foreign Missions was a powerful lobbying group, and had backing from Olyphant & Co., one of the few foreign *hongs* in Canton who would not participate in the drug trade, restricting themselves to silk and fancy Chinese articles. Peter Parker, a missionary and doctor at the hospital in Canton, travelled back to America to speak to the American Board about the problems with opium in the Canton population, and went to Washington 'to call the attention of the men in power to the relations of America to China'.[49] He was persuasive and influential in shaping American policy towards China during the Opium Wars and subsequently. The reduction of the opium trade to a basic 'good versus evil' argument had begun in earnest.

The mercantile reality across China was somewhat different. In a cash-poor rural society, where opium poppies could now be grown practically if not legally – the central government would not remove the ban until 1890, but turned a blind eye to production – opium latex was as good as money, and something that had previously had to be imported was now available in the fields outside. Crucially, for a government ever desperate for money, it could also be taxed. Levels of addiction were also rising rapidly. At the outbreak of the First Opium War in 1839, imports of opium into Canton stood at 2,500 tons, but by 1880, this had risen to 6,500 tons. When domestic production was legalized in 1890, imports fell dramatically, but opium cultivation and consumption boomed until, in 1906, China was producing a gargantuan 35,000 tons per year and an estimated 25 per cent of the male population were not only users, but addicts, and it was consumed at every level of society.[50] British and American missionaries wrote ever more impassioned tracts on the nature of the opium trade, never mentioning that, back at home, trouble was brewing.

Chapter Six

THE AMERICAN DISEASE

Pioneers and Patent Medicines

'From sea to shining sea'[1]

North America's relatively brief relationship with opiates is as short and dramatic as its history, and as wide as its geography. Absence of records make it difficult to know if the earliest settlers travelled with laudanum or opium, but it seems unlikely that they would make such a perilous journey without a reliable painkiller to hand. And it seemed somewhat unwise to rely upon doctors like John Cranston of 1663, who was granted a licence to 'administer physicke and practice chirurgery' after paying the appropriate fee to the General Court in Rhode Island.[2] It is much more likely that people purchased their drugs from someone like Mr Russell at the Galen's Head, before setting out for their new homes.

Doctors arrived in America with degrees from respected international medical schools, but America did not have its own formal medical institutions until the College of Philadelphia opened in 1765, and King's College in New York two years later. Based on European models, they established themselves rapidly as centres of learning and turned out practical, knowledgeable doctors (if rather young at twenty-two) for a growing nation.

Nathaniel Chapman was born in Virginia in 1780 and studied both in Edinburgh and under Benjamin Rush in Philadelphia, where he was later in charge of materia medica. He regarded opium as essential to the physician, 'there being scarcely one morbid affection or disordered condition, in which, under certain circumstances, it is not exhibited, either alone, or in combination'.[3]

There had been shortages of opium in America, as the earlier Dr Thaddeus Betts observed in the *Connecticut Journal* in 1778: 'opium is an article which no physician ought ever to want . . . no substitute will supply its defect'.[4] Betts grew his own poppies so that he could ensure a steady supply.

Connecticut was particularly prone to outbreaks of smallpox and other diseases, and Dr Vine Utley – practising in Lyme County from 1798, and who introduced America to the idea of vaccination – recommended the liberal use of opium in cases like the 1812 typhus epidemic. But in more rural areas, it seems it was far harder to obtain. Elias P. Fordham was an English immigrant and the original surveyor of Indianapolis, and he recorded on his travels in Chesapeake, Virginia around the same time that 'The fever and ague are very common here. I gave away in these visits all my bark and laudanum. They would send a negro five miles through the woods, and as far with a canoe on the water, for one or two doses.'[5]

For Thomas Jefferson, who was growing white opium poppies in the flowerbeds at Monticello in the year of the Connecticut outbreak, there was presumably no shortage of opium, should it be required – although visitors to the estate were not always complimentary: 'There are few plants whose flowers are so handsome, but having an offensive scent and being of short duration, they are not much regarded.'[6]

Regardless of Jefferson's offensive ornamental *Papaver som-*

niferum, early America relied on patent medicines, and English ones, such as those imported by Mr Russell, were the most popular for a long time. In the eighteenth century, Europe had experienced a rise in luxury goods and standards of living, but for many who moved to America, particularly those who settled in the centre of the continent, luxury was not a part of everyday life. For the cash- and time-poor settlers, patent medicines offered a way to treat the ills of all the family from one handy and easily available bottle. Advertisements for English patent medicines become regular after 1750 in the small East Coast newspapers, indicating the availability was increasing, and patent medicines are one of the very earliest products advertised in America.

Supply stopped with the American Revolutionary War in 1775, and afterwards the patent medicines returned, although in much smaller quantities. In a move that shadowed China's isolationism, revolutionary Americans argued that America had all her people needed, and to boycott goods from Britain. But people still wanted their trusted English brands, and American manufacturers, known as nostrum makers, stepped into the breach. In 1824, a twelve-page pamphlet appeared with the title *Formulae for the preparation of eight patent medicines*, adopted by the Philadelphia College of Pharmacy, the first professional pharmaceutical body of America, founded in 1821. All of the recipes were English, and they included the famous Godfrey's Cordial.

With a large number of Americans living in extremely rural circumstances, with little or no access to healthcare, they had come to rely on folk remedies and home cures. Many used Thomsonian Medicine, created by Samuel Thomson in the first part of the nineteenth century, who came from a Unitarian pig-farming background and was raised in remote circumstances. Having spent time with a root or herbal doctor as a young man, he used plants to cure himself of an ulcerated ankle injury, strengthening his belief in plant remedies. He published the *New Guide to Health; or Botanic Family Physician* in 1822, and practised in New Hampshire, although his influence was far more widespread as it seemed perfect for people living in the wilderness, with access to plants but not expensive doctors. Ohio's *Botanico-Medical Recorder* even claimed excitedly in 1839 that the Cherokee Nation had abandoned their ancient botanic practices and adopted Thomsonian Medicine, although this seems unlikely. Thomson's system was regularly jeered at by medical professionals, and the debate often divided around class issues – due to his farm-labouring background – and jealousy of his obvious success. However, Thomson was highly influential in the way many early nineteenth-century Americans regarded medicine: simple, allegedly safe and cheap.

One element of frontier individualism was a scorn for education and sophistication, so Thomson's method of self-medication, and therefore self-reliance, held a special appeal. This was also true of the patent medicines, which were sold as safe, family friendly and increasingly had comforting images and words on the bottles. Now manufactured on a large scale in America, these home-made medicines contained opium as often as the British ones. (Opium shortages in America appear to ease almost exactly in line with the American involvement in the Chinese opium trade.) The most famous of all of them was Mrs Winslow's Soothing Syrup. Sold by Curtis and Perkins of Bangor, Maine, this patent medicine was supposed to have been invented by Mrs Charlotte Winslow in the 1830s, although there is no evidence she existed. Despite containing over sixty milligrams of morphine per fluid ounce, it was marketed directly at fraught mothers. As with Godfrey's Cordial, it was recommended for teething children, to relieve 'the little sufferer at once', and 'produces a natural, quiet sleep by removing the child from pain'. It also promised to relieve wind and stop diarrhoea, and after all this the child would awake 'as bright as a button'.[7]

Mrs Winslow's Soothing Syrup appeared in the 1830s, just as the advertising industry was starting in earnest in America, and Curtis and Perkins exploited this to the full. Images of beautiful, relaxed mothers and happy, round-cheeked children feature on each ad. Many of the nostrum makers saw the potential of this new, dynamic advertising industry to open up new markets. The distances involved meant that mail order was on the rise. Men were moving from the land to factories, leaving wives in the home looking after the children. Busy, yet bored, Mrs Winslow's Soothing Syrup was soon not just for children. It was also notorious amongst the medical community for being responsible for a significant number of infant deaths, as the superintendent of health for Providence reported in 1873:

> The decedent from poisoning in March was a child killed by a dose of Mrs Winslow's Soothing Syrup. It has long been well known to physicians that the soothing properties of this medicine are due to opium in some form, and that the quantity of opium is so large to make it a decidedly dangerous nostrum. There is no doubt that a considerable number of deaths each year should be recorded 'Mrs Winslow's Soothing Syrup'.[8]

Another 'dangerous nostrum' native to America was Ayer's Cherry Pectoral. James Cook Ayer, one of nineteenth-century America's success stories, was born in Connecticut in 1818, and attended the University of Pennsylvania Medical School. He never practised medicine but went straight into compounding medicines, working in Lowell, Massachusetts. At twenty-two, he purchased an apothecary shop with $2,486.61 borrowed from his uncle, and managed to return the money in three years. His success came not from the effectiveness of his medicines, but the almanac he put together and distributed widely, and the reputed $140,000 he spent on advertising. The *Ayer's Almanac* announced proudly that it was aimed at 'Farmers, Planters, Mechanics and All Families'. Around 5 million almanacs were printed, with editions in English, French, German, Portuguese and Spanish. His most popular products were sarsaparilla, which he claimed purified the blood, Hair Vigor, which was equally useless, an Ague Cure containing cinchona bark, which was helpful in cases of malaria, and the Cherry Pectoral, containing three grams of morphine per bottle. Ayer's Cherry Pectoral's entry in the almanac of 1857 declared that 'Every comfort, encouragement and support that can be afforded, should be provided. The mind should be cheerful, free from depressing cares. Courage helps to conquer.'[9]

Ayer is clear that Cherry Pectoral is an emotional cure as well as a physical one. One charming undated advertisement in black and white shows a small girl in her Sunday best and a bonnet, trying to reach into a giant bottle with a spoon, and announces, 'It is in every sense An Emergency Medicine'. It was hugely popular, and helped Ayer amass a fortune of $20 million.

Ayer was not America's first quack, nor the last, but he was the most successful. The almanac was a superb piece of advertising that hit all the right notes with bone-weary, lonely farmers, worried housewives and factory workers. He had also industrialized the nostrum business, and perfected mail order, providing a model for the many who followed him, although few with his rapid success. With his plain, printed book and comforting tones, Ayer was perfect for the emerging Middle America, a million miles from the barking sideshow snake-oil men who were rampant at the time. Yet, seemingly, the one person in America who Cherry Pectoral couldn't help was James Ayer himself. 'Anxiety and care brought about a brain difficulty, and for some time prior to his death he was confined in an asylum.'[10] He died there on 3 July 1878.

At the time of his death, America's medical advertising was at a peak. From the 1850s onwards, agencies had sprung up in Philadelphia, Boston, Chicago and in particular in Lower Manhattan. Advertising was suddenly big business, and it was moving away from adorable pictures of little girls and upright wholesome mothers to women dressed in negligees lounging on a bed with a giggling child, all in lush colours, or bold catalogues of the new farm machinery. Brighter and more promising in every sense, America was changing into a land of efficient consumers.

The Rise of Morphinism

The isolation of morphine had been a huge commercial success, although sadly not for Friedrich Wilhelm Sertürner. It was soon available across Europe and America, most often as a powder. Yet it wasn't perfect, and doctors knew that administering morphine solution under the skin with minimal damage would be infinitely preferable for the patient, preventing 'the subcutaneous cellular tissue being torn up with a common probe to make room for the reception of a drachm of solution of morphia.'[11]

The invention of the hypodermic needle was the answer. Syringes had existed since Galen used them to inject cerebral vessels with fluid, and da Vinci used them to inject the blood vessels of corpses with wax. They had no needle, but were used to flush wounds or apply medicines in hard-to-reach places. Crude but effective, they were an essential part of the physician's hardware. The Dutch doctors of the late Renaissance, around 1600, coined the term *inject*, meaning to drive in, and referred to their attempts at blood transfusions using tubes and bladder systems. Christopher Wren had used an animal bladder to push opium into the dog's vein in 1657. Dominique Anel (1679–1730), a French surgeon who studied under the royal physician, began to refine the syringe at the turn of the eighteenth century. In 1713 he began to publish on his small syringe, which he used to treat eye problems. The 'Anel syringe' is immediately recognizable, and although Anel never used it with a needle, it was the start of the hypodermic revolution.[12]

Throughout the eighteenth century, physicians refined syringes and began to use them more widely, but manufacturing had yet to create a hollow needle fine enough to inject through the dermis. From the 1820s, the most common form of administration was for a small cut to be made through the skin and a flap lifted, often with trocars and lancets, into which the powder was sprinkled. This obviously carried the risk of local infections through irritation, or total systemic infection through blood poisoning. Morphine powder, however, had the great advantage over opium in that it didn't have to be ingested, thus bypassing nausea or cramps, or smoked, and it could be applied to the whole system through one or two small cuts. The method had been invented in France, and was soon popular across Europe and America, particularly for neuralgia, such as the case John Locke had encountered.

By the middle of the nineteenth century, needles could be made fine enough to break the skin and deliver medicine. This development was taken up by various scientists and doctors, but three came to the forefront, two of whom were Irishman Francis Rynd (1801–61), and Alexander Wood (1817–84), a Scot. Rynd probably invented the hypodermic as we know it today in 1844, but he was so secretive he only revealed his findings after 1855, when Wood published 'New Method of Treating Neuralgia by the Direct Application of Opiates to the Painful Points', in the *Edinburgh Medical and Surgical Journal*.[13] Both were using hypodermics to treat patients with morphia for pain, and Rynd was treating a woman with neuralgia. The third doctor, Charles Gabriel Pravaz (1791–1853) in Lyons, was also an early developer, and his design became the default in Europe.

Although there are many squabbles over which doctor first used the modern hypodermic, it's likely that many doctors were working on similar lines, but didn't publish or achieve any fame. What secured the lasting notoriety of these three men was the instant uptake of their new invention. By the time Charles Hunter (1835–78), a London surgeon, first used the term 'hypodermic', meaning under the skin, in 1863, the apparatus was already being manufactured on a large scale. Hunter had realized that introducing a drug into the bloodstream meant that injections didn't need to be administered at the exact site of the malady, which was particularly helpful for neuralgia patients who couldn't bear their head to be touched, let alone injected.

Pain theory, so important to the history of opium, was also central to the development of the hypodermic needle. Neuralgia, although well known before, had first become a much debated concern around 1800, when it was described as 'a modern disease' because it was a nervous problem with no obvious cure or cause. The pain in the head, jaw and teeth for a neuralgia sufferer is almost unbearable during an attack, and it is a condition associated with suicide in sufferers who can no longer endure it. So it seems natural that Wood, and others, would be trying to find a way to relieve the pain of neuralgia sufferers. Hypodermic administration of morphine for unidentified pain became an instant success, and crucial early papers in respected medical publications such as the *British Medical Journal* all refer to the hypodermic treatment of neuralgia with morphine.

The hypodermic had the great advantage on many fronts. Many of the first patients found the immediacy of the effects of subcutaneous morphine injections nothing short of miraculous. As important as patient experience was the dosage control the hypodermic gave to doctors. The small, relatively simple piece of equipment allowed for a measure of preparation and theatre before the magic medicine was delivered, which then brought instant relief.

By 1857, American firm Fordyce Barker was manufacturing in the United States where, in the middle of the nineteenth century, the finest medical instruments in the world were being made. For the discerning buyer, it was soon possible to purchase hypodermics with gold needles and shagreen cases. But not all medical professionals were convinced the hypodermic was the right route to take with morphine solution in particular. Regulatory bodies in the UK, the US and Germany all preached caution in the face of this new cure. One warning voice in America was that of the physician Robert Bartholow, who wrote a manual on the safe use of hypodermics and said that 'The possibility of communicating disease by inoculation of specific matter should not be overlooked.'[14]

Yet, such was the perception that only the oral consumption of morphine or laudanum created an addict, because it stimulated an appetite, injecting below the skin seemed a straightforward way of stopping the problem: 'When long-continued use of morphia is required, the danger of the habit of opium-eating will be avoided if we inject the opiate.'[15]

Thus, doctors in the first few years thought that hypodermic injection did not create morphine tolerance. Their error was soon apparent. Such was the demand for this new, efficient method of delivery that doctors were soon discussing what might be done. Firstly, it was recommended to 'Never under any circumstances teach a patient how to use a hypodermic syringe.'[16] This had been a sticking point for some doctors, who, when treating middle- and upper-class patients, particularly women, would hand over medicines or treatments to a carer or a husband.

Furthermore, doctors were using it too much, said German physician Felix von Niemeyer: 'I know many physicians who never go out to their practice without a Pravaz's syringe and a solution of morphine in their pocket, and who usually bring the morphine-bottle home empty.'[17]

Lack of proper sterilization and injecting in dirty conditions was also becoming an obvious problem. One doctor wrote about the morphine addict who had come to his office: 'The entire surface of the abdomen and lower extremities was covered with discoloured blotches . . . the marks of injections. He was spotted as a leopard. For four years he averaged three or four a day – an aggregate of between five and six thousand blissful punctures! The right leg was red and swollen, and I discovered a subcutaneous abscess extending from the knee to the ankle and occupying half the circumference of the limb.'[18] Niemeyer had written about the dangers of such addiction to hypodermic injections of morphine in his manual on practical medicine: 'If injections of morphia have been made for some time . . . the patients begin to feel an absolute need of the injections.'[19]

It had taken less than twenty years for the medical profession to realize the potential for harm the hypodermic presented, whereas previously they had seen the invention as one of the most important of the nineteenth century. 'It is no exaggeration to say this abuse is becoming a gigantic evil, to the extent and dangers of which the medical profession should be fully aware,' wrote Robert Bartholow, whose manual had helped not only doctors, but users to self-administer.[20]

The instant pain relief offered by the hypodermic injection of morphine was something neither doctors nor patients had experienced before. Freedom from pain, particularly chronic pain, had suddenly become possible through the simple prick of a needle. The dual nature of the hypodermic was now as stark as that of the morphine it contained, and by 1880 doctors across Europe and America had realized that 'no therapeutic discovery . . . has been so great a blessing and so great a curse to mankind as the hypodermic injection of morphia'.[21]

Civil War

'You don't mean he must die, Doctor?'[22]

The Civil War of 1861 to 1865 put a brief halt on America's headlong rush towards the future. In Louisa May Alcott's *Hospital Sketches* of the time she spent as a night nurse at the Union Hospital at Georgetown, Washington DC, she writes extensively about the bravery of the men who arrived there, shattered by the new inventions in artillery and firearms. Particularly touching is the tale of John, the Virginia blacksmith with the beautiful face, who had been shot but appeared unwounded. Alcott asked the surgeon about his fate: 'the poor lad can find neither forgetfulness nor ease, because he must lie on his wounded back or suffocate . . . It will be a hard struggle, and a long one.' No mention is made of pain relief for John, only God, cleanliness and love. There is a brief mention earlier of the 'merciful magic of ether', but none for John, who ended up in the anonymous burial ground known as the Government Lot.[23]

The reality of the Civil War was that a soldier was eight times more likely to die when wounded than a soldier in the First World War, but ten times more likely to die of disease.[24] An estimated 620,000 men died in the war, representing 2 per cent of the male population, and more than half died of disease while in prison or in hospital. The first Civil War field hospitals were tents or even open fields, soon moving into requisitioned houses or any building large enough to hold the grotesque number of casualties. Walt Whitman, the American writer, remembered visiting a field hospital in Fredericksburg, Virginia, after the battle there: 'Out doors, at the foot of a tree, within ten yards of the front of the house, I notice a heap of amputated feet, legs, arms, hands, &c., a full load for a one-horse cart. Several dead bodies lie near, each cover'd with its brown woolen blanket.'[25]

The new technology deployed in the Civil War meant that loss of limbs and shattered bones were the common injuries. On arrival at the field hospital, the surgeon or assistant's first job was to tourniquet what was left of the limb in an attempt to stop the bleeding. Drinking water was supplied and, as Federal surgeon W. W. Keen remembered, 'Powdered morphine was adminis-tered freely, doled out with a pocket knife [sprinkled directly into the wound] without worrying about superfluous exactitude in doling out the blessed relief that morphine brings to men in pain.'[26] They were often also offered whiskey.

Morphine powder was used liberally throughout the Civil War, with one Federal surgeon so hard pressed during a battle that he diagnosed from horseback, tipped it into his hand and had the men lick it from his palm. Medical science had not begun to catch up with the types of injuries that men could now inflict upon each other with heavy artillery, and the best that could be hoped for post-amputation or gunshot was a ready supply of morphine powder or pills, or opium for plasters. Any of these would also have helped with the terrible dysentery that was rife in both the camps and the hospitals. For the army surgeons, quinine for fevers and chloroform for anaesthesia were also vital.

The Union army was far better equipped in almost all ways than the Confederate forces, which were often reduced to smuggling in medication such as opiates. John S. Cain, a chief surgeon of a division in Tennessee, admitted they were 'frequently overdrawn' in the field.[27] Not so the Union army, which issued almost 10 million opium pills and 2.841 million ounces of other opiates in 1865. And by the end of the war, the Union army had issued 2,093 syringes to about 11,000 surgeons, though probably fewer actually used the instrument, which was probably quite impractical in the utter chaos of a battlefield hospital, when a steady hand was needed to draw up solutions and concentration required to ensure the correct dosage.[28]

Experiencing the Civil War hospitals, with holes drilled through floorboards to catch the pints of blood that flowed from amputations and surgeries, the gangrene, the overcrowding, misery and despair, must have been horrifying.

In the years that followed the Civil War, doctors across the country noticed a striking rise in the number of morphine addicts they were treating, and many of them had one thing in common: they were all veterans. Many had lost limbs that had been removed at speed and sometimes with little skill, badly healed and agonizing; the need for pain relief was obvious. But for others, there were no visible wounds at all, such as the anonymous writer who published *Opium Eating: An Autobiographical Sketch* in 1876. He had been sixteen when he had enlisted as a Union army drummer in 1861, but was soon carrying a gun. In 1863 at Chickamauga, his second battle, he was captured and forced to march to Richmond in Virginia. With 5,000 others he was kept in terrible conditions at Danville prison, then moved to the dreaded prisoner-of-war camp at Andersonville, Georgia. He was transferred once more and finally released in February 1865 as part of a prisoner exchange. Cared for by Union doctors, he suffered insomnia and was given a sleeping draught. At home, he suffered stomach cramps and ongoing headaches, and eventually went to see a doctor who was keen to inject him with morphine, which miraculously cured his ailments but cast him into the 'wretchedness' of addiction.

This story is by no means uncommon, and reflects the emotional hardship that many of the Civil War veterans had clearly been through. As late as 1919, at the morphine maintenance clinic in Shreveport, Louisiana, doctors treated an eighty-two-year-old Civil War veteran who, after being shot in the head, had been treated with morphine, and had taken it ever since.[29]

These stories are numerous, and morphine addiction came to be known as 'the army disease', which refers not only to the amount of narcotics that were administered during the war, but also the fact that hypodermic syringes were available for the first time. However, quite when it took that name is not clear, although it emerged in the early twentieth century when America was attempting to justify involving itself in opium prohibition. The first mention appears in 1914, in a paper by Jeanette Marks, a Yale historian, on the 'Curse of Narcotism in America', when she asked, 'Did you know that there is practically no old American family of Civil War reputation that has not had its addicts? Did you know it was called "the army disease" because of its prevalence?'[30]

The ordinary doctors who saw these patients were certainly not unsympathetic, and many were mostly concerned to see the veterans maintained on the correct pension, as is echoed by the physician Thomas Crothers in his book on drug addiction: 'The sufferings and hardships growing out of the perils of war often react in illness, nerve and brain instability, and feebleness, and the use of morphine is a symptom of the damage from this source which should be recognized as its natural entailment and sequel by the Pension Bureau.'[31]

Another soldier, but one only suspected of opiate addiction, was the Confederate veteran 'Doc' Pemberton. He was wounded at the Battle of Athens, Georgia, and later became a chemist in Atlanta, where he created a recipe of kola nuts and cocaine to try and prevent people drinking alcohol. It is known today as Coca-Cola.[32]

It has long been a popular myth that the Union and Confederacy demobbed an army of addicts, and estimates have been anywhere from 100,000 up to 300,000. Some argue that there was no such thing as lingering morphine habits after the war, let alone an epidemic of addicted soldiers, but the sheer number of morphine pills handed out, probably for self-administration, would indicate otherwise, as would the amount of morphine bottles thrown down the latrines of the Civil War prison on Johnson's Island, where they appeared not just in the hospital block. In addition, it took doctors until the early 1870s to make the association between the hypodermic and morphinism, and they were usually specialists in the needles themselves or in addiction. From the existing accounts, it seems the addicts came out and became opium eaters or remained dependent upon morphine. As Horace B. Day wrote in his 1868 book *The Opium Habit*, 'Maimed and shattered survivors, from a hundred battle-fields, diseased and disabled soldiers released from hostile prisons ... have found, many of them, temporary relief from their sufferings in opium.'[33]

The liberality with which doctors dosed their patients was addressed one year before the war had broken out, by the eminent doctor Oliver Wendell Holmes, in a speech to the Massachusetts Medical Society, in May, 1860, when he said that the population was 'overdosed', one of the first recorded uses of the word. 'How,' asked Holmes, 'could a people ... which insists on sending out yachts and horses and boys to out-sail, out-run, out-fight and checkmate all the rest of creation; how could such a people be content with any but "heroic" practice? What wonder that the stars and stripes wave over 90 grains of sulphate of quinine, and that the American eagle screams with delight to see three drachms of calomel given at a single mouthful?'[34]

Welcome to Dai Fou

The word coolie comes from the Chinese word *k'u-li*, translated as 'hard strength', from their traditional work as physical labourers. These workers who came aboard the merchant ships bound for America after the end of the Second Opium War were often indentured, and, having left the money for selling their labour with their families, emigrated for a set period of time, often a considerable number of years, to another country. Peru, America and Australia were the main destinations for them in the middle of the nineteenth century, and many were deceived about just how long they would be away from home. Many were also kidnapped and placed in *barracoons*, or holding centres, until the ships were ready to sail. Mortality rates, for which there are no reliable figures, were high enough to make perishing on the journey a genuine risk.

Their main point of entry was on the West Coast of America at San Francisco, which they called Dai Fou. By the time many of the first Chinese immigrants arrived there, the California Gold Rush was beginning and there was work to be had in the mining communities, or in large San Franciscan construction companies. The San Francisco Chinatown was the first and most significant on the West Coast, and well established by the 1850s, when it had over thirty general merchandise stores, more than a dozen apothecaries, several restaurants and herb shops and three boarding houses. It had been put aside by the city as an area where the Chinese could own land, so had become an obvious place to settle, as well as providing the comforts and ties of home. The level of immigration was incredibly rapid, with only 325 Chinese recorded in San Francisco in 1849, but 25,000 by 1852.[35] This was partly because ordinary workers, now free to leave China, booked their passage on the Pacific Mail Steamship Company boats. They soon made up 10 per cent of California's population, and were making their way east to work not only in mining towns but other settlements, although many remained on the West Coast.

The Chinese presence was almost uniformly resented by the American press and the American people. It did not matter that they had been pressed out of their own country, either by force or financial necessity, by people who then charged them for their crossing. One of the problems was the Chinatowns, which created an alien presence inside large, predominantly white settlements. Another was the sheer difficulty of the cultural barrier. Another was that the Chinese workers brought with them their prime means of relaxation at the end of a long day: opium.

Soon there were opium dens in San Francisco, causing both social and political problems, 'where heathen Chinese and God-forsaken women and men are sprawled in miscellaneous confusion, disgustingly drowsy, there. Licentiousness, debauchery, pollution, loathsome disease, insanity from dissipation, misery, poverty, profanity, blasphemy and death are there. And Hell, yawning to receive the putrid mass is there also.'[36]

Authors of this type of writing, such as B. E. Lloyd produced in 1870, had plenty to say on the unsavoury habits of the Chinese, and on the evils of opium smoking, and Lloyd dwells for a page and a half on a scene within an opium den in the same book. Mark Twain is less salacious in *Roughing It* (1872):

Smoking is a comfortless operation, and requires constant attention. A lamp sits on the bed, the length of the long pipe-stem from the smoker's mouth; he puts a pellet of opium on the end of a wire, sets it on fire, and plasters it into the pipe much as a Christian would fill a hole with putty; then he applies the bowl to the hand and proceeds to smoke – and the stewing and frying of the drug and the gurgling of the juices in the stem would well-nigh turn the stomach of a statue.[37]

There were various attempts to stop Chinese immigrants bringing in opium or serving it to white people, but none of them worked. The habit for the Chinese was so ingrained that they would obtain the drug from whatever source necessary, although there were so many entering San Francisco it was unlikely they would have to venture out of the community. America was, by this time, in the grip of early morphinism and its attendant problems, and opium was seen as the root of the issue. This disregards the fact that few Chinese smokers changed from the pipe to another method of achieving the same effect; most tended to reach a plateau of use from which they did not increase or deviate. This is in direct contrast to morphine, which causes the user to crave an increased dose as tolerance is established. These facts were known at the time, but the chemical mechanism was not understood.

Also mentioned repeatedly were the Chinese prostitutes, who sat behind closed doors on various streets in Chinatown, only their faces visible, and the proportion of Chinese female immigrants who engaged in prostitution. Because Chinatowns contained drugs, women, drink and gambling, they had long been haunts for sailors and labouring white men, further denigrating them in the minds of middle-class Americans such as Lloyd. Later in the century, when young white men and women began to visit opium dens to smoke, the San Francisco and New York authorities were barraged with complaints. San Francisco's attempt in 1880 to get a grip on the problem was to make a detailed map showing every opium den and brothel in the fifteen-square-block territory of Chinatown. How effective this was in solving anything is dubious, but it was an attractive way of displaying San Francisco's sharp racial divides. The population had boomed after workers had returned from the finished Transcontinental Railroad in 1869 and things were reaching a crisis. 'Thus, in San Francisco, it is but a step from the monuments of the highest type of American civilization, and of Christianity, to the unhallowed precincts of a heathen race,' railed Lloyd.[38]

Part of the problem was that America had spent over a century placing enormous emphasis on the importance of family, home and domesticity. The advertising industry thrived on depictions of wives and mothers, or the moment father returns from work to be greeted by his loving children. The Chinese population had none of that. The men had left their homes and families and come to America, willingly or unwillingly, to earn money. From necessity they lived alone or in boarding houses, and they lived in the same area as each other because there was no possibility of integrating and there was comfort in familiarity, and because, mainly, they went where they were put. The majority of women who came at the beginning were indeed prostitutes, or involved in opium dens, or both. They were unfamiliar and their culture was alien. And the drug culture was a large part of their daily lives. All these things were ostensibly true, but ultimately, the reasons for American resentment of the Chinese immigrants were economic. The acute labour shortages that had seen the Chinese arrive on the West Coast in the 1840s had changed with the Gold Rush, demobbing, and then the railroad. The railroad almost immediately attracted large numbers of

Chinese labourers, for the single reason that few white people were prepared to do the physical labour required to build it.

In 1865 the Central Pacific Railroad Company of California hired fifty Chinese workers, of whom the company superintendent said, 'They prove nearly equal to white men in the amount of labor they perform, and are much more reliable.' By 1867, the company employed 12,000 Chinese workers, 90 per cent of the entire work-force.[39] The railroad meant that Chinatowns, no matter how small, spread along the western arm of the Transcontinental Railroad under construction, and the Midwestern press reported on Chinese men taking away launderessing work from local white women, and in what conditions they lived, and how cheaply, which did not benefit local economies. As Lloyd had remarked, 'So well do they understand how to make each cent extend their lease of life, that how they succeed in doing so is a matter of surprise and wonder to Americans.'[40] Taking into account how little they were paid, this was not necessarily a matter of choice.

Another outstanding thorn in the side of the Americans heading up the anti-Chinese movement was that because they were single men they could afford to live and work so cheaply. This was also true, because they were not allowed to bring in their wives or families unless they were wealthy, and even then there was no guarantee of immigration being granted. As single men, they also represented a threat to the family unit, particularly when they were gathered together, as in opium dens. When young white women began to be seen entering or leaving opium dens, the San Francisco Board of Supervisors passed an anti-opium-smoking law in 1875. Still, the anti-Chinese feeling gathered. Henry Grimm's 1879 racial drama 'The Chinese Must Go': A Farce in Four Acts caught the mood: 'By and by white man catchee no money; Chinaman catchee heap money; Chinaman workee cheap, plenty work; white man workee dear, no work –

sabee? . . . White man damn fools; keep wife and children – cost plenty money; Chinaman no wife, no children, save plenty money. By and by, no more white workingmen in California; all Chinamen – sabee?'[41]

In 1858, state legislature in California, today regarded as one of the most liberal states in America, made it illegal for anyone of Chinese or Mongolian appearance to enter the state, but it was thrown out of the Supreme Court. After the Civil War, the economy went into decline and the Chinese were even more reviled. Dennis Kearney, the racist labour leader who gave long, ranting speeches against the Chinese, and his labour organization the Workingman's Party of California, were responsible for stirring up huge anti-Chinese sentiment, and finally the state tried exclusion again in 1878, but President Rutherford B. Hayes refused. So California passed an Act that meant the state could let in who it wanted, and forced the Chinese Exclusion Act through in 1882. The Act was repealed in 1943, but it took until 2014 for California to call upon Congress to apologize for passing it in the first place.

'Trixie!'*: Deadwood, South Dakota

Opiates were not just a fixture of the West and East coasts of America in the late nineteenth century. They also moved inland with the workers who travelled along the railroads and into the mining towns, and it was not only the Chinese who controlled

---

* In the critically acclaimed HBO series *Deadwood*, which aired between 2004 and 2006, Al Swearengen is frequently heard to call for his trusted confidante, the prostitute Trixie. Trixie was depicted as one of the few women to escape Swearengen's employ, finding a job and a partner, and is later revealed to have overcome an opium addiction.

the trade in it, or consumed it. In the winter of 1875, in a ravine between two rocky outcrops over two and a half miles long and initially full of dead trees, the mining town of Deadwood, South Dakota, was established at the end of the Gold Rush, 'at the centre of the last and richest gold field on the globe'.[42] The year before, Colonel George Armstrong Custer had struck gold in South Dakota, and there were still plenty of people who wanted to try their hand at mining. In early 1876, Charlie Utter led a wagon train to the new settlement, carrying notorious gambler Madame Mustache, as well as others determined to live a new life in what was essentially a large camp.

Deadwood had a small Chinese community from the start, which in 1880 numbered 116 out of around 5,000 miners, business and townspeople, according to the census, although archaeological evidence points to a far bigger community of around 400.[43] They established a Chinatown at the lower end of Main Street, creating the necessary infrastructure to house a large group of men aged sixteen to eighty-six, including a Joss House, which served as a temple and meeting place. Estelline Bennett, a resident of Deadwood during its earliest time and well into its most established phase, and also the judge's daughter, described it as 'painted brown with little red embellishments pointed and peaked and squared itself in unexpected ways and places . . . The inside we were never permitted to see. A peculiar and intriguing odor of incense came to meet you a block away'.[44]

On 7 April 1877, the Gem Variety Theater, owned by Al Swearengen, opened its doors. Martha Jane Burke, best known as Calamity Jane, worked for him as a dancer and procuress, but she lived in Chinatown. Swearengen not only had the bar and brothel, he also ran the town's opium trade. This strange reversal of roles was down to three things. Swearengen was a career pimp and drug dealer, and also had the monopoly on the supply chain through Charlie Utter and his brother Steve. Lastly, the nearest Chinese community and potential source of supply was 300 miles away in Wyoming.

Wing Tsue, a Chinese grocer of high standing in the camp, was also involved in the opium business and was fined for it at least once in the early years of the settlement, presumably to push him out of the trade. His main business rival in the Chinese community was another grocer known as Hi Kee, and the two rarely spoke and were suspected to be leaders of rival Triads.[45] On 4 July, they held what was known as the firehorse race, where the employees of each man would drag a fire engine through the street by the hose to a finish line. Deadwood is conspicuous for the Chinese community joining in the American and Christian celebrations and vice versa, including Chinese New Year. The local doctor was invited to Chinese funerals and carried a spoon with him for the wake because he couldn't use chopsticks. Wing Tsue's grocery advertisements, which included the finest Chinese silk scarves, were embellished at the bottom: 'Americans as well as Chinese are invited to call and inspect my goods.'[46] Having learned English at the Congregational School, Wing Tsue (whose real name was Fee Lee Wong) once decorated a wedding cake with 'God made the world but Wong made this cake'.[47]

In November 1883, three opium dens were operating in Dead-wood, corroborated by archaeological evidence of pipes, bowls and paraphernalia found in the early 2000s on a four-year dig there. Also discovered were a selection of bottles, including American and Chinese patent medicines, and 'beer, wine, cham-pagne, whiskey, gin, brandy, soda and mineral water, and soda pop'.[48] The cost of a pipe of opium in one of the dens was twenty cents, and for a dollar the customer could smoke as much as he liked until he fell into a slumber. Estelline Bennett said the judiciary, which included her father, were uninterested in

Deadwood's opium trade. 'If a Chinaman wanted to smoke, who cared? They were rarely any trouble about anything else.'[49]

The only people who seemed to care about either the close communities or the opium consumption were the newspapers, who regularly sent reporters to Deadwood to try and tease out a story or an angle. The *Black Hills Daily Times* reported on 6 May 1878 'that thousands of dollars a week is taken from circulation here by the Chinese smoke houses. Every dollar which drops into their coffers is salted. Something should be done to root out those institutions. They not only gobble a large portion of our floating cash but demoralize and destroy a large portion of our citizens. Opium smoking is a greater evil than whiskey drinking.'

Owing to this sort of pressure, the Territory of Dakota finally passed a law in 1878 to make it illegal to own a den or handle opium. It did not make much difference. What did stir public feeling, though, were the reports of suicide attempts by Deadwood's prostitutes. Of the three connected with Al Swearengen reported in the local press, Hattie Lewis (his mistress), Emma Worth and Eva Robinson had all tried to take their lives with opiates.

Ultimately, however, the press failed to have much effect on Deadwood, despite nipping persistently at its heels. The close alliances between communities of American and Chinese are doubtless not unique to Deadwood, though it is recorded there in a uniquely detailed fashion because of the amount of famous characters of the Old West who passed through – or didn't, in the case of Wild Bill Hickok, who was murdered there in 1876, just as the town got on its feet. Charlie Utter, Seth Bullock, Al Swearengen and Calamity Jane were all involved with the Chinese community on Lower Main Street, where the Chinese loved the white American bread of the baker there, Bob Howe, so he baked to the Chinese dinner hour.[50] This level of integration was a far cry from the anti-Chinese sentiments of coastal America, where drugs, and therefore the Chinese, were rapidly being demonized. Life at the edge of civilization had brought disparate groups of people together in a way that, for better or worse, absorbed the opium trade as an accepted fact of life.

Al Swearengen was found dead in Denver on 15 November 1904, of a blow to the head with a blunt instrument.

From the Gold Rush to the Gold Cure

Deadwood, and many places like it, were completely without law up until the 1880s, but elsewhere, such as in Pennsylvania, New York, London and European cities, attempts to regulate the medical profession had begun in the middle of the century. In 1858, Britain passed the Medical Reform Act, attempting to ensure that doctors were licensed medical practitioners, and then in 1868 the Pharmacy Act meant that finally the two disciplines were separate. The Pharmacy Act was particularly significant as it limited the sale of certain drugs over the counter without a doctor's prescription. There was an immediate and significant drop in the death rate caused by opium preparations, from 6.4 per million in 1868 to 4.5 per million in 1869. More significantly it meant that deaths amongst children under five dropped from 20.5 per million (1863–7) to 12.7 per million in 1871. Owing to the removal of opiates from most patent medicines, it continued to fall in the 1880s to around 7 per million.[51]

There were, however, a rising number of addicts. Leading members of the medical communities of Britain and America began to study groups of opiate addicts in particular, to find out the demographic and, crucially, try to find out why people became addicted.

Dr Alonzo Calkins, a specialist in narcotics, collated 360 case studies of opiate addicts in 1871, and judged that many wealthy women who spent their days 'idly lolling upon her velvety fauteil' waiting for the hours to pass were most susceptible to fall prey to opiate addiction.[52] 'Uterine and ovarian complications cause more ladies to fall into the habit, than all other diseases combined,' remarked another doctor.[53] In *American Nervousness: Its Causes and Consequences* the neurologist George Miller Beard noted that, 'The general laws are that the more nervous the organization, the greater risk the susceptibility to stimulants and narcotics ... Woman is more nervous, has a finer organization than man, and is accordingly more susceptible to most of the stimulants.'[54] Even worse, Gaillard Thomas, president of the American Gynecological Society, confided that 'for the relief of pain, the treatment is all summed up in one word, and that is opium. The divine drug over-shadows all other anodynes ... You can easily educate her to become an opium-eater, and nothing short of this should be aimed at by the medical attendant.'[55] There were even arguments for the education of women being the culprit, something self-proclaimed addiction expert Dr Leslie Keeley also agreed with.

As cases of escalating drug use presented themselves, and women who had been treated with laudanum for period pains ended up injecting morphine, these arguments seemed increasingly arrogant and dangerous.

The invention of the hypodermic had been so groundbreaking it had been a catalyst for the squabbling British medical community to pull itself into a coherent unit, and they were keen to see the Pharmacy Act passed, and control over morphine injections returned to the doctor. Thomas De Quincey, who reissued *Confessions of an English Opium-Eater* in 1856, also issued a challenge to the British medical community: that they knew nothing about the true experience of opium upon the individual, so therefore they were in no position to regulate such

matters. Two doctors, James Russell and Francis Anstie, rebuked
him, Anstie especially on the subject of self-injecting, but with
regulation looming, most doctors did not want to be involved.

Research into the potentials and dangers of the hypodermic
and morphine intensified over the next two decades as, particularly, wealthier patients presented with more related problems,
despite the apparent new difficulties getting hold of morphine.
Harry Hubbell Kane was an American doctor who conducted
much research into both opiates and cannabis – the latter he
tried personally and wrote up the experience in 1883 – and he
attacked De Quincey as 'hand[ing] down to succeeding generations a mass of ingenious lies', and condemning them to
bondage.[56] Alonzo Calkins was another to attack De Quincey
on the grounds that the doctor knows best.

Amongst the majority of the professional medical community,
it was firmly believed that women in their thirties were the most
likely to abuse opiates. Stay-at-home wives were especially vulnerable. Therefore, it was quite a shock to the reputation of the
medical community on both sides of the Atlantic when, in 1883,
prominent American physician J. B. Mattinson made the claim
that the majority of United States doctors were morphine users,
and that between 30 per cent and 40 per cent were addicts.[57] A
later study reinforced this, taking different countries around the
world and gauging that, of all addicts, doctors comprised 40 per
cent and their wives 10 per cent. The recently formed body of
medical professionals, now in both Britain and America, looked
like hypocrites in the new debates on addiction and therapies.

In the midst of this, Dr Leslie Keeley established himself in
Dwight, Illinois, where he opened a sanitorium charging 'inebriates'
$160 per day to take tonics including his 'Gold Cure'. His injections
contained a solution of strychnine and boric acid, with the alkaloid
atropine. The Keeley Institutes were an enormous success.

PART THREE

Heroin

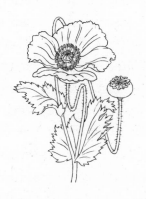

Chapter Seven

A NEW ADDICTION, PROHIBITION AND THE RISE OF THE GANGSTER

Narcomania and the Birth of Addiction Therapy

Just as morphinism truly took hold in America during the 1870s, the next chapter in the history of opiates began across the Atlantic, in a research laboratory near Paddington Station. The massive edifice of St Mary's Hospital, operating since 1851, is one of London's great Victorian monuments to public health and social improvement. It and the associated medical school, based on 'Christian and genteel values', were in a rough area known for prostitution, vagrancy and a high immigrant population. Initially they took in around forty students and taught basic sciences, medicine and surgery, as well as materia medica or the early study of pharmacology. It is often, rightly, lauded for being the place where researcher Alexander Fleming returned from holiday in 1928 and found penicillin infesting one of his neglected petri dishes, but in 1874 it was also the place where diacetylmorphine was first synthesized by Charles Romley Alder Wright (1844–94), whilst working under chemist Augustus Matthiessen (1831–70).

Matthiessen had started at St Mary's in 1862, focussing on the alkaloid components of opium. He was joined by the young Alder Wright, a physicist and chemist working primarily on codeine and morphine. Matthiessen and Alder Wright had been charged with finding a form of painkiller that wasn't as addictive as morphine.

Matthiessen had studied under Robert Bunsen in Heidelberg, and the Bunsen burner was part of the equipment at St Mary's. His and Alder Wright's experiments seem precarious, consisting as they did of sealing potent chemicals inside test tubes and then heating them with burners, but they produced a range of compounds that included apomorphine, which is now used to make dogs vomit when they eat something poisonous. Then, in 1870, Matthiessen killed himself owing to 'nervous strain' aged thirty-nine, after he was accused of indecently assaulting a young man, leaving his colleague Wright to continue alone. Alder Wright went on experimenting with alkaloids, particularly with a process known as acetylation. Acetylation is the chemical process of introducing an acetyl group of atoms into a compound, substituting them for an active hydrogen atom, and even the most basic of explanations about how this works open with the qualifying phrase 'extremely complicated'. The physical process, though, is not so complicated, and as Matthiessen had discovered previously, acetylation made alkaloid compounds more potent.

As his main equipment consisted of test tubes and a Bunsen burner, a common misconception is that Alder Wright simply boiled morphine and ended up with heroin. Instead, Wright used acetylation to 'cook' diacetylmorphine from morphine base in 1874. The physical process of making diacetylmorphine from morphine base is not that complicated, although it requires precision, skill and some degree of patience. The process that Alder Wright used is also the process that has been used for cooking legal and illegal diacetylmorphine ever since: the only thing that varies is quantities of scale. The blocks of high-grade morphine base that could be freely ordered by a research laboratory were broken down and reduced to small chips, sometimes simply by hammering or grating them. The chips were then heated slowly to remove all moisture, then put into a steel vat and acetic anhydride added. This created a reaction that gave off a reeking gas, and when it had finished reacting, water was added to convert any remaining acetic anhydride to harmless acetic acid. Impurities found at this stage were removed with chloroform, and then sodium carbonate was used to neutralize the acetic acid. Then, as now, this is the second dangerous part of the process, when the mixture can 'boil' and explode. Litmus paper was used continuously to make sure all the acid was gone, and then the resulting precipitate was dried, ready for use.

Alder Wright handed this product over to the London doctor F. M. Pierce to be tested on a dog and a rabbit, along with codeine, as he and Matthiessen had done before. Pierce failed to make comparative tests with standard morphine, so diacetylmorphine didn't seem any more or less effective, and was thus discarded as yet another failure. Wright went back to work in his laboratory.

In the same year, 1874, the largely Quaker-led and catchily named Anglo-Oriental Society for the Suppression of the Opium Trade set up its headquarters in King Street, Westminster, to be near both the India Office and the Houses of Parliament. Its intention was to lobby the government to stop selling opium to China, and to see legislation passed to that effect. Previously, it had been a well-organized but dispersed group of businessmen who believed the British government was responsible for the deliberate degradation of the Asian peoples through the opium trade, although they drew the line at abolishing the British Empire altogether, preferring instead to lobby for more missionaries to convert those Asian peoples. Their focus was almost exclusively on China, rather than India, where the opium habit was not perceived to be a problem in the main, and the population was already sufficiently exposed to mission-ary culture.

The 1870s and 80s saw a distinct shift towards legislation by the 'improvement societies'. Largely, they were modelled on the temperance movement, which had always been in the vanguard of ways to ban intoxicants. The British temperance movement had gone down the legislative route as early as 1853 with the formation of the United Kingdom Alliance in Manchester. Inspired by the American state of Maine's legislative lead in 1851, the purpose of the Alliance was 'to call forth and direct an enlightened public opinion to procure the total and immediate suppression of the traffic in all intoxicating liquors or beverages'.[1]

It is difficult to overestimate the strong feelings that develop-ed towards social order and intoxicants in the late nineteenth century amongst the middle classes of Britain and America. Rising wealth and standards of living had resulted in a class of people for whom maintaining a constant and comfortable steady state was all, and who were alarmed by the social disorder visible in towns and cities when working men and women celebrated payday, rather than by the long-term debilitating effects of alco-holism. Their answer was to attempt to extend the control and order present in their own lives, out to wider society. These social-improvement movements had their detractors: John Stuart Mill, the utilitarian philosopher, attacked the Alliance, and prohibition in general, in his 1859 essay *On Liberty*: 'And though the imprac-ticability of executing the law has caused its repeal in several of the States which had adopted it, including [Maine], an attempt has notwithstanding been commenced, and is prosecuted with consid-erable zeal by many of the professed philanthropists, to agitate for a similar law in this country.'[2]

Mill saw trade of any commodity as a natural extension of society, but his views were in direct opposition to those who wanted to push towards a politically enforced utopia, rather than an individually chosen one. Because the changes in society brought about by urbanization and the Industrial Revolution had both concentrated certain problems, and made them more visible, the need to deal with them was more urgent. In 1879, the Habitual Drunkards Act was passed through the British Parliament. Although the Act was largely unsuccessful – because it required a patient to surrender themselves to enforced rehabilitation for up to one year, and also to be able to pay for that year's treatment – it did address one fundamental issue: voluntary admission and the desire to seek help.

The Drunkards Act was at the very beginning of true understanding about addiction. Seeger, the otherwise anonymous pioneer who wrote to the *Boston Medical Journal* in 1833, was far ahead of his time: 'Sir,—I observed in yesterday's *Northampton Courier* an article from your Journal upon Opium Eating, in which you acknowledge not to know a remedy against that fatal practice; and any one acquainted with such a thing, is invited by you to communicate it . . . I consider this practice generally a real and complicated disease'; and the doctors and social commentators of the 1870s were rapidly coming to similar conclusions.[3] Two camps were set up: those who believed that addiction was not only 'bodily deterioration, [but] lapsed moral sense as well' and those who believed addiction was both symptom and cause of some greater imbalance within the individual.[4] These two camps persist today, in both society and legislation.

Unlike America, where the addiction of women and the dangers this presented to society were front and centre in the debates surrounding morphinism and alcohol, Britain and Europe focussed largely on working people of both sexes. The European

Industrial Revolution had changed the way people lived so dramatically, in a way not yet seen in America, that opiates had
become the drug of the masses in ways that were intimately tied
to their working lives. The need to understand this relationship
between the functions of working people and their addictions,
rather than the need for oblivion pursued by prostitutes, the destitute or those harmed by war, led to a very different approach to
addiction on the European side of the Atlantic.

The Society for the Study and Cure of Inebriety was founded
in Britain in 1884, as activists saw the need for an understanding
of addiction because 'We know but too well, much of the evil
that arises from intemperate drinking; but of the origin and
development of intemperate habits in the individual, we know
next to nothing.'[5] It was formed largely as a pressure group to
lobby the government over the inadequacy of the Drunkards
Act, and the inaugural address of 25 April by Norman Shanks
Kerr included an extraordinary opening that went to the heart
of the study of addiction, listing 'constitution and temperament',
mental and psychological 'susceptibilities', 'environment' and
'inherited predilections' as key areas for investigation.[6]

The same year, Kerr presided over the programme of the
Dalrymple Home for Inebriates in Rickmansworth, Hertford-
shire, 'prettily situated on the banks of the Colne', with sixteen
beds available.[7] Other rehabilitation centres existed in Derby-
shire and Scotland, and also one specializing in the treatment of
women in Kennington, London, but Dalrymple was properly
funded and well organized.

Kerr was the leading British addiction doctor of the late
nineteenth century, advocating complete abstinence from all
intoxicants. He was chair of the British Medical Association's
Inebriates Legislation Committee, the BMA's lobbying arm, and
in 1888 they campaigned successfully to get the Inebriates Act

through Parliament. Strong political agitation had also seen the Truck Act the previous year, which stopped workers receiving payment in alcohol. The Inebriates Act was an amendment of the Drunkards Act, 'inebriates' referring to drug addiction as well as alcoholism, and allowing for compulsory detention of the patient. Kerr, whose contribution to the field of addiction is undeniable, in 1890 coined the term 'narcomania' during a lecture in Christiania, Norway.[8]

Kerr's general demeanour is, to put it politely, Victorian. His strict rules, unfortunate terminology for those he deemed morally inadequate, and lifelong abstinence from all substances except large meals, in particular turtle soup, can make him seem pompous, even objectionable, yet the best of his writing reflects his understanding of the nature of addiction:

> The continuous and victorious struggle of these heroic souls with their hereditary enemy – an enemy more powerful because ever leading its treacherous life within their breasts, presents to my mind such a glorious conflict, such an august spectacle, as should evoke the highest efforts of the painter and the sculptor.[9]

Friedr. Bayer et comp.:
'Plenty of natural curiosity and two kitchen stoves'[10]

In the same year that Kerr gave his lecture in Norway, two Scottish doctors reported to the British Medical Association at their grand headquarters at 429 The Strand on the results they had seen using diacetylmorphine on frogs and more unfortunate rabbits, which acted on the spinal cord and respiratory system. Although interesting, neither the doctors nor the BMA seemed to find anything of particular value in the research, and the opportunity to claim the 'invention' of diacetylmorphine for Britain was passed over again.

Charles Alder Wright continued his work at St Mary's, although he had moved onto acetylating camphor in the hopes of making more effective soap, stern stuff no doubt, as well as experimenting with fireworks. Like Matthiessen, he died young, in 1894, from the complications of diabetes.

Then, in 1897, a research chemist named Heinrich Dreser took a job with a company called Bayer in Germany. Bayer, founded on 1 August 1863 in Elberfeld, had originally specialized in dyes, but soon diversified into the manufacture of medicines. They were, as their own website proudly proclaims, 'a 19th century startup with tremendous potential'.[11] Quite how much potential, none of them could have known at the time.

Dreser, who is most often credited – wrongly – with the invention of heroin, was in charge of a development team including Arthur Eichengrün and Felix Hoffmann, who were in contact with both Edinburgh and London and watched developments there and elsewhere with interest.

Eichengrün in particular was, like Dreser, a shrewd manipulator of teamwork to his own ends, and arguably the pivotal character in the process. It is disputed whether he or Hoffmann synthesized diacetylmorphine, and then aspirin from salicylic acid, in the same fortnight in 1897, but Eichengrün was the senior chemist, and Hoffmann a technician. Eichengrün was rightly famous: a prolific scientist who held forty-seven patents. In his lifetime he was best known for creating a silver proteinate marketed as Protargol, the go-to gonorrhea treatment for fifty years, until penicillin. When he left Bayer soon after the discoveries of 1897, it was to establish his own company. When the Nazi Party came to power in 1933, Eichengrün, who was Jewish, was running a successful business but had to take an Aryan associate. He was forced into selling the company five years later, and then imprisoned in Theresienstadt concentration camp forty miles outside Prague in 1944, aged seventy-six. From there, he wrote to Bayer detailing his work in the development of aspirin, by then one of the world's most successful drugs, and asking for help. Bayer filed it neatly in their archives, and left the most successful research chemist they had ever had exactly where he was. Although released soon afterwards, dying peacefully aged eighty-two in 1949, Eichengrün's place in the creation of aspirin and heroin had been supplanted in the official histories by Hoffmann and Dreser, and is rarely mentioned now.

Of the two drugs, aspirin was regarded as the most dangerous at the time, mainly because of the risk of bleeding in the stomach. Thus, in a single fortnight, three men were responsible for the world's most successful legal drug, and its most successful illegal one.

Dreser tested both drugs on himself, and some of Bayer's workers, before the products went for animal testing. Amongst his many achievements, Dreser has the dubious credit of introducing large-scale animal testing to the pharmaceutical industry. He also published two papers in 1898 which ensured his lasting association with diamorphine's early days. One was on the pharmacology of derivatives, and the other on 'the effect of some morphine derivatives on respiration', revealing that, specifically, in the diacetylmorphine experiments, he had been looking for a drug that would treat advanced lung disease, and in particular tuberculosis, which was rife at the time.[12] Studies on sufferers indicated that it really did stop them coughing, made them feel calm, and as a sedative, helped them get a good night's sleep: diacetylmorphine seemed almost miraculous in its effects. Even better, the patients liked it, and almost always asked to continue the treatment. Dreser, following the trend for 'heroic' medicine in the late nineteenth century, named Bayer's diacetylmorphine preparation 'diamorphine', gave it the brand name Heroin, and put in for the patent, granted the following year.

It is an indicator of how intense experimentation and competition were between these large industrial chemists in the late nineteenth century that Joseph von Mering, working for E. Merck in Darmstadt, also produced diamorphine in the same year as the Bayer team. Yet Mering thought other derivatives would be better at treating lung disease, and so passed over diamorphine in their favour. He published on the subject for *The Merck Report*, but it was only later that he came to see the error of his decision.

Heroin was a tremendous success, marketed across Europe and the United States by 1900. Tubercular patients, and others suffering advanced lung disease, could not pronounce themselves cured, but their symptoms were reduced dramatically and instantly. They *felt* well.

Originally, there were two main preparations of heroin. The first was the pure diamorphine synthesized by Eichengrün and Hoffmann, $C_{21}H_{23}NO_5$, a bitter, white, crystalline powder soluble in alcohol, or to be mixed with sugar to be sold as pills.[13] Heroin hydrochloride – made by the addition of hydrochloric acid at the end stage of the cooking process, and with the molecular formula $C_{21}H_{24}ClNO_5$ – was available by 1899, and soluble in water. These two versions of heroin are still the main starting points for the ways the drug is consumed now, and their properties dictate how.

Pure diamorphine is quite volatile, with a low melting point of 173 degrees centigrade, making it more suited to smoking. As a 'salt', heroin hydrochloride has the advantage of being more stable, but has a higher melting point of 243–4 degrees and decomposes with heat rather than releasing the powerfully intoxicating vapours of the pure diamorphine. It is, however, water-soluble, making it more suitable for injecting, taking orally, or sniffing, where it will pass across the mucous membranes of the nose very quickly.

Heroin is converted to morphine in the body almost instantly, but the initial feeling is much more intense, which made it more popular with patients. Early marketing was aimed squarely at those with serious lung conditions, and they tended to remain on the medicine until they died, so the addiction issues were not marked until use spread into the general population. Heroin pills, ridiculously cheap and easy to make, were retailing over the counter in packets of a hundred, some of them flavoured with rosewater and coated with chocolate. One cough syrup was marketed as 'suitable for the palate of the most discerning adult or capricious child'. My personal favourite is the idea of Syrup Toluheras, each dose comprising: 20 mg heroin, 150 mg cannabis, tartar emetic, chloroform, alcohol and, naturally, syrup of tolu from Colombia. Letters from concerned doctors were soon appearing in medical journals on both sides of the Atlantic, but the genie was out of the bottle, or at least in millions of bottles on thousands of chemists' shelves. Multitudes of proprietary medicines, similar to the original soothing syrups, were soon in shops and catalogues, most of them sold as cough mixtures and containing combinations of heroin, strychnine, quinine and terpin, a popular expectorant at the time. Owing to the bitterness of heroin itself, sugar featured heavily in almost all of them.

By 1900, Bayer were retailing Heroin, Heroin Hydrochloride and Aspirin in the United States by mail order, 'samples available' from Bayer's outlets at 40 Stone Street, New York. The same advertisement also features Eichengrün's Protargol, as well as a variety of worming preparations, and a treatment for piles. The essential human ailments vary little over the centuries, it seems.

The synthesis of heroin happened at a key moment in history. Although it was largely overlooked for some two decades, the discovery of its potential could hardly have been better timed to ensure its global success. Then in 1901 heroin overdose begins to appear in the *British Medical Journal*. The following year, leading American specialist Thomas D. Crothers introduced the term 'narcomanias' in his work on opiate addiction. In 1903, London junior doctor Sophie Frances Hickman sparked a nationwide manhunt when she disappeared from her post at the Royal Free Hospital. Hickman was found dead in Richmond Park some months later, next to intravenous morphine paraphernalia. The worst fears of the medical community had been realized, and all too late: world events were conspiring to create a climate that brought heroin to the forefront of medical science, and forced it underground in a way that birthed a new kind of organized crime, the like of which had never been seen before.

The American–Philippine War and Bishop Brent

At exactly the same time as Bayer's Heroin met the world market, from 1899–1902 America was involved in a war with the Philippines. It seems now like the preposterous escalation of a bar brawl, but it had serious consequences for the people of the Philippines, and also on US drug policy and the international trade in opium.

Cuba was fighting for independence from Spain, a long, wearisome campaign of spats and wars, the latter phase of which started in 1868. Ordinary Americans, sick to death of their own war and the depression that followed, did not want to be involved in another, particularly a foreign one. In order to be seen to protect its interests, America deployed the rather feeble warship USS *Maine* to Havana in late January 1898. She had been a long time in the shipyard, and when she was launched, technology had moved on. On 15 February, an internal explosion resulted in the sinking of the ship with the loss of 258 crew members.

The mysterious sinking of the *Maine* caused a wave of outrage across America, fuelled by myriad newspaper reports featuring spurious stories about how and why the ship had gone down – Mines! Spies! Sabotage! – and of Spanish atrocities against the Cuban people. On 19 April, Congress passed joint resolutions supporting Cuban independence. A US force would be stationed there, it stated, and removed as soon as the Spanish were out, because as the amendment named after Colorado Senator Henry Moore Teller stated, 'the island of Cuba is, and by right should be, free and independent'.[14] The Americans declared war on the Spanish on 20/21 April 1898.

Even now, the true motives for America entering the Spanish–American War remain unclear. Some maintain that it was as a result of a propaganda battle between the print empires of Joseph Pulitzer and William Randolph Hearst. Others point to America's intention to take from Spain the island they had already tried, and failed, to buy. Wars rarely happen for one reason alone, but America's war with Spain did have remarkable and unintended consequences. The Teller amendment, stating as it did that Cuba would not be occupied by America after Spanish withdrawal, did not mention the Spanish colonies of the Philippines, Puerto Rico or Guam. America promptly invaded Cuba, the Philippines and Puerto Rico, and Spain conceded the war on 17 July 1898.

Guam was visited by a US warship that fired warning shots on entering the harbour, which the locals thought was a cheerful greeting. They were informed about the war, news of which had not yet reached the tiny Pacific outpost, and the Spanish soldiers stationed there promptly acquiesced, and the whole business was despatched with minimal fuss.

The Filipinos, however, were not going to make things so easy. In over 300 years of Spanish rule, the Philippines had developed a complex social structure and a solid, Spanish-speaking middle class. They were exposed to European ideas, but remained firmly rooted in their Eastern geographical identity. In particular, their strong trading culture with the Chinese went back to the tenth century, and many layers of Filipino and Chinese interactions existed: from simple business to intermarriage, as well as class distinctions and particular names for people originating in different parts of China, Canton, Fujian and Guangdong especially. From the beginning of Spanish rule, the Chinese had been troublesome in the Philippines, and marked out for special consideration, particularly as far as trading was concerned. First they were pirates, then tricksy merchants, then general traders. *Sangley* was the common term applied to those of pure Chinese origin, and *mestizo de sangley* to those of mixed heritage. Over the centuries, although almost all of these Chinese-Filipinos came to regard themselves as simply Filipino – specializing in manual trades such as building and agriculture, food industries and in some cases money-lending – to outsiders such as the Spanish, British and Americans, they were a different and very useful group, trading as they did, continually, with China. During the nineteenth century, and the Chinese diaspora, many more Chinese arrived in the Philippines, and the government began to regard them as a social problem. And with them, of course, they had brought that particularly Chinese habit: opium.

In 1815, the Spanish galleon trade with Mexico had been abolished, followed by Mexico's declaration of independence in 1821.

The Manila–Acapulco galleons that had hoved back and forth so reliably for 250 years were suddenly a thing of the past. In centuries of trade, Mexico had received mangos, rice, water buffalo, silk, tea and fireworks; the Philippines, the avocado, guava, papaya and pineapple, and above all, silver. Spain had gone from one of the ocean-going Titans of the Renaissance to a country in deep financial trouble, in the space of just a few years. By 1843, the Spanish Bourbon government had realized that the opium trade was not only profitable, it was confined largely to the Chinese and Chinese-Filipino population as a habit. They were desperate to boost the Philippine economy and to pacify the Chinese element of the population, and so auctioned the rights to an opium monopoly.

The effects of what was happening in the Philippines were amplified by the fact that they weren't only a magnet for Chinese immigrants and traders. Many European merchants and businesses had seen the opportunity to work with, or exploit, a nation that was emerging from the age of galleons. British and American businesses, and often individual merchants working hand in hand with those businesses, already so dominant in the East, were innovating at a remarkable speed and keen to collaborate across the world in the interests of making money, and the Philippines presented an excellent proposition. Two prominent British firms, Ker & Co. and Wise & Co., were trading items such as alcohol, knives and combs, as well as tobacco, salt and essential oils, but all from within the British possessions. Spain also allowed British merchants into the Philippine sugar trade, and in return received new technology developed at the beginning of Britain's Industrial Revolution, such as steam power for mills, and iron-working, all of which improved Philippine agricultural practice significantly.

Rich Chinese merchants were subject to government policy.

Historically, the main trading market for luxury goods was the Alcaiceria, or silk market, of San Fernando, the southernmost of the two San Fernandos in the northern Philippines. The Chinese were allowed to unload and warehouse their goods there, and take lodgings for as long as it took to sell on, but it was all for a price, and in 1756, restrictions on business had become tiresome in San Fernando. Don Fernando Mier y Noriega offered to put a substantial sum towards the costs of building a new exchange, in return for him and his descendants reaping the benefits in perpetuity, and it passed on 15 July 1758. But the new Alcaiceria had proved a chaotic, criminal disaster. Not only was it full of gambling establishments, ruffians and houses containing 'opium divans', it had been burned down twice in a short space of time.[15] The Philippine government came to associate this kind of dissolution with both the Chinese and opium smoking, and after the first fire in 1810, passed a law on 1 December 1814 by Madrid Royal Decree that banned opium smoking. The Madrid decree is interesting because of the three-strikes aspect to it: caught once and it was fifteen days in prison; twice, thirty days; the third time was four years of hard labour. Those caught with intent to deal were instantly in for six years of hard labour.[16] But by 1828, the government had experienced a surprising change of heart when they allowed the cultivation of opium. They realized they were missing out on the revenue reaped by other South-East Asian governments from the institutionalizing of opium smoking, particularly those with a large Chinese immigrant population.

Chinese agricultural workers were an important part of Philippine society, and the move towards opium cultivation was not only about helping the economy, but was also about creating a social system of recreation in more remote areas. In 1835 the Chinese community asked the government to build a centre

A scene in an opium den depicting a Chinese man offering a pipe to an American woman. The caption read, 'He often made an honest dollar teaching American women how to smoke "hop"'. 1900.

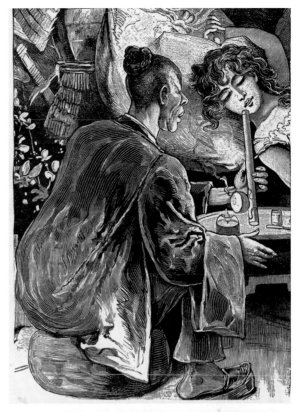

Studio portrait of Fee Lee Wong, his wife, six children and their maid (standing behind them), 1889–1907.

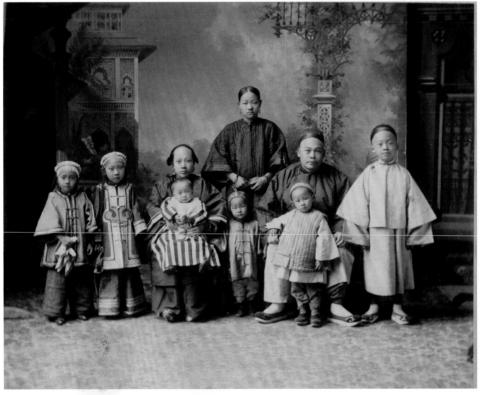

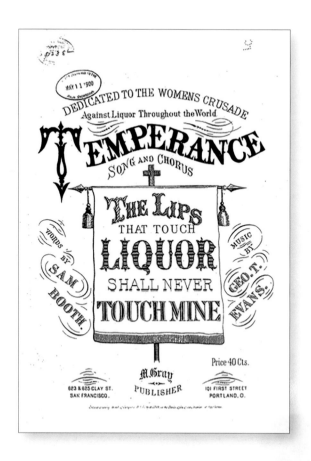

The molecular structure of diacetylmorphine.

Songs of the Temperance Movement and Prohibition (M. Gray, 1874).

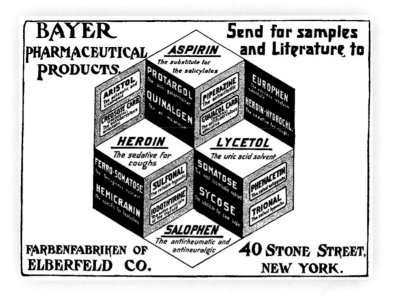

Advertisement for Bayer Pharmaceutical Products
by mail order, *c.*1900.

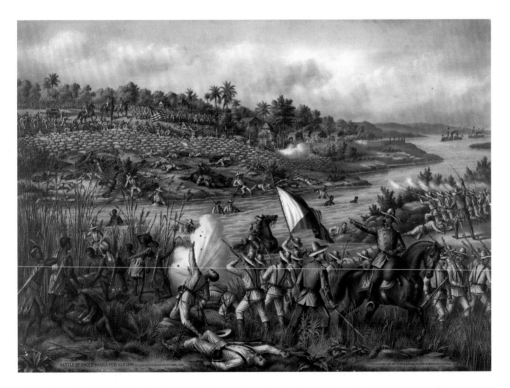

The Battle of Manila, the first and largest battle fought during the Philippine–American
War, was fought on February 4–5 1899 between 19,000 Americans and 15,000 Filipinos.

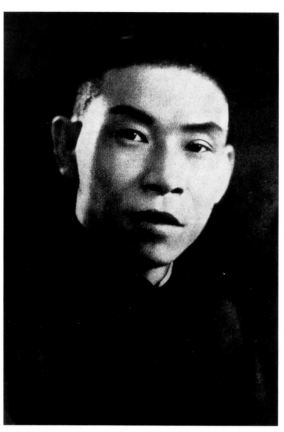

Du Yuesheng, Green Gang
mobster and Shanghai
godfather (1887–1951),
as a young man.

The opium man of
Mehrangarh Fort, Jodhpur.

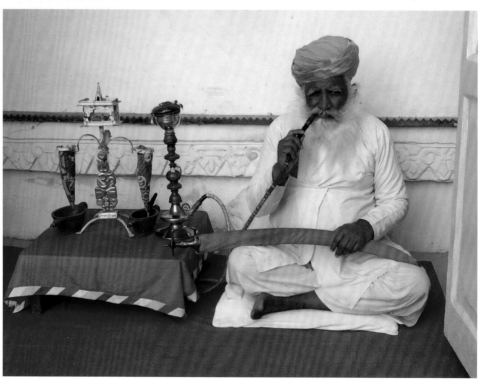

Mugshot of 'Lucky' Luciano as taken by the NYPD on his arrest for running a prostitution racket in 1936.

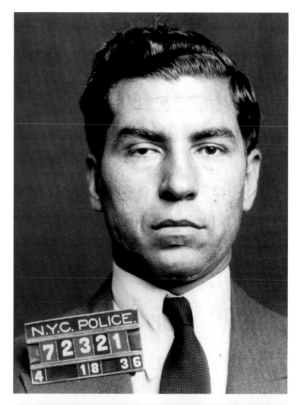

Frank Lucas wearing a chinchilla coat and hat outside Madison Square Garden before the Muhammad Ali vs Joe Frazier fight in New York.

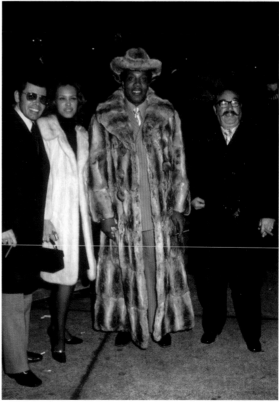

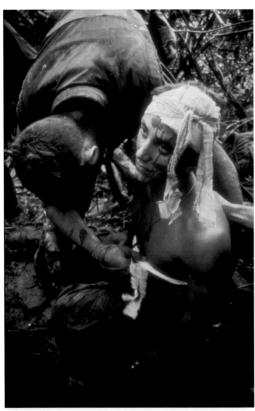

A shell-shocked, wounded marine being bandaged in a muddy jungle during OP Prairie, South Vietnam.

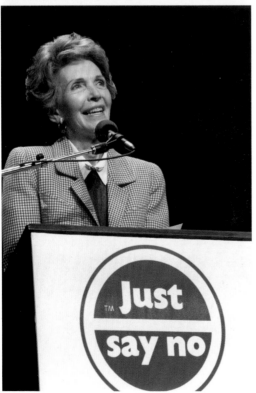

First Lady Nancy Reagan speaking at a 'Just Say No' rally, Los Angeles, 1987.

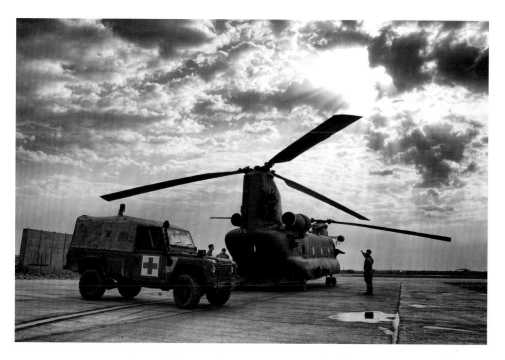

An ambulance waits to receive a casualty from a
Chinook helicopter at Camp Bastion, April 2011.

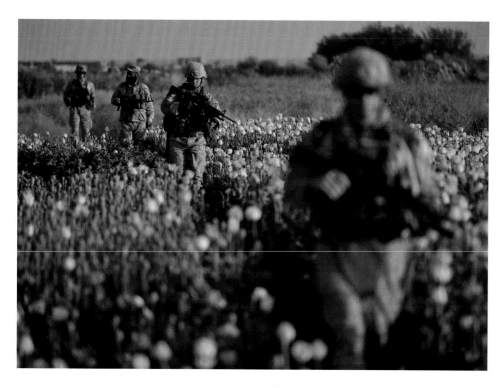

US Marines walk through a poppy field in Helmand Province, 2011.

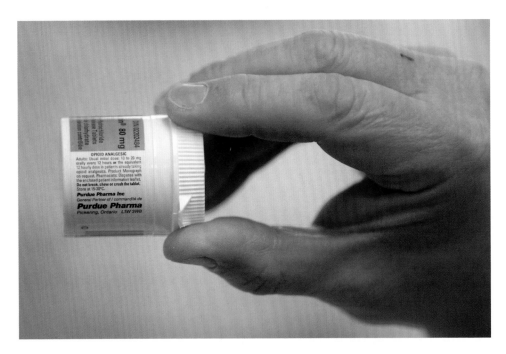

OxyContin tablets at a pharmacy in Montpelier, Vermont, 2013.

where they could manufacture decent quality opium and requested that it had an attached venue for smoking it. But home-grown opium wasn't nearly enough to supply the demand, and this resulted in the 1843 monopoly auction.

The high level of organization rapidly implemented in the Philippine opium importing, manufacture and smoking culture indicates how deeply entrenched it was. The taxation system was detailed and highly structured, and it appeared to work efficiently with only minor infringements, such as a Spanish tavern owner, Luis Velasquez, who withheld his payments because he believed that his establishment, the Alhambra, was being blighted by the stench from a local opium den. The owner of the den was instructed to sort out his chimney, which was done within twenty-four hours, and order restored.

Two key points to the opium-smoking culture and laws of the Philippines were that the Chinese were banned from smoking in their own homes, or outside of the government-approved houses, and that no Spanish or Filipinos were allowed into the opium dens. Gambling and drinking were banned, and the opening hours were late in the evening so that smoking had minimal effect on the working day.

The scale of the opium trade in the Philippines is shown in the records for 1867 when sixty-two ships brought in 13,027 kilograms of opium purchased from Chinese, English and German merchants.[17]

As the century progressed, there was an increasing amount of agitation for Philippine independence. The sophisticated Filipino middle classes wanted a progressive, self-determining nation, and saw Spain as an ageing force, reliant on old glory.

The revolution began in August 1896. Emilio Aguinaldo was a sensible twenty-eight-year-old revolutionary, and assumed leadership on 23 March 1897. The following August, with the

Philippines still in turmoil, the Americans invaded and captured Manila. It was an extraordinary situation: just as it seemed the Filipinos had extricated themselves from centuries of colonial rule, they were landed with an invading nation that had no notion of what it was to be a colonial power. Compared to later American deployments, the US campaign to the Philippines was modest: no more than 70,000 troops at its height, and later no more than 40,000. The extensive Philippine archipelago had a population of over 7.5 million at the time.[18] Its scattered, yet intense trading communities are what made it both vulnerable, and allowed it to subvert colonial authority. In addition, the young US troops were born of parents who had witnessed a land war, they had been raised well versed with guns, and they were supplied with copious ammunition. The Filipino troops, such as they were, were none of these things: two-thirds of them fought with traditional bolo knives and the large American cavalry horses frightened them.

On 10 December 1898, the Treaty of Paris saw Spain hand over the Philippines to the US for $20 million. Aguinaldo and his revolutionaries were not consulted in the negotiations. However, they were undeterred, and continued to rouse their fellow Filipinos with the reasons they needed, and must have, independence. Aguinaldo was also convinced of the necessity to keep the opium dens going, not least because they would be a precious source of revenue for a government in its infancy.

Between the Treaty of Paris and the beginning of the American–Philippine War, there was a lull in which US President William McKinley published the charmless proclamation of 21 December 1898, that became known as Benevolent Assimilation. Theoretically, it was meant to placate the Filipinos 'by assuring them in every possible way that full measure of individual rights and liberties which is the heritage of free peoples, and by proving to them that the mission of the United States is one of benevolent assimilation substituting the mild sway of justice and right for arbitrary rule'.[19]

America's prior record of assuring the full measure of individual rights and liberties of free people, let alone benevolent assimilation, is hardly something that could be expected to comfort the Filipinos. Hostilities were kept just about under control, until the night of 4 February 1899 when an American shot a Filipino sentry, known as the San Juan Incident, triggering the American–Philippine War.

Aguinaldo fled, and skirmishes continued throughout the summer, but on 7 August the Philippines – with the exception of some notable guerilla fighters – handed over power to a new colonial master.

In terms of the opium trade, the American–Philippine War presented America with a unique conundrum. Domestically, it was facing a level of morphinism that was threatening to run out of control. Yet it had taken control of a foreign nation with a highly sophisticated and entrenched opium culture, and crucially for America, it was a Chinese opium culture. The American hostility towards Chinese migrants, and their proclivities, was already written into the US constitution by the Chinese Exclusion Act, yet now they were in charge of a brisk, Chinese-run colonial opium trade. Politically and morally, it was a mess.

Yet the money was a concrete fact, and the tax revenues payable to Manila continued to rise under American occupation, quadrupling in the first four years.[20] Contrary to their alleged ideals, American free-spending and capitalist culture was bringing more Chinese migrants to the Philippines, despite the problematic international relations.

Added into this potent mixture was the concept that empires owed it to their primitive charges to civilize them. In South-East Asia at the time, the main powers were French, Dutch,

British and now the USA. America had yet to coin a term for their self-imposed obligation, while the French termed it, charmingly, their *mission civilisatrice*; the Dutch, pragmatically, *ethische koers*; and the British, 'the white man's burden'.

Charles Brent, the ambitious American bishop of the Episco-pal Church in the Philippines, revealed the global extent of the opium trade to the American government, and the impossibility of controlling it without international cooperation. A series of meetings were organized, culminating in the Shanghai Conven-tion of 1909, in which Brent played a prominent role on behalf of the US, along with United States Opium Commissioner and anti-narcotics zealot Hamilton Wright, at the beginning of the global attempt to control the opium trade. And like the mission-ary Peter Parker in the Opium Wars, it was also another important moment in the involvement of religion in American foreign policy, where it has continued to play a part ever since. Brent's rise to success played a large part in the organization of the Shanghai Convention and the consequences. The world had moved on after the Opium and Arrow wars, and Great Britain was no longer the force it had once been: her empire was shrinking.

Harrison and Volstead

'The opium and morphine habits have become a National curse, and in some way they must certainly be checked, if we wish to maintain our high place among the nations of the world and any elevated standard of intelligence and morality among ourselves.'[21]   Hamilton Wright, 1911

The International Opium Commission, proposed by the United States and 'accepted by Austria-Hungary, China, France, Germany,

Great Britain, Italy, Japan, the Netherlands, Persia, Portugal, Russia, and Siam', met on 1 February 1909 to discuss what to do about their respective, and common, opium problems.[22] The USA also proposed to impose a special tax on all persons who 'produce, import, manufacture, compound, deal in, dispense, sell, distribute, or give away opium or coca leaves, their salts, derivatives, or preparations'.[23]

The USA had also attempted to steal a march in public relations with China by banning opium smoking during the conference. The Opium Smoking Exclusion Act came into force during the commission on 9 February 1909. In reality, the 1875 Act against smoking opium, aimed at the San Francisco Chinese population, was more or less the same thing, and the 1909 Act had the effect of turning younger white smokers onto heroin instead, whilst the Chinese carried on smoking opium as they always had; it was now just illegal, again, to do so.

James Martin was a prime example of a typical young white opium smoker turned onto heroin by the Act. In 1908 he was a music-hall worker on Coney Island who smoked about $4 of opium a week, but the Act put his 'can of hop' up to an impossible $50, which made him look to morphine for a cheap fix, then heroin for an even cheaper one.[24]

In Shanghai, the combination of Hamilton Wright and Charles Brent must have been powerfully persuasive if unappealing, both of them so anti-narcotics and so sure of their own righteousness. Wright, however, was accurate in a lot of what he said, laying the blame primarily at the door of the patent-medicine manufacturers, and over-prescribing physicians. The 1906 Pure Food and Drug Act may have removed opiates from over-the-counter medicines, but morphine, heroin and hypodermic kits were still freely available for a few dollars.

The meeting was little more than a series of proposals, although

China did propose to support existing addicts, while preventing new ones from taking up the habit. The meeting led to the International Opium Convention in The Hague in 1912. For Great Britain, this must have been a somewhat awkward interlude, having as it did three major pharmaceutical companies in the form of T. Whiffen & Son, T&H Smith and J. F. Macfarlan Ltd, who were exporting morphine and heroin straight to China. Macfarlan's was, apparently, the connoisseur's choice of morphine in China: 'the Chinaman buys his morphia by the pound, and it must be Macfarlan's, which he must have in the original pound bottles'.[25] Even more embarrassing was that nine years later Whiffens' were stripped of their licence for smuggling.

The outcome of the meeting was that all 'The contracting Powers shall use their best endeavours to control, or to cause to be controlled, all persons manufacturing, importing, selling, distributing, and exporting morphine, cocaine, and their respective salts, as well as the buildings in which these persons carry such an industry or trade'.[26]

The US were quicker to act than most, owing in part to agitation by groups similar to the Society for the Suppression of the Opium Trade. There was also a racially motivated series of articles run in the *New York Times*, designed to both prey on and drum up anti-Black American feeling associated with cocaine in order to win over the South to the Act. The paper published stories about 'negroes' on cocaine, written by one Edward Huntington Williams, MD. One story from 18 February 1914 ran:

a hitherto inoffensive negro ... was 'running amuck' in a cocaine frenzy, had attempted to stab a storekeeper, and was at the moment engaged in 'beating up' various members of his own household ... Knowing that he must kill this man or be killed himself, the Chief drew his revolver, placed the muzzle over the negro's heart, and fired – 'Intending to kill him right quick,' as the officer tells it, but the shot did not even stagger the man . . . He had only three cartridges remaining in his gun, and he might need these in a minute to stop the mob. So he saved his ammunition and 'finished the man with his club'.

All the stories involve violence, and most involve the idea of an unstoppable, raging, cocaine-fuelled black man. They were very successful in helping to get the Harrison Narcotics Tax Act (named after its proposer Francis Harrison) and the Opium and Coca Leaves Trade Restrictions Act through, and they were both passed on 17 December 1914, with them becoming totally prohibitionist by 1922 through a series of amendments, ultimately called the Jones-Miller Act. Maintenance for addicts was banned by the Supreme Court in 1919. A further convention was held in Geneva in 1925 to update the rulings from The Hague, which the League of Nations would uphold and enforce. Britain had introduced the Dangerous Drugs Act in 1920, and over the next couple of decades, the signatories of the League of Nations and other countries followed. Turkey was a notable exception.

The ceaseless voices of the lobbying missionaries, as well as America sending its young troops into war overseas, played a significant role in driving the international drugs network underground, almost overnight. The medical fraternity continued to use heroin but began to call it medical diamorphine, and the term heroin came to mean the illegal product, except in the US, where the terms are routinely confused.

Logically, the Harrison Act and the National Prohibition Act – also called the Volstead Act (after Andrew Volstead, the chair of the committee that oversaw it), which enacted the Eighteenth Amendment prohibiting intoxicating beverages – were a natural part of vice reform during what is known as the Progressive Era of the United States, from the late nineteenth century to 1920. On the surface it was a good thing, a cleaning up of a society at the end of one century and the beginning of another. Yet the reality of these laws was far different. America – which, after Keeley's absurd Gold Cure, led the world in terms of addiction research under Dr Lawrence Kolb, head of the US Public Health Service's experimental hospital for treating drug addicts in Lexington, Kentucky – began to shut down its public health services. By the time 'junkie' had passed into American dictionaries in the early 1920s, referring to the ever-growing hordes of young male addicts who used to scavenge scrap metal in Manhattan to sell in Brooklyn yards in order to get high, New York's first and best public clinic had been shut up. Research into addiction was handed over to bodies such as J. D. Rockerfeller's Bureau of Social Hygiene, which cast addiction as part of criminology and over the course of the 1920s increasingly aligned itself with federal drug policy. Attempts to clean up prostitution saw women forced from houses with a matriarchal system to end up working for pimps on the streets. These men, post-Harrison, sold drugs because it was cheap and easy to get into, and addicted women were easier to control, thus establishing an indelible link between heroin and prostitution. On the day the Harrison Act was passed, the opiate ward of Philadelphia Hospital had to turn dozens of people away.

Another deliberate effect of Harrison was to pave the way for prohibition of alcohol. The passing of the Volstead Act delighted the temperance movement, and swathes of organized criminals across America and Mexico.

According to the Federal Bureau of Investigation, organized crime is 'any group having some manner of a formalized structure where the primary objective is to obtain money through illegal activities. Such groups maintain their position through the use of actual or threatened violence, corrupt public officials, graft or extortion, and generally having significant impact on the people in their locales, region or the country as a whole.'[27] This definition is an oversimplification of the complicated nature of global organized crime, and underplays the deeply tribal and specialized nature of the biggest and most powerful gangs. These groups often operate on both sides of the law, and have far-reaching networks that cover not only narcotics, but also human trafficking, gun-running and political corruption. In each part of the world, the structure of organized crime, as it emerged globally in the early part of the twentieth century, was as individual as the countries from which it emanated. As the century has progressed, organized criminals have been some of the first to respond to economic and political change all over the world. In looking at the history of some of these gangs, the most impressive elements include adaptability and speed of action. Organized crime is a large part of the hierarchy of any society, larger than any law-enforcement body or politician in any country wishes to admit, and inside that hierarchy, heroin is at the very top.

The Rise of Sinaloa

Geographically and circumstantially, Mexico was in the perfect place to respond to Harrison and Volstead. The USA shares a 1,989-mile border with Mexico. The Mexican states most involved with drug production traditionally (and now) are Baja California, Sonora, Chihuahua, Sinaloa and Nayarit.

In Sinaloa, in the Badiraguato area, the people had close ties to California, through Mexicali and Tijuana and also Arizona, where they sold their agricultural produce. Sinaloa had been growing opium poppies since at least 1886, courtesy of the Chinese who had arrived there in the late nineteenth century, allegedly when their boats were turned away from the United States. High in the mountains, villages are remote and close-knit, and families work together, as in every opium-growing region in the world. Domestic drug use, particularly of opium, was not tolerated. Marijuana was deemed more medicinal than recreational. What began in the late nineteenth and early twentieth century as supplementary income on what would have been a necessary journey anyway, morphed into full-time occupations, which then became dynastic businesses. Unlike almost every other Latin American drug-producing country, they do not involve themselves in politics, as this is judged too precarious, but maintain relationships with officials and the police. After all, everyone is in the business in some form or another. This is the reason behind the longevity of their leaders and family businesses. At this stage, they were not termed 'cartels', which came into use in the second half of the twentieth century.

Mexico had traditionally imported considerable quantities of opium for smoking, for which it had a limited domestic market, leading US officials to believe it was then exported up the West Coast of America through Baja California, along with home-grown marijuana. The border, however, was so vast and so porous that there was no way of controlling it and Mexico had a negligible home market for drugs. Soldiers smoked marijuana, the Chinese smoked opium, artists and the middle classes took cocaine or morphine, which needed to be refined. There was not enough money to be had domestically, and demand from the north was far higher, particularly for opium. This suited the Sinaloans perfectly, and they even coined a term for the opium traffickers: *gomeros*.[28]

With the 1909 Opium Smoking Exclusion Act, there was more demand for the Mexican opium than ever, and with the

Harrison Act, there was also an immediate demand for morphine and heroin. Poppy planting spread rapidly to the other states, particularly when President Carranza stopped opium imports in 1916, and banned marijuana cultivation in 1920 in what was essentially a sop to America's campaign to ban the drug. The ban made little impact on Mexico's marijuana culture. But in 1920 the Mexican government also prohibited opium, opium derivatives and cocaine growing and handling, with a potential seven-year prison sentence if caught. The following year, the Mexican newspaper *Excélsior*, which ran a stern anti-trafficking campaign, informed its readers of a man caught with a kilo of heroin, which he declared was for personal use, and he was let off with a fine. Curiously, he had been caught coming *into* Mexico from the US, and not vice versa.

In the border areas, many American brewers, who had seen prohibition on the cards for a long time, and faced with the complete loss of their livelihood when Volstead passed in 1919, had already been moving over into Mexico, bringing brewing knowledge, skills and employment. They also had legitimate ties back in the US, and so had reasons to move between the two countries.

In 1922, when the amendments to Harrison tightened opium prohibition to a stranglehold, the Federal Narcotics Control Board was founded to oversee the import and export of opiates and coca. In the State and Treasury departments were a number of like-minded individuals who were not satisfied with Harrison alone as a means of ending the opiate and cocaine problem of the United States, but were concerned with shutting off supply at source. These departments had, to an extent, been working with Mexico at cutting off some of the larger drug routes into the United States, but the implementation of the extreme version of the Harrison Act had created a huge black market in America instantly, one the Mexican traffickers were ready to exploit.

All of this happened in the midst of the Mexican Revolution, making it far easier for the traffickers to exploit the unrest and inattention of the authorities. Border raids by the US authorities, mainly in Baja California, were the main opposition to what was an increasingly lucrative trade, but there were still hundreds of miles of porous border to take the goods across.

Prohibition in the US caused a large spike in demand for drugs: they were easier to conceal and transport than bulky liquids, and as they were not all illegal anyway, people took what they could get. The ruined Mexican economy was given a huge boost by the brewing businesses, and by the business of smuggling alcohol and drugs back across the border. The Southern Pacific Railways newspaper vendors handled smaller shipments, passing them up the line to California, and soon the Mexican traffickers were making so much money they were investing in air transport. The most famous of the early traffickers was Enrique Fernández Puerta, the 'Al Capone of Ciudad Juárez', who was often escorted around the city in the 1920s by the police, although not at the time he was shot dead.[29] It was so lucrative that before long Sinaloa had dozens of small, secluded airstrips. Alcohol prohibition only lasted thirteen years, but in that time a whole new drugs infrastructure was set up, one that had gone from a simple import and export smuggling business, to a production, refining and trafficking business on a grand scale, and people were making millions of dollars. At this time, the violence was relatively contained, and mainly involved standoffs between police and traffickers, and was done out of the way in suburban areas.

Mexico's narcotic cartel culture is relatively young in terms of organized crime, but it is enormously successful owing to a cluster of events that all happened within half a century: a war that created an effective yet corruptible military infrastructure, the arrival of the Chinese, a revolution and its largest neighbour declaring prohibition on drugs and alcohol.

Ironically, Mexico City had been the first place to introduce opiate control in the Americas, in 1878, when a prescription from a doctor was required to obtain morphine.

The Young Turks

Arguably, Turkey has one of the oldest organized-crime histories in the world, based principally upon smuggling. It stretches back to the bandit gangs of the early Ottoman Empire, and then progresses through groups of rural gendarmes and the police force and the disbanded janissary corps. In addition, the Turkish population was traditionally highly mobile on a seasonal basis, so crime was associated with this vagrancy. The ethnic cleansing in Macedonia during the First Balkan War (1912–13) added to this displacement. This movement of approximately half a million people into a land where the existing population already had little led to struggles for power and security. Albanians, Chechens and the Laz Muslim group were all strongly associated with criminal behaviour. The Laz Muslims in particular had a large presence in the Istanbul heroin trade. When the Young Turk dictatorship was established in 1913, these ethnic groups were not allowed to form ghettos but dispersed among local populations, where they could not make up more than 10 per cent.[30] Still, the violence and general criminal behaviour got out of hand during the lawless days of the First World War refugee crisis, as Turkey's many different peoples clashed. There was a strong incentive to band together and use violence if necessary to gain control over scarce resources, or to protect established smuggling activities.

With its refusal to enter into the Versailles or Hague negotiations, when it became a republic in 1923 Turkey was still producing
opium legally, and was soon the most important post-Hague
supplier in Europe, with the best product. It also had miles of
infrastructure and factories dedicated to the production of morphine and heroin. The republic's first president, Mustafa Kemal
(later given the surname Atatürk – 'Father of the Turks' – by the
Turkish Parliament), attempted to use this to secure power over
the now extremely lucrative morphine market, before Ankara
would consider discussing the Hague Convention. The US, in the
form of drug czar Harry Anslinger, first head of the newly formed
Federal Bureau of Narcotics (1930), attempted to pressure Turkey,
saying they knew that people in power in Turkey were profiting
from opium smuggling, thereby implying that the organized crime
in Turkey was at the top rather than the bottom, and that a total
ban would convince people of the honesty of the regime. Ultimately, on Christmas Day 1932, Kemal announced that Turkey
would abide by the Hague Convention and reduce Turkey's opium
fields to no more than was needed for medicinal purposes. Despite
the accession, and the US's satisfaction with their inspection of
closed factories, Turkey's output of illicit heroin appeared to
remain unchanged, no doubt owing to the 'not tens but hundreds
of small, clandestine drug plants operating in Turkey without fear
or interference'.[31]

The most well-known man of the period to take advantage of
these plants was not, in fact, Turkish, but a Greek using the
Turkish criminal network to build one of the largest narcotics
empires of the time. Elias, or Elie, Eliopoulos was born into a
privileged family in Piraeus in 1894. He and his younger brothers
George and Athanasius were well educated and well travelled,
and in 1943 in New York, Elie and George were charged with
smuggling $2 million worth of morphine into Hoboken in 1931.

They had, in 1927, been searching for a new place to invest their money, and were impressed by the efforts of the League of Nations to limit the world's supply of opiates. After trips to Paris and Tientsin, they 'decided that the narcotics business had a sound future with impressive profit in prospect'.[32]

They set up in Paris and established the 'biggest share of the world's illicit trade in opium, morphine and heroin ever organized in one system',[33] before things became too tight with the law and they had to leave for Turkey. There, they found it was not a gentleman's game, and thievery and double-crosses were rife. A Grecian shipping agent blackmailed them into using his services by telling the brothers that he and his company were 'informants of the League'. Adapting to this new way of business, the Eliopoulos brothers attempted to charge an American dealer twice for 1,000 pounds of morphine and were hoisted by their own petard when the Hoboken shipment was impounded. Tired of their losses, they took their money out of opiates and put it into gold and bauxite mining. Their great mistake was to visit New York, imagining that they were protected by the statute of limitations. They were tried and convicted, much to the delight of the federal prosecutors, but on appeal it was found that the timeframe for prosecution had indeed expired and they were free to go. Elie returned to Greece and the family business, which was mainly arms dealing.

Shanghai's Green Gang

Opium trading has always had one foot either side of the legal line, but nowhere was it done in such style as in Shanghai, with its beautiful colonial architecture, exclusive clubs and smart parties. Before 1910, the most powerful figure in opium, both legal and illegal, in Shanghai was Edward Isaac Ezra, a Chinese-born Jewish businessman. Born in 1883, he was already making a fortune at seventeen from construction and later hotels, but it was opium that made him truly rich. In 1913, he became chairman of the Shanghai Opium Combine and amassed a legal fortune of around $20 million. He may have gained much more, running illegal opium to San Francisco with his younger twin brothers, Judah and Isaac, had it not been for the work of one woman: the remarkable American codebreaker Elizebeth Smith Friedman (her forename was down to her mother, who detested the idea that she would ever be called Eliza). Born in Indiana in 1892, Friedman graduated with a degree in English literature, but found an interest in secret writing when she met her future husband in her first job at Riverbank Laboratories cryptography centre, and she was very young when she began to work for the US government on intercepting and breaking messages that were to do with drugs, and later rum-running during prohibition. She was soon onto the brothers' operation, for which they used an increasingly complicated messaging system. Her codebreaking skills revealed the illegal side of the business and they were exposed. She went on to have a great career breaking other opium rings in the US and Canada, and was later the security advisor for the International Monetary Fund. Upon his arrest, Ezra gained immunity by turning in business associate and fellow crook Paul Yip, but it was his brother Judah's gambling habit that saw Ezra leave Shanghai public life. A remarkable businessman, Ezra died of a cerebral haemorrhage aged only thirty-eight, leaving the way clear for the rise of Shanghai's Green Gang.

The Triads are, as already stated, a political movement as well as a collection of secret societies and criminal gangs. In Shanghai in the late 1920s and the 30s they were so enmeshed in the political movements operating at the time that they were pivotal to the Green Gang's success. Between 1910 and 1930, the population of Shanghai trebled to just over 3 million, bringing many unskilled workers and Green Gang society members, which led to racketeering, extortion and anything that would turn a profit. The Green Gang was, in fact, many gangs under an umbrella name, and competition was fierce. In terms of controlling Shanghai revenue, control of the supply of heroin to the French Concession area was crucial. Three men, Huang Jinrong, Du Yuesheng and Zhang Xiaolin, joined together to take over this supply, which they hoped would allow them to dominate the other Green Gangs. To do this, they decided to cultivate the new Guomindang regime, which had just come to power in China. The charismatic Du Yuesheng met with the party representatives and offered to keep all the other Green Gang members in line, as long as their opium supply system was not interfered with. The men were also concerned that, as the government was poor, it was going to try and co-opt the opium business with an official monopoly. To do that, it had to come to an agreement with the Green Gang.

What followed was a power struggle in which the government repeatedly asked for loans, which the 'Three Prosperities Company' (the official trading name that Huang Jinrong, Du Yuesheng and Zhang Xiaolin had adopted) refused, as the government had no security, and the government threatened to shut off their opium supply. By 1933, the Three Prosperities were controlling and refining a significant proportion of the opiates that passed down the Yangtze River.

Because of the instability of the political situation, it was necessary for Du Yuesheng, as the frontman, to maintain good relations with an almost endless parade of warlords and political figures. Operating out of the French Concession gave them a measure of safety and they had extended their interests into gambling, with much success. By this time, the authorities in Paris had been informed of the level of influence the Three Prosperities had built up and decided they needed to scour the French Concession of their influence, and organized crime. So, in 1932, the gang ended up back in Shanghai.

The Japanese invasion of Manchuria after the Mukden Incident in 1931, essentially an attempt to create a Japanese-sponsored opium monopoly for the crops they were growing in Korea, destabilized Shanghai, creating opportunities for rival Green Gangs. The governance of Shanghai was taken over by members of the bourgeois community until order was restored. Months later, they sent a telegram to the government demanding they be allowed to offer advice on the situation. In such chaos, the Green Gangs were thriving.

The Three Prosperities played a prominent role in setting up relief for the Manchurian refugees and assisting in aid efforts. Such charitable works gave them ample opportunity for extortion and embezzlement. Then, Du Yuesheng decided to try and legitimize the opium sale, owing to being under enormous pressure from the French authorities to get out of the business. He applied to hold opium auctions in return for a kickback to the government of three million Chinese silver dollars and set up the Shanghai Peace Preservation Corps for the purpose of protecting his shipments.[34] The Guomindang government agreed, and the Three Prosperities was no more. Du Yuesheng had become legitimate.

Du Yuesheng worked closely with the bourgeois organization, which now had a strong political voice, and instead of two partners he appointed two deputies, one involved in labour unions and one politically and socially active. This brought the seamen's union and the river under his control, and kept him well connected. He then created the Endurance Club, an elite network for politicians, governors and business. With the cooperation of the minister of finance and the mayor of Shanghai, Du Yuesheng had achieved his goal of creating his own opium monopoly whilst still remaining a member of the Shanghai Civic Society.

The Corsican Mafia

The French Connection was another scheme using Turkish heroin, but this time it was the Corsican Mafia, under Paul Bonnaventure Carbone, Francois Spirito and Antoine Guérini. They came to dominate Marseilles over a twenty-year period beginning in the 1920s, transforming the city's organized-crime scene. Spirito was born the rather less romantic Charles Henry Faccia in Marseilles in 1900 and never became fully literate. His first job was as a transatlantic drug smuggler and he was convicted twice in Boston, the second time for smuggling fifty-five pounds of opium out of the SS *Exeter*.[35]

Spirito and Carbone established a French brothel in Cairo in the late 1920s and then returned to Marseilles with the same model, eventually reorganizing the Marseilles prostitution scene. In 1931, they made an agreement with Simon Sabiani, Marseilles' deputy mayor, who made Carbone's brother director of the city stadium and appointed various associates of Carbone to civic posts. In return, Carbone organized violent street protests in the name of fascism to support Sabiani's political stance, and eventually his men opened fire on a genuine fascist riot of dock workers and the time had come to seek new opportunities.

The Harrison and Volstead Acts had given new impetus to organized crime in America, and a Jewish racketeer named Arnold Rothstein had taken an iron grip on the narcotics business on the East Coast from his base in New York, but he had been shot in 1928 and the market was suddenly opening up. Seeing a gap in the market, Carbone and Spirito opened a heroin laboratory in the early 1930s, and later began dealing arms during the Spanish Civil War.

When the Germans arrived in Marseilles in 1942 they needed informants against the Resistance. Carbone and Spirito were more than happy to help, and handed over a list of names and details. A year afterwards the Resistance blew up a train Carbone was on and Spirito fled to America. He later returned and ran a restaurant in Toulon, but continued to deal in heroin. The business passed to the next generation.

If Carbone and Spirito were not exactly loyal Resistance members, their hitmen the Guérini brothers were. Antoine Guérini was an agent for Anglo-American intelligence, who hid English agents in the basements of his nightclubs, and his younger brother Bartélemy won the Legion of Honour for his work for the Resistance. After the war, Marseilles was a shambles and the Central Intelligence Agency (CIA) intervened to topple the Communist Party from power, leaving the Guérinis and their socialist connections in power for the next two decades.

In 1947, France had not only not recovered from the war, people were poorer than ever, and the Communist Party of France was organizing labour strikes throughout the country. The newly formed CIA began to pay the Socialist Party $1 million a year to promote itself to voters and lead the attack on Communism. For the USA, it was essential that the Communists did not take control of Marseilles, the second largest city and the largest port. The CIA sent a 'psychological warfare unit' to the city to work with the Corsican Mafia and the Guérini brothers to break the general strike on Marseilles docks. It lasted for a month, with the CIA delivering food, then threatening to take it away if the dock workers would not unload it. The strike was broken, and the Guérinis were firmly connected to the CIA. From that moment, they became one of Canada's and America's main suppliers of high-grade heroin refined from Turkish opium in Marseilles, as the CIA and French intelligence used them as and when.

For the Guérinis, from then until 1965, it was a rising market in line with demand from the USA, and the Corsicans ended up with more than twenty laboratories around the city. The brothers banned the rest of the Corsicans from dealing inside France, on principle.

It came to an end in 1967 when the Francisci syndicate shot Antoine at a petrol station in Marseilles over a feud, and Bartélemy went to prison for twenty years for avenging him.

The Five Families of New York's Cosa Nostra

Of all of the Italian crime organizations involved in heroin, the Cosa Nostra (translating literally as 'our thing' but meaning 'our family') is probably the most famous, along with the 'Ndrangheta of Calabria and the Neapolitan Camorra. The New York Cosa Nostra's heroin trade, at one stage responsible for 90 per cent of the heroin in America, has consisted, since 1931, of the five families: Bonnano, Columbo, Gambini, Genovese and Lucchese.

All of these families originated in Sicily, and were brought together by one boss, who declared himself *capo di tutti capi* – the boss of all bosses – Salvatore Maranzano. Beneath him was the boss of each individual family (*capofamiglia*), the boss's assistant (*sotto capo*), the counsellor (*consigliere*), the line manager (*caporegime*), the foot soldier (*soldato*), and finally the associate who is the gopher for everyone else. At the time, this structure was unique to the Sicilian Mafia, and its military organization played a strong part in the steady rise of the five families of New York. Their style of business also came from Sicily, beginning in the nineteenth century, when the first true Mafia gangs emerged there.

The end of feudalism on the island, beginning in 1812, and the acquisition of smaller parcels of land by the people, meant the start of modern property rights there. Without the protection of a large estate, and living on poor land where resources were precious, the Sicilians were prone to raids and attacks by violent gangs of bandits. And with a police force of only around 350 for the whole island, the gangs were free to act with impunity. Landlords and citizens were therefore better off paying a small set of thugs whom they trusted, both to protect their belongings and property, and in addition their businesses, by seeing off incoming competition, known as cartel protection. These were the two mainstays of the earliest Sicilian mafiosi. Many had been armed guards on the large feudal estates, and so were not only accustomed to firearms, but were also professionals with aristocratic connections, giving them status when it came to hiring themselves out to the new, anxious landowners. Yet even towards the end of the century, the Sicilian Mafia had little formal structure.

Aware of the need to understand their growing problem with organized criminals, the Sicilian Parliament ordered two inquiries: the Bonfadini Report of 1876, and the Damiani Report of 1881–6. Bonfadini found that 'The Mafia is not an association that has established set forms or special structures; neither is it a temporary grouping of criminals with a transitory or precise aim . . . it does not have leaders.'[36] It also recorded that mafiosi worked in gangs called *coshe*, who were strongly territorial.

The Damiani Report is the more intriguing of the two, and marks the Mafia's move into business: primarily, the Sicilian citrus market. Towards the end of the eighteenth century, the discovery that citrus fruit cured scurvy, initially noted by Scottish physician James Lind in 1753, meant a sudden high demand for the fruit from the maritime industry. Sicily was the dominant force in the citrus market, and so, when feudalism ended, those who were suddenly in a position to supply a lot of oranges and lemons were making a considerable amount of money.

This did not escape the notice of the emerging mafiosi, who began to gather in the towns and villages producing the most and best lemons, offering their services to prevent lemon-rustling. Because the landowners had little or no faith in public protection, another of the key Mafia elements emerged, that of personal trust.

By the time the Damiani Report was published, it showed the Mafia were firmly entrenched in the best citrus-producing towns and villages. The link to New York emerges soon after that, when Sicily began exporting millions of dollars' worth of citrus to the US, most of it through New York. In 1898 and 1904, 100 per cent of US lemon imports came from Sicily, and in 1903, 100 per cent of its limes.[37] And the US was not only importing lemons and limes into New York, but the Sicilian Mafia too, who were soon dominant in the market in the city. The armed guards and protection racketeers had moved into business. In Sicily, by the second decade of the twentieth century, the Mafia had become so powerful that Fascist leader Benito Mussolini initiated a crackdown in 1924, driving many of the island's Mafia to New York and wider America, where by now they had established family ties. The mafiosi of New York, many of whom arrived only a few years after Harrison had created such demand for heroin, soon realized how profitable the trade was, although

many of the older ones would not take part in either the drugs
trade or prostitution owing to Sicily's 'honoured society' code.
The East Coast heroin and bootleg liquor trade was largely
controlled at the time by Jewish gangs, headed up by Meyer
Lansky, nicknamed The Mob's Accountant, and also a young
Sicilian immigrant who had arrived in America at the age of
nine, Charles 'Lucky' Luciano, who had close ties with the
Genovese family, and was not so influenced by the 'honoured
society' ideal. When a war broke out within the American Mafia
in 1930–1, resulting in more than sixty deaths, Luciano was in a
prime position to come to power at the head of the Genovese
family. He had already forged close ties with the Jewish gangs,
and with Meyer Lansky in particular, and at a conference in
Atlantic City in May 1929, just before the Mafia war broke out,
Luciano, Lansky and other notorious American gangsters such
as Al Capone and Bugsy Siegel met to form the National Crime
Syndicate, and carved up America between them. After the massacres of the following year, the Italian-American Mafia formed
what was known as The Commission, to strengthen ties between
the families and enforce the hierarchical structure. It was controlled by the five families and also had connections with Al
Capone in Chicago and the Buffalo crime families.

Luciano began to build up a prostitution racket, bullying
small-time pimps out of the action and taking over the girls
forcibly. He discovered that they were more pliant when addicted
to heroin, and began to run it as a side business, which grew
rapidly. Five years later, he oversaw 200 of New York's brothels
and more than 1,200 prostitutes, bringing in an estimated $10
million a year.[38]

He was also beginning to dominate the heroin trade. The
Jewish gangs had largely brought in skilfully cooked high-grade
heroin from China, made in Shanghai or Tientsin, which could

be snorted. However, the Sicilians began to forge links with the Corsicans of Marseilles and the Eliopoulos brothers, and by the late 1930s, Luciano was largely in control of the city's street distribution. Heroin purity dropped significantly, leading to a boom in the use of the hypodermic needle. As one dealer complained, 'the Jews were businessmen, they gave it to you the way you wanted it . . . Then the wops started to get in it . . . These sons of bitches were so hungry for money that they cut it half a dozen times.'[39]

By now, the Federal agencies were mobilizing against the mobsters and, in 1936, the strongly anti-Mafia District Attorney Thomas E. Dewey had enough on Luciano to imprison him either for drugs trafficking or forced prostitution. Luciano chose the latter, and on 7 June 1936 was convicted on sixty-two counts of forced prostitution, with three of his prostitutes testifying against him. He was sentenced to thirty to fifty years in state prison.

In Sicily, the Mafia had also taken a serious blow when, in the 1920s, Mussolini, offended by a local Mafia boss during a visit to western Sicily, once again went to war with the Mafia. Arrests and torture became common, and by the time of Luciano's arrest, the decimated Sicilian Mafia were surviving only in the mountain villages.

The saviour of the Sicilian Mafia, like that of the Corsican Mafia in Marseilles, came with the Second World War. Ships on the New York waterfront were being sabotaged, and the Office of Naval Intelligence (ONI) decided to step in. They were unable to penetrate the tightly knit labour unions and gang networks there, and when their initial attempts to recruit the Mafia failed, they turned to Luciano, who was interned in an upstate New York prison.

The ONI was also hearing rumblings about the Allied invasion

of Sicily, named Operation Husky, planned for 1943. The invasion was intended to establish a US base in Europe for
the Italian Campaign, but prior to that they hoped to win over
the natives and gain information. It was suggested that Luciano
was the man to do both. The Office of Strategic Services (OSS),
forerunner of the CIA, was becoming increasingly alarmed
about the rise of the Communist Party in Italy, and the US army,
which had been conducting weapons drops to the Italian resistance fighters, scaled back their efforts to help. Luciano's connections enabled the OSS to penetrate both Sicily and Naples
through Vito Genovese. A Mafia member who had fled to
Naples in 1937 to avoid the law in New York, Genovese worked
for the Allies as what was coyly termed an 'interpreter', while
running the black market in military-issue weaponry across the
south of Italy. By the end of the war, the Mafia had not only
made a return to power, they were well connected and often on
friendly terms with American secret services. And, in Sicily, the
Allied bombing, which had left 14,000 homeless, allowed them
to become firmly entrenched in the construction trades, which
were soon exported to New York, just as the lemons had been.

In 1946, Luciano was deported to Italy as a parting gift, never
to return. His exile from the United States resulted in the establishment of one of the largest heroin-trafficking empires in
history. In America, the near collapse of the large Mafia drugs
businesses, and tightened border surveillance, had seen heroin
consumption and addiction drop dramatically, perhaps to as low
as 20,000 addicts. Twenty years later, the boom in heroin trafficking, owing largely to Carbone's French Connection and Luciano's
operation, saw it rise to 150,000.[40]

Left alone by the authorities for a decade, Luciano brought
heroin in from Turkey through Beirut using the influential narcotics dealer and Beirut socialite Sami El Khoury. At first

Luciano refined it in laboratories he had constructed on the coast of Sicily, but later he relied more on the better quality result from the Marseilles chemists. Teaming up with Meyer Lansky, who ran the finances and directed part of the traffic into the US through Cuba (where Luciano and Lansky had secretly gone to organize the route in 1946, and to watch Frank Sinatra sing, Lansky alleged) and the Caribbean, their operation was dominant in the American heroin trade until Luciano's death in Naples airport in 1962. Naples remains scourged by heroin, the city's heroin trade now controlled by the powerful Camorra mafia. The Mafia's return to power after the Second World War was remarkable, aided as it was by US complicity in its determination to fight radical leftist politics, but it came at such great cost for so many American addicts.

These are only a few examples of the many stories of organized crime based on the illegal demand generated worldwide by the Harrison Act, which meant that after 1914 opiates were inextricably linked with the trafficking of weapons and people, and, increasingly, government collusion in criminal activity. An Act that was supposed to make the world black and white had increasingly fragmented it into shades of grey, populated by figures who operated all the way through the spectrum, from corrupt politicians to mob bosses and street pimps. And at no time were there more shades of grey than when the very states which signed the Hague Convention had to go cap in hand to the countries which didn't, so that they could send soldiers to war.

Chapter Eight

FROM THE SOMME TO SAIGON

The First World War

'A war benefits medicine more than it benefits anybody else. It's terrible, of course, but it does.'[1]
Mary Merritt Crawford, surgeon at the American Hospital,
First World War

It's safe to say that Britain and her Allies were unprepared for the medical needs that the First World War would present to them. When war broke out on 28 July 1914, the Harrison Act was in motion, although it would not be passed until December. Instantly, the price of pharmaceuticals rocketed as supplies dwindled. For the previous two decades, Europe had relied upon Germany, primarily Bayer and Merck, to supply them with the highest-grade medical products. Now that this was not an option, Britain found herself woefully unprepared. It wasn't only supply issues, either. Hydrogen peroxide, which was used to propel German rocket motors and is also a disinfectant for minor wounds, was usually shipped in from the USA, and the price rose 75 per cent four to five weeks after the declaration of war.[2] This was not so much a case of profiting from war, as outright profiteering by pharmaceutical companies.

At the first battle of the war, the Battle of the Marne on 6–8 September, 2 million men in total fought and the dead on all sides amounted to around one in four. It was hailed as a victory for the Allies, but four years of trench warfare ensued. Initially the wounded were dragged from the battlefield by horses or mules with carts, placed in boxcars and taken off down the railway tracks to the nearest town. At the Marne, this primitive system was overwhelmed; 'things were badly organized and the conditions were shocking', recorded Harvey Cushing, an American volunteer doctor. 'One of these trains had dumped about five hundred badly wounded men and left them lying between the tracks in the rain, with no cover whatsoever.'[3]

The US ambassador, Myron T. Herrick, assembled a group of friends with cars and began to take the wounded to the American Hospital in Paris. They retrieved thirty-four on the first run before returning to save as many as they could. By 1915, the American Field Service, a small corps of volunteers, were driving motor ambulances for the French army, one of the revolutionary innovations of the First World War.

In the field hospitals, however, things were still little better. Harvey Cushing watched with dismay as a colleague attempted to dress war wounds. 'Dr Dehelly did a number of dressings – very badly I thought – unnecessary pain and bleeding from the extraction of adherent gauze. It was awful, wicked indeed, to see the poor devils, one of whom chewed a hole in his coverlet rather than utter a groan.'[4] This was in April 1915, when Britain and the Allies were coming to realize that the Harrison Act had put them in a very difficult position. They did not have the almost bottomless supplies of morphine and diamorphine that were going to be needed for the number of casualties involved in fighting a land war on such a scale. No one had anticipated that the trench warfare would last so long, and stocks were in short supply. Even such basics as aspirin, which might have offered a little relief, had shot up to 'more than 20 times the prewar price' by the following year.[5]

Cushing's diary entry for April 1915 continued, 'When we got back to the Ambulance the air was full of the tales of the asphyxiating gas which the Germans had turned loose on Thursday – but it is difficult to get a straight story. A huge, low-lying cloud of greenish smoke with a yellowish top began to roll down from the German trenches, fanned by an easterly wind.' This was, of course, the beginning of the German use of mustard gas, causing terrible burns, as well as eye and lung injuries. 'The smoke was suffocating, and smelled to some like ether or sulphur, to another like a thousand sulphur burning matches . . . [the men were] either suffocated or shot as they clambered out of the trenches to escape'.[6]

Mustard gas, a new invention by German chemists, would have horrific consequences for those fighting. The First World War introduced many technological and scientific innovations to the theatre of war, and mustard gas, flamethrowers and tanks were only a handful of them. Shellfire accounted for many of the more horrific injuries, and Cushing relates the story of trying to save a young man whose spinal cord had been severed by a piece of debris. Gunshot wounds, burns, and other such injuries must have presented many dilemmas in the face of dwindling pharmaceutical stocks. In the same month Cushing was writing, it was reported that there were limited holdings of Turkish opium left, but they were being offered to the market 'at a greatly inflated price'.[7] The British authorities deemed that neither Indian nor Chinese opium were of sufficient quality to convert into morphine successfully, and attempted to source it from Iran.

In the meantime, the need for other drugs that Germany had produced so well was becoming pressing. Salvarsan, used to treat syphilis, was no longer available, and as German trademarks had been suspended, British pharmaceutical companies were busy trying to create a copy. It was soon available under the trade name Kharsivan and rapidly shipped to the front lines.

It wasn't only large British pharmaceutical companies like Burroughs & Wellcome & Co. that contributed their expertise to the war effort. Forty of Britain's universities and technical colleges were called upon to take a wide range of German pharmaceutical and chemical branded products and find their active ingredients. This was done by students, postgraduates and staff, 'freely and cheerfully'.[8]

Voluntary medical staff were vital in this war, from doctors and nurses to stretcher-bearers. There were no field medics, and immediate comrades were forbidden from helping the fallen, but ordered to press on. One stretcher-bearer, known only as Tom, remembers watching the men go over the top at Arras, 'Wave after wave in perfect order, marching into the jaws of death.'[9] The wounded had to make their own way if possible, or wait for help from the stretcher-bearers who would give rudimentary care then haul them back to the dressing station or waiting ambulance. It could be between one and four miles from the front line back to the rendezvous, often on impassable terrain. They carried minimal pain relief with them, and their golden rule was not to jolt or drop the stretcher. This was not always easy, as 'We had to step on these dead soldiers to keep from going in the water and mud so deep and throwing the [wounded] off the stretcher.'[10]

By 1917, medical care had vastly improved, but morphine supplies were still low. Not so low, however, that it had been reserved only for human patients. At the Battle of Gallipoli, Jack McCrae and his dog, Windy, were both wounded in the leg by the same shell and brought into the shelter together. Windy was granted a medical card and patched up at the hospital, and after that, they were inseparable. Perhaps somewhat too inseparable: Windy would whine outside the medical tent when his master was working, and attacked anyone who wasn't in khaki. One day Windy was poisoned, and he suffered for two days, until Jack and Harvey Cushing euthanized him with 'two or three hypos of morphia'. Windy was buried in the grounds of an old Jesuit college with full military honours.[11]

The treatment of leg wounds was one of the areas of huge improvement during the war. In the first year, 80 per cent of soldiers suffering a broken thigh bone died, but thanks to Robert Jones bringing his uncle's invention, the Thomas splint, to the battlefield, where the thigh is stretched then held by traction, by 1916, 80 per cent of the wounded survived.

Other notable innovations were in antiseptic practice and anaesthesia. Dysentery and other gastric diseases were endemic in trench warfare, which, when living thigh-deep in water, could turn a scratch into blood poisoning rapidly. Better understandings of infection, and the liberal application of antiseptics made from coal tar, improved chances of a healthy recovery in a time before penicillin. Anaesthetic came as either nitrous oxide, ether or chloroform, and through the war, delivery methods improved markedly, so that there was far less chance of the patient dying on the table. Britain was the main producer of chloroform during the war. Also in use for the first time were battlefield blood transfusions, and the design and resilience of the hypodermic needle had improved dramatically, with graduated glass syringes encased in metal for accurate dosing and safety, and easily changeable needles. By the end of 1917, the Ford factory in the US had built and shipped to France 2,350 newly designed ambulances.[12]

In 1918, just as the war was coming to an end, Britain secured a new line of opium, from Iran, although there was some uncertainty as to exactly where it was coming from. Requirements for a sufficient quality seem to have fallen by the wayside, as Britain marched into its fourth year of war with casualties that had been unthinkable in 1914. Germany too was now suffering shortages, not of chemical and synthetic drugs, which it was still producing in huge quantities, but of most botanicals, and there's some evidence they were trying to grow opium poppies during this time.[13]

The conclusion by pharmacists regarding First World War shortages is that the Allies were woefully underprepared for the medical needs of the wounded, and understocked with medicines of all kinds. But the decision to suspend all Germany's medical trademarks early, the voluntary help given by British chemists in universities around the country, and the money poured into development of synthetic drugs meant that by 1917, most battlefield medical needs could be taken care of. The one shortage, which mirrored Germany's own, was the lack of opiates.

Harvey Cushing's war ended in November 1918, after the Armistice. He returned home to the US to practise neurosurgery, using techniques he had invented at war. He also identified what is now known as Cushing's disease, won the Pulitzer Prize, and is one of the fathers of neurosurgery. His last days in France were full of relief, as, 'In the farmyard courtyard below chanticleer crows, guineas and geese cackle, porcs grunt and the beagles bark excitedly', but he admitted he would miss the war and the opportunity to learn that it granted him: 'There is nothing quite like this combination in civil life – no comparable incentive.'[14]

The Great War is perhaps only great in terms of numbers, with approximately 18 million dead and 23 million wounded on all sides. While no country could have prepared itself for such prolonged carnage, the opium question remains: whether the prohibition ultimately had a significant effect on supplies, and whether the decision not to use Indian and Chinese opium was a sensible one. There are few sources regarding shortages from the time, and most of the pharmacological records are believed to have been pulped to make paper in the Second World War, a scant twenty-one years later.

Other records, however, survived, such as the diary entry by Private Daniel Sweeney of the 1st Lincolnshire Regiment, on surviving the Battle of the Somme: 'These are places where hundreds of men have said their prayers who have never said them before ... I was wet to the skin, no overcoat, no watersheet ... I was in an open dugout and do you know what I did – I sat down and cried.'[15]

The Second World War

'We sewed up orange peels as they were supposed to be a realistic substitute for human flesh. At least we learned how to thread a needle properly and could bring the edges of the orange peel together even if they were a bit mismatched.'[16]

On the battlefield, the one great difference in terms of medical care between the First and the Second World Wars was the field medic. As it had in the First World War, America took its responsibilities in this department very seriously, and established Camp Campbell (which became Fort Campbell in 1950) on the Kentucky and Tennessee border, where medics were trained to a high standard, orange peel notwithstanding. They were exceptionally well equipped in terms of ambulances and personal supplies. A typical medic's kit would consist of morphine tartrate syrettes, iodine swabs, ammonia inhalants, bandages and adhesive tapes, safety pins, tourniquets, and myriad other anti-

septics and coagulants, all of which had been thoroughly explained at Camp Campbell. One medic wrote that 'We learned
which injury to treat first and how to stop the flow of blood, how
to sew and protect damaged tissue, and how to administer morphine and blood plasma.'[17] Contrary to popular belief, ordinary
soldiers did not carry morphine in the Second World War unless
they were in parachute regiments, and then only a single dose.

Things were different off the battlefield as well. Before the
war began on 1 September 1939, Winston Churchill on behalf of
Britain, and the US army on behalf of America, had been stock-
piling medical supplies, taking note of the lesson from the First
World War. The American army had even produced a handbook
about how they were intending to make sure each theatre of war,
such as the Pacific, was to be supplied. Manufacturing facilities
were set up to last five years, or 'the course of the emergency',
whichever was shorter.[18] Britain had made similar, if not quite so
lavish arrangements.

Advances in medicine had been astonishing. Alexander Fleming had accidentally discovered penicillin in 1928, and although
his work was lost for a decade, a group of students at Oxford
University rediscovered it. Then, in 1941, experiments with
penicillin were shown at a symposium attended by Pfizer representatives, and the company picked it up for trials and mass
production between 1941 and 1944, when the war was underway.

Sulfanilamide, patented in Austria during the First World
War but not used, was an anti-bacterial powder – 'sulfa powder'
– that could be sprinkled into wounds to stop infection instantly.
These two drugs, along with morphine, were the mainstays of
medicine during the Second World War.

Between the wars, Germany had gone through a golden age
of pharmaceutical production. In 1926, they were the top
morphine-producing country in Europe and the top heroin

producer in the world, in terms of both quality and quantity. Between 1925 and 1930 German companies produced 90,620 kg of morphine, more than 41 per cent of the total global production.[19] The pharmaceutical giant Merck was now the leading business in the world in both opiates and cocaine, which it had first extracted in 1862, and the Nazi government even had an expert policy group for the two drugs, the Fachgruppe Opium und Cocain. Like the rest of Europe and America, Germany had adopted a much sterner attitude to opium and cocaine in the first part of the twentieth century, but it had a remarkably relaxed attitude to synthetic drugs, probably because drug companies were innovating faster than the legislature of the fragmented governments of the Weimar Republic could keep up.

The vast majority of these drugs were stimulants. Dr Fritz Hauschild, who developed Benzedrine for IG Farben, had been hugely impressed with its effect on the athletes at the 1936 Olympic Games. First synthesized as an asthma cure in 1929, amphetamines had proved a popular stimulant. Hauschild wanted to design an even better form, and synthesized a very pure methamphetamine, branded as Pervitin, which became tremendously popular throughout Germany when it was released to the market in 1937. In wartime, though, Pervitin tablets had a different and very efficient use, promoting aggression whilst lessening fatigue. Air crews took them on flying missions and they became known as 'Stuka tablets'. There were reports in the media of 'heavily drugged, fearless and berserk' German paratroopers.[20] The German military's peak period of methamphetamine usage was during the Blitz, when the Wehrmacht issued 35 million 3-mg methamphetamine tablets in three months.

British stretcher-bearer and medic Tom Onions may have wished for some methamphetamine on the day of the Normandy landings on 6 June 1944, when he recalled coming in on an amphibious vehicle towards the beach: 'I had all my medical stuff, a stretcher, 600 rounds of ammunition for the machine guns and two mortar rounds. When the ramp went down, there was none of this Iwo Jima stuff running onto the beach in light order ... We were struggling.'[21]

At the time, the British government was carrying out extensive testing on depression and fatigue in soldiers, hoping to avoid the appalling psychological fallout of the previous war. They took a keen interest in amphetamines, particularly Pervitin. The RAF, concerned by the rising number of flight crews consuming stimulants, conducted various long-range bombing trials using both amphetamine and methamphetamine, and found that pilots responded slightly better on the former because they had a greater sense of well-being. In late 1942, each member of the flight crew on bombing missions was issued with two 5-mg Benzedrine pills. Amphetamine use was rolled out across the army in the same year, although it was never implemented in the navy.

After the First World War, when morphine and diamorphine were in such short supply, there had been extensive testing on finding a powerful, yet non-addictive painkiller. In 1939, Otto Eisleb of IG Farben discovered dolantin, which is less potent than morphine, and they were soon mass-producing it, but subsequently found out that it was as addictive as morphine. Between 1937 and 1939, chemists working for Hoechst AG, Gustav Ehrhart and Max Bockmuhl, working towards the same aim, synthesized methadone. The disruption of the war meant that methadone was not tested or developed much further immediately, but it was approved for use in the United States in 1947.

The Allies, having suffered shortages before, were well supplied this time, and there had been one significant breakthrough: the syrette. Invented by the Squibb Corporation, it was a sealed unit of one dose of morphine with a small, fine needle. It had been pioneered by the company in the 1920s as a single half-grain dose insulin unit for diabetics, but was particularly suited to warfare as it was small, sterile and disposable. After use it was pinned to the wounded soldier's collar or clothing so that they were not accidentally overdosed on arrival at the clearing station.

Not everyone, however, wanted pain relief. Henry Beecher, an anaesthetist, was at the Battle of Anzio in 1944, and observed that three-quarters of the wounded declined pain relief when offered and reported little or no pain. Beecher later surveyed male patients after surgery and found that 83 per cent of patients reported pain and requested pain relief. He recorded that it seemed 'the intensity of the suffering is largely determined by what the pain means to the patient' and that 'the extent of wound bears only a slight relationship (if none at all) to the pain experienced'.[22] This is now referred to as the Anzio Effect.

There were many, though, who did need large amounts of morphine, and, unlike in the First World War, when hope was gone it was freely given. On one occasion, a doctor noted that 'Despondently I arranged for him to have a large dose of morphia to ease his pain and instructed the stretcher-bearers to place him in a corner to die.'[23] When the doctor arrived the next morning, however, the soldier had lived through the night and recovered.

Before America entered the war in December 1941, it had been making extensive preparations to make sure that there were no morphine shortages, despite continuing to formally ask Mexico to cease growing opium poppies: 'Both the Treasury Department and this Department regard the illicit production of opium poppies in Mexico and the recent trend towards increased production as a menace to the health of our people. It would appear that Mexico, replacing the Far East, from which supplies are no longer available, is fast becoming the principal source of opium entering the United States.'[24] However, Edward Heath of the

Drug Enforcement Agency was 'concerned our supply of opium or morphine would be cut off because the world was at war. So we needed a supply close by.'[25] The US government came to an agreement with Mexico to open up the Sierra Madre Occidental mountain range to poppy cultivation, and even sent over advisors to help the local people get started. 'The Sinaloan mountains were crowded with unofficial instructors from both countries, who taught the local people how to grow poppy.'[26] The US returned to its position of superiority after the war, and continued to pressure Mexico to stop producing heroin, but by then it was institutionalized in the Sinaloa mountains, funded in part by the American war machine.

The Camp Campbell medic's war ended soon after the liberation of Dachau. He recorded that, on 26 April 1945, 'strange people wearing ragged clothing began straggling to the 12th Division's rear ... Up close we saw that they were emaciated; their bodies were just skin over bone. They spoke in high-pitched, almost birdlike voices. They carried nothing. They could hardly put one foot ahead of the other. Their only clothing was thin, striped rags although the air was cold.' A fortnight before, the medic had attended a downed spotter plane that had been hit with a shell just behind the observer's seat. He treated the observer for a 'sucking chest wound', plugging it as best he could with a vaseline bandage, and attended to the pilot's severe head injuries. This had been the medic's daily experience for the past year. As he approached Dachau he could see smoke: 'The German guards had herded a bunch of captives into a barracks and set it on fire only minutes before.'[27] The German soldiers were not only destroying prisoners, but evidence of all that went on at Dachau, including the medical testing on inmates without consent. The doctors working at Dachau specialized in developing drugs geared towards the immune system and aimed at eliminating malaria, typhus and typhoid, amongst others.

The most terrifying of their operations was based at the notorious Auschwitz camp in southern Poland. The Auschwitz III Camp, known as Monowitz, was a satellite labour camp of the IG Farben factory, a gigantic gasoline and rubber factory. Compulsory medical testing of new drugs by IG Farben doctors was designed to see if different races responded in different ways; some drugs were therapeutic, and some were biological weapons. At Auschwitz, where Dr Joseph Mengele subjected 1,500 sets of twins to genetic experiments, the project was on a terrifying scale, as was the complicity of IG Farben employees. Dr Fritz ter Meer in particular, who helped design the Monowitz camp, was involved in the testing. Outside testing was performed by other companies in the IG Farben fold, such as Bayer Leverkusen, which ordered hundreds of prisoners, many of them women, for testing. Bayer had to pay for these women, and haggled with the superintendent over the price, considering 200 Reichsmarks too high, offering 170 instead. These 150 were to be subjected to the testing of a new 'sleeping drug'. Bayer confirmed receipt of its human cargo, and, 'Despite their macerated condition they were considered satisfactory.'[28] Bayer later reported that all the women died. As inhuman and incredible as these tests are, what is almost more incredible is that after the trial of twenty-four IG Farben employees at Nuremberg on 30 July 1948, Dr Fritz ter Meer, after serving two years in prison, was appointed chairman of AG Bayer in 1956. The actions of the IG Farben group during the war are a prime example of the extremes of which the pharmaceutical industry is capable. In his opening statement against them at the trial, Telford Taylor, the US chief prosecutor, was damning: their 'purpose was to turn the German nation into a military machine and build it into an engine of destruction so terrifyingly formidable that Germany could, by brutal threats and if necessary by war, impose her will and her dominion on Europe and later on other nations beyond the seas. In this arrogant and supremely criminal adventure, the defendants were eager and leading participants.'[29]

These tiny glimpses of those camps are reflected in the Camp Campbell medic's descriptions of Dachau, which are markedly more impassioned than his retelling of battles, blood and chest wounds, and when confronted with the true horrors of the camp he says only, 'We were not prepared for this.'[30]

Korea

'One great irony of warfare is that the more humanity increases its ability to inflict injury on human beings – through technology, tactics and psychological manipulation – the more humanity must advance its capability to deliver emergency medical care to the swelling number of casualties.'[31]

Unfortunately, for many young men who served in the Second World War, the call-up to Korea in June 1950 was not that far away. Korea had been ruled by Japan from 1910 until the end of the Second World War. Under Japanese rule, Korea emerged as a major producer of opium in the 1920s. At the time of the Manchurian Incident in 1931, the International Military Tribunal for the Far East identified Korea as the 'principal source of opium and narcotics'.[32] In addition, they deemed that emigrant Koreans played an extensive role in drug trafficking in China, particularly Manchuria, but as Japanese citizens, Koreans were immune from prosecution by the Chinese authorities owing to extraterritoriality. During its time as a Japanese colony, Korea had developed a substantial domestic drug problem. Japan ruled that opium smoking would be punished as it was in Japan, but that Korean addicts could wean themselves off on a reducing dose, before it was prohibited altogether in 1914. As with all prohibitions, this seemed to fuel the problem. Japanese pharmacists were allowed to issue substitute morphine injections in Pyongyang, but this only created another type of addict. In 1924, the Korean newspaper *Toa Nippo* reported there were 4,000 morphine addicts created this way in Seoul alone.[33] As of December 1930, all addicts had to be registered, but the problem was still out of control, and the Korean Society for the Prevention of Drug Abuse was formed in 1934.

Poppy growing in Korea had been undertaken in response to the worldwide shortage of opium resulting from the outbreak of the First World War, but in Manchuria, Japan had found a ready market for opium and had established an opium and narcotics monopoly. After creating 1.5 million addicts, the demand upon Korea's opium supply was enormous. (Japan is one of the few nations in the world that has almost zero domestic market for heroin: amphetamines are far more popular.)

After the Soviet Union liberated Korea north of the 38th parallel in August 1945, Japan withdrew, poppy farming was banned and farmers were urged to return to planting food and plant crops, with limited success. US forces moved into South Korea, and as a result, Korea was split into two regions, governed separately. Four years later, on 1 October 1949, Mao Tse-tung declared the foundation of the People's Republic of China.

Chairman Mao remains the only leader to successfully eradicate poppy farming and the opium trade in any country in the world, and he achieved it within a few years of coming to power. Poppy production simply moved elsewhere, however. Remnants of the Chinese Muslim Kuomintang Army, the KMT, fought their way into Burma and hid out in the jungles of Burma's Shan states. There, the Wa and the Acka people have grown opium as part of a subsistence existence for hundreds if not thousands of years. Like the Japanese, the Wa have almost no levels of opiate addiction, despite farming it themselves for medical use. What was left of the KMT seized the opium fields and expanded production, making a commercial alliance with General Phin, prime minister of Thailand, who had taken control of the Thai opium trade after the Second World War. From Shan state, the KMT undertook to put in place a transport network to Thailand. This was no mean undertaking: there are few roads in and out of the Shan states, and those there are often become washed out during monsoons, so to guarantee regular movement of goods would not be easy. As they were a distinctive thorn in the side of Chairman Mao and his Communist Party, the CIA, through its Sea Supply Company, funded the KMT with about $35 million worth of equipment between 1950 and 1953, during the years of the Korean War.[34] The CIA's involvement with the KMT had a practical benefit that the organization did not need when dealing with the Corsican Mafia in Marseilles: opium is a currency on its own. Funding covert anti-Communist operations in the Far East is not easy, but, much as in the old Silver Triangle, opium opens a ready line of credit.

In June 1950, with the support of Russia and China, the North Korean People's Army crossed the 38th parallel into South Korea, and open warfare began. Two days later, on 27 June, the United Nations authorized the deployment of troops to address the North Korean invasion.

In South Korea, the vast majority of troops were American, forming the 8th Army. They were assisted by the Republic of Korea Army, the Commonwealth Division and other UN forces. Supporting all of these assorted soldiers were the Mobile Army

Surgical Hospitals, or MASH. Made famous by the television show starring a world-weary Alan Alda as Hawkeye, and his equally jaded companions, the reality was that most of the MASH teams were very young, 'perhaps too young', writes Richard Hooker in his book that inspired the film and television series. Although a gifted surgeon, Otto Apel, who arrived from Cleveland as chief surgeon for a MASH team, was only twenty-eight, and had left a wife and three young children at home. Many of the surgeons had less than three years' experience.

American casualties in Korea were high, with the official death toll at 33,629 and 103,284 wounded. Despite these numbers, the comparative death toll from Korea is far lower than in the two world wars, where in the First World War 8.5 per cent of US troops died, in the Second World War 4 per cent and Korea 2.5 per cent.[35] The last figure would have been significantly higher without the MASH units, which were conceived in 1945 as a go-between from the front line to the field hospital, and first deployed effectively in Korea.

The core MASH team or auxiliary service group (ASG) was tiny compared to military field hospital units, consisting of a chief surgeon, an assistant surgeon, an anaesthetist, a surgical nurse and two enlisted technicians. A pilot and a medic operated in a precariously small Bell helicopter, ferrying the wounded back from the front line to the ASG station on stretchers or 'skids' mounted on the sides of the helicopter. This had the disadvantage that the casualty could not be treated in flight, but the advantage that they were tightly strapped in and immobile. Back at the ASG hospital, treatment was administered, including surgery if necessary, before the casualty was moved out to a large army hospital. The living conditions for the ASG teams were hard, often in mountainous terrain with extremes of temperature, moving several times a month to keep up with the combat units – the tent had to be down and ready to go in six hours – coupled with long hours of tedium followed by frantic activity. It was not unusual for a MASH team to treat over 3,000 patients in one month.[36] Otto Apel performed eighty hours of non-stop surgery as soon as he arrived at his first MASH assignment, and wrote a letter to his wife to say he wouldn't care if he never saw another surgery. But unlike previous field hospitals, if a wounded soldier made it to a MASH unit, he had a 97 per cent chance of survival. The quick and efficient establishment of a blood bank by Far East Command was crucial in this success rate, as the shelling injuries patients often presented with were horrific, involving the loss of whole hips and buttocks. Despite this, the amputation rate from the Second World War dropped by two-thirds owing to improvements made in ligation techniques, rather than just a straight tying off of the artery and removal of the limb.

In the Korean War, there were no shortages of opiates. The army even sent a specialist out to trial methadone compared with morphine, finding the results 'favourable'.[37] The army was, however, having some problems with drug use amongst the troops. It continued to dole out amphetamines, but heroin and marijuana were both so freely available that there was no way to regulate use. Heroin was also cheap, 'between eighty and ninety cents for 65 milligrams', and surgeon Albert Cowdray thought it was used socially, 'similar to the ordinary use of alcohol'.[38] Cases of addiction were more likely to happen in troops stationed further from the front line with less to do, as were cases of venereal disease, which ran rife in downtime. Around the port cities some officers reported that about half of all their men were involved with drugs, especially heroin. And it was during the Korean War that the first mentions appear of the practice of mixing amphetamines with heroin and injecting it intravenously. There were some deaths from overdoses. Because of the difficult fighting conditions, there were also numerous cases of self-inflicted wounds, which at one stage reached epidemic proportions in the New Zealand ranks, with up to 75 per cent of wounds presented being self-inflicted.[39]

The Korean War ended on 27 July 1953 in a stalemate. An armistice was called and the UN, US and Commonwealth troops withdrew. Yet the adage 'Medicine is the only victor in war' held true for the Korean War perhaps more than any other. The young MASH teams had achieved extraordinary things and made advances in the fields of vascular reconstruction, the use during surgery of artificial kidneys and ligation, and they also researched the effects of heat and cold on the body. From the Korean War we now have lightweight body armour and cold-weather gear. They tested the anti-coagulant heparin, and the sedative nembutal. In-depth records were kept, allowing for the best battlefield data comparisons that had been made to that point. The list goes on.

North Korea still insists it won the war.

Vietnam

'Public enemy number one, in the United States, is drug abuse.'[40]   Richard Nixon

Vietnam is America's longest war, lasting from 1 November 1955 to the fall of Saigon on 30 April 1975. As with Korea, the Vietnam War was fought between the north and south, with Russia and China backing the north, and the US with allies – South Korea, Australia and Thailand – backing the south.

In the south, the Viet Cong was a Communist group who wanted to reunify Vietnam, and engaged in guerilla warfare with the US and its allies. They fought with mines, booby traps and snipers, attacking mainly in the jungle. For infantry with an average age of twenty-two, the mental pressure, coupled with the physical pressure of the climate, was exhausting. They were assisted in Vietnam not by MASH, but by MUST, the Medical Unit Self-Contained Transportables, which were tents with inflatable ward sections and expanding parts for radiology, laboratory, pharmacy, and other areas. Because of the jungle warfare in southern Vietnam, the front line was not defined as it had been in Korea, so no one knew where to set up the hospitals. MUST solved that problem, coupled with the large UH-1D Huey helicopters carrying six to eight casualties with an average evacuation time of thirty-five minutes. High-velocity missile wounds were common, involving burns as well as injury, and the Vietnam War saw innovation in their treatment, and a 50 per cent drop in fatalities from the Korean War.[41] By 1968, the air force was evacuating over 6,000 casualties per month.

Films and media have often perpetuated the idea of the junkie soldier in Vietnam, high on heroin and marijuana. This stems largely from a 1971 report to Congress about levels of drug addiction in soldiers serving in Vietnam. It claimed that 15 per cent of US troops serving in Vietnam were addicted to drugs, especially heroin. The media went into a frenzy, and President Richard Nixon created a new office called the Special Action of Drug Abuse Prevention, headed up by drug czar Jerome Jaffe. The president called a press conference where he announced a 'new offensive' on the drugs trade, for which no expense would be spared.

What wasn't mentioned in the press conference was the role that America itself had played in creating what was a new heroin-producing cradle of the world, called 'the Golden Triangle' by Vice Secretary of State Marshall Green in a press conference the same week. He was referring to the triangle of Laos, Burma and

Thailand, which by 1968–9 was harvesting 1,000 tons of raw opium a year, which was refined into morphine base, mainly in Laos, and exported straight to Europe or to the US through Hong Kong. The heroin they produced was known as No. 3, a chunky, low-grade heroin that looks a little like broken sugar cubes, meant for smoking. No. 4 is high-purity, high-grade white heroin powder, produced from opium often orginating in Afghanistan, intended for rendering into an injectable solution. In late 1969 and 1970, Chinese heroin cooks had been brought in from Hong Kong to try and chemically render the cheaper No. 3 production of the Golden Triangle into something more like Afghan heroin. This heroin was then sent to southern Vietnam with the express intention of selling it to serving troops there. It became very popular almost immediately and many divisions were reporting high rates of both use and addiction. Packaged in small, neat phials that cost around $3 each, many of the bored, anxious soldiers in Vietnam turned to it for relief.

The My Lai Massacre of 16 March 1968 had only fuelled the controversy. My Lai, where US soldiers killed approximately 500 elderly men, as well as women and children, was a key moment in how Vietnam veterans came to be viewed by those back home. Photographs of the incident, taken by US army photographer Ron Haeberle, were not published until November 1969, after Haeberle's discharge, and when panic about the narcotics situation amongst serving soldiers was taking hold of the American establishment. Evidence of the rape and mutilation of the female victims caused further outrage.

There have been many explanations for the My Lai Massacre, including collective madness (at least thirty soldiers took part in the killings), as well as drug abuse and addiction. The reality is that My Lai took place before the heroin crisis among US soldiers in Vietnam, and that the American government had underestimated the mental strain of fighting a prolonged guerilla war in a hostile and alien environment.

Meanwhile, at the end of the Korean War, and funding the KMT, the CIA decided it needed to set up a transport hub somewhere in the South-East Asia area, and chose Laos, conveniently the place where Burma and Thailand refined their opium into morphine for export. Air America ran the CIA's covert operations in Laos for nineteen years, their longest ever disclosed covert operation. There are credible allegations that the CIA ran heroin and morphine out of Laos during these years, using it to fund their work in South-East Asia, which it denies. Nevertheless, there is the inescapable fact that it was present and using Air America as a front, dealing with the Hmong who used opiates as hard currency, and hence in all likelihood the US was involved in establishing the Golden Triangle on which President Nixon declared war on 17 June 1971.

It seems unlikely to be a coincidence that Nixon's war was declared just as America began to experience one of its cyclical heroin epidemics. With the Golden Triangle on the rise, and the Asian gangs organizing their operations to aggressively target Western users, in addition to the enormous growth of international travel and shipping, bringing heroin to the West was becoming easier and more lucrative. This created excellent opportunities for men like Frank Lucas to build empires from Vietnam. Lucas was born in North Carolina in 1930, and as a child watched as his twelve-year-old male cousin was murdered by the Ku Klux Klan for looking at a white woman. Lucas claimed later that this drove him into a period of delinquency that resulted in him leaving for New York in fear of his life. He fell in with a criminal memorably named Bumpy Johnson, and worked for him for over a decade. When Johnson died in 1968, Lucas decided to take a risk. The New York heroin business was at the

time run by the Italian Mafia, namely the Lucchese family, out
of Harlem, with a seven-man African-American group called
The Council and a drug dealer known as Mr Untouchable –
Nicky Barnes. Until he was touched by arrest in January 1978,
Barnes had an astonishing career that saw him running significant parts of the eastern seaboard and Canada. Another
drug-runner from North Carolina, Frank Matthews, was making
a fortune with acquaintances he had made in South America,
bringing in huge quantities of both cocaine and brown heroin.
Inspired by these two operations, Frank Lucas had his own ambitions. Knowing he had no chance of getting into the heroin
scene in Harlem without bypassing the Mafia somehow, he decided
to visit Bangkok, and in a bar ran into Leslie 'Ike' Atkinson.
Atkinson – a former US army sergeant who was well connected
with serving soldiers in Vietnam, and in Bangkok – was also
from North Carolina, and the two men were distantly related by
marriage. Through his bar – Jack's American Star Bar – he had
come into contact with a Chinese-Thai man named Luchai
Rubiwat, who had contacts in the Golden Triangle heroin trade.
Atkinson and Lucas began buying straight from the manufacturers, bypassing the Italian families back in New York. They
employed American servicemen returning to the US to carry
heroin for them, arriving home usually through Fort Bragg,
North Carolina. But they also had other, less aware mules: dead
servicemen, in whose coffins they secreted the drugs.

Perhaps the New York branch of the Black Panthers, the
Marxist black rights group, had one eye on Lucas when they
published a paper in 1970 about the heroin that was ravaging
their Harlem community: 'Drug addiction is a monstrous symptom of the malignancy which is ravaging the social fabric of this
capitalist system.'[42] Nevertheless, it was a hugely successful
system for Lucas, and GIs both living and dead made him a very

rich man, with a several-thousand-acre ranch, numerous properties, both private and investment, and millions of dollars in
Cayman bank accounts. The fall had to come, and in January
1975, he was arrested at his home in Teaneck, New Jersey and
later sentenced to seventy years in prison, although he only
served five and was put on lifetime parole. Three years later, he
was caught doing a drug deal, and served another seven years.
His assets either confiscated or gone, his biographer Mark
Jacobson recalls him 'living in a beat-up project apartment and
driving an even more beat-up 1979 Caddy with a bad transmis-
sion'.[43] Frank Lucas, in his heyday, served as a direct link between
the East Coast of America and the Golden Triangle heroin
trade, forging business ties with associates across the world.

Back in Vietnam, the US government instigated a testing programme for heroin, where GIs had to prove they were clean
before they were allowed to return home. Jaffe helped establish
methadone clinics in response to the perceived need following
Vietnam. Yet the test results were surprising for everyone who
imagined that the US troops had become feral junkies in Vietnam: almost all of them gave up instantly in order to return home.
The government monitored them for the following year, and most
did not relapse. The idea of the drug-crazed GI in the jungle was
simply not borne out by the results of the testing. Yet there
was no doubt many hundreds of thousands of young men were
psychologically damaged by the war.

Philip Caputo, a young GI who graduated from college and
went straight to war, served for three years. On returning to the
US he realized that he could strip an M16 rifle with his eyes
closed, but that he did not know how to do anything in civilian
life. Vietnam had taken a generation of American boys and
equipped them only for war. 'I came home with the curious

feeling that I had grown older than my father, who was then fifty-one.'[44]

When President Nixon made that speech on drugs in 1971, America was worried about shipping back an army of addicts, but it is a sad irony that it is far more likely they were busy creating one at home. Before the War on Drugs, Vietnam was the only war America had ever lost.

Chapter Nine

AFGHANISTAN

'There is no such thing as joy there. There is no such thing as peace, or comfort, or rest or ease . . . Life is serious from the start to the close, and the very children who act as messengers learn to gossip and intrigue from their infancy.'[1]
    Lillias Hamilton, doctor to the emir Abdur Rahman Khan

There are few places as untouched by modernity as Afghanistan. Marco Polo would still recognize the Roof of the World in Badakh-shan, almost unchanged in 800 years. To understand how and why Afghanistan became the producer of 90 per cent of the world's heroin, it is necessary to understand the history of this 'harsh, beautiful, and brutal land'.[2] Dynasties such as the Persian Ghaznavids, who ruled at the turn of the first millennium, made Afghanistan a centre of the Muslim world during Islam's golden age, home to 400 poets and 900 scholars. A summer residence and the military training academy was at Bost, now Lashkar Gar, which means 'Place of the Soldiers'. The modern Afghan people romanticize this time of literature, science and music, although they are an almost completely non-literate society.

The devastation wreaked by the Mongols, in particular destroying the Islamic focus of culture and learning that was Herat, returned Afghanistan to a rural society, which it has remained for centuries. It is home to over twenty different ethnic people including the Pashtun, Tajik, Hazara and the nomadic Kuchi people. These people fight fiercely amongst themselves, but unite under the Afghan identity with just as much determination. The two official languages are Pashto and Dari, a Persian dialect. They are almost all proud Muslims, yet outside the main cities most villages practise folklore rituals that hark back to the Buddhism and Zoroastrianism that was displaced by Islam. Dependent on herbal and plant remedies, they have used the opium poppy for millennia. The children drink poppy tea made from the exhausted seed capsules steeped in boiling water. The men often carry a piece of poppy capsule between their cheek and gum, and the women eat the latex to ease their aching backs as they pound grain on work carpets, seemingly oblivious to the bitterness. As a herbal remedy the opium poppy is an integral part of their daily lives. Those who farmed it lived mainly in the Afghan mountains, where the conditions conspire to create a poppy with a particularly powerful alkaloid yield, superior even to the Egyptian poppy. There, they would make their flat cakes of opium, wrapped in the poppy petals, stamp them with their own identifying mark, pack them onto a donkey or a mule, and send them off to the closest market town like a farmer's wife sending her butter to market. Prior to the 1970s, much of this opium went to Iran to supply the illegal market after the shah's 1955 ban.

Afghans feel that they are ground between a huge set of millwheels, comprising Russia to the north, Pakistan to the east and south, and Iran to the west. But to invade Afghanistan is a painful fool's errand, as Britain, Russia and the United States have discovered. All relationships in Afghanistan are based on kinship, and based around a patriarchal village model. There is no transparency in personal or business transactions, and it is widely regarded as one of the most corrupt countries in the world.[3] Over 90 per cent of the population are subsistence farmers, a figure unchanged from a century ago. Before the opium poppy, the country's main export for centuries was the wool and skins of the Karakul sheep.

Afghanistan's first national interactions with Europe began with France's invasion of Egypt in 1798 and Napoleon's determination to restore a French presence in India, which would mean coming straight through Afghanistan. Russia's invasion of Kazakhstan in 1734 had already caused alarm in Afghanistan as the threat from the north came closer. The fractious relations between Persia and Russia broke down during the Napoleonic Wars when the French encouraged the Persians to engage with their Russian neighbour. The French influence in the area from the late seventeenth century meant Afghans had absorbed some French ideas, including romantic notions of the Revolution. This influence ended with Waterloo in 1815, when Napoleon's eastern ambitions were curtailed abruptly.

The nineteenth century was a pivotal time in Afghan history which could have brought the country towards a modern existence, but British and Russian imperialism ended up driving it further back into its entrenched rural existence. In an ongoing series of battles with the Sikhs in the early part of the century, Afghanistan lost territory and prestige. Dost Mohammad Khan proclaimed himself emir in 1826, determined to stop the Sikh encroachment in the east. He applied to Lord Auckland, governor general of British India, and asked for assistance in settling the Afghan–Sikh dispute. Auckland replied crisply that the British government followed a policy of non-interference in the affairs of independent nations, preferring to maintain the British alliance with the Sikhs. Meanwhile, the Persians were attempting to retake Herat in the west, now with the support of Russia.

In response, Auckland gathered the Army of the Indus in 1838 and made it clear to Persia that they saw the invasion of Afghanistan as a threat to British India. The Persians withdrew, but Britain decided Dost Mohammad Khan was too troublesome, invaded Kabul and placed a puppet on the Afghan throne, Shah Shuja. This was, with hindsight, a mistake of mammoth proportions.

British thinking was that this would protect India, and also stop Russia reaching the warm-water ports in the Persian Gulf and the Indian Ocean which Peter the Great (1682–1725) had begun to covet a century before, feeding into Russia's greedy delusions of relentless expansion. Britain, now well established trading opium out of India, did not want Russia arriving on the shores between the mouth of the Persian Gulf and the Gujarat coast.

Initially numbering around 25,000 British and Sikh soldiers, the Army of the Indus invaded in 1839 and suffered heavy losses at the hands of the Afghan tribes. The Afghans had managed to stop the Sikhs at the Khyber Pass two years before, and did not take kindly to this new mass of men marching into their country. So confident were the British of success in Afghanistan that they took their wives and children with them. In Kabul, the British troops endured the privations of the hard Afghan winters, and the incompetent if well-meaning leadership of William Elphinstone. In the winter of 1841–2, the Afghans rose up and Elphinstone was forced to negotiate safe passage to the British garrison at Jalalabad. Unable to comprehend the level of double-crossing endemic in Afghanistan, the British began the retreat with wives and children in tow, and were massacred in their droves at the Gandamak Pass, with few survivors. The only soldier to reach Jalalabad was William Brydon, although some of the women and children made it out. Others were absorbed into the Afghan tribes, such as the wife of a Captain Warburton, who married her captor. Many of the surviving children were adopted locally. It was a catastrophic and tragic defeat, brought about by British hubris.

This, however, did not stop the British invading again in 1878. Again, this was ostensibly to protect British India from Russia. At the Treaty of Gandamak in 1879 Afghanistan became a British protectorate and Kabul was opened up to a British mission, something Afghans still consider to be an appalling loss of face. The mission lasted less than two months before it was massacred by outraged tribesmen from Herat. Britain invaded again, expelled the emir, and placed on the throne Dost Mohammad Khan's grandson, Abdur Rahman Khan (1844–1901), who became known as the Iron Emir.

Abdur Rahman Khan was not known as the Iron Emir for nothing. He saw his chief task as putting 'in order all those hundreds of petty chiefs, plunderers, robbers and cutthroats'.[4] He established many of the infrastructure systems that still dominate Afghanistan today. He was a vicious, underhand, utterly controlling and callous despot, but he also created departments for education, public works, posts and communication, medicine, public records, as well as a board of treasury and a board of trade, things that had previously been beyond the rigidly feudal and backwards-looking tribespeople. But the real source of his power was the Afghan army, through which he controlled the people absolutely whilst seeking to undermine them at every step by means of espionage, pitting everyone against each other. He was an extraordinary man who was tutored in military tactics as an adolescent by an Anglo-Indian named William Campbell. Campbell was first a soldier in the Sikh forces of Ranjit Singh, then switched sides and fought for the exiled Shah Shuja when he was displaced by Dost Mohammad.

Wounded in Kandahar in 1834, he changed sides again, and became quasi-commander-in-chief of Dost Mohammad's Afghan army. He converted to Islam and took the name General Sher Mohammad Khan as a show of loyalty. When the British placed Shah Shuja on the throne as their puppet king, he abandoned his post and returned to Shuja's service. When Dost Moham-mad was returned to Kabul, such was Campbell's apparent value, he was allowed to remain a general in the Afghan army. As wily and ingenious as any Afghan, he made a lasting impression on the young Abdur Rahman Khan, whose approach to ruling remained firmly military. Abdur Rahman Khan was, however, surprisingly enlightened on certain matters: he suppressed repres-sive religious leaders and had a female British doctor, Lillias Hamilton, as his personal physician, and Mrs Kate Daly was his harem's medical advisor. He also employed another English doctor, John Gray, as well as Messrs Pyne, Stewart and Myddleton as engineers, and the well-known mining engineer Arthur Collins.

However, he also continued the long Afghan tradition of committing genocide against the Hazara people of central Afghanistan. The persecution of the Hazara, like that of the Yazidis of Iraq, is based on an inexplicable tribal hierarchy that has over centuries forced the Hazara to the bottom of the pile, to the point that now no defilement or insult is too grotesque. Even the otherwise sensible Lillias Hamilton described them memorably as 'broad, squat little persons, with faces like full-moons and heads like rugged bullets'.[5] They were 'cheaper to feed than donkeys, and can carry almost as much', so they were often kidnapped for slaves.[6]

Two historic events marked the Iron Emir's rule: the Panjdeh Incident, in which Russia captured an Afghan fort on the north-ern border in 1885, and the drawing of the Durand Line between Afghanistan and Pakistan in 1893.

The Panjdeh Incident took place when Britain and Russia were negotiating the north-west Afghan border and Russia captured Panjdeh Fort, killing 900 Afghans, while only eleven Russians died. The Iron Emir, in Rawalpindi at the time for a meeting with the British, chose to see it as a skirmish rather than an invasion, to avoid Russia and Britain squabbling over his country, and Britain backed away from war. However, when Britain ceded the Panjdeh Fort to maintain peace rather than supporting Afghanistan against Russia as they had pledged at the Treaty of Gandamak, the emir lost any faith in their promises.

The Anglo-Afghan relationship was further undermined in 1896, when Sir Mortimer Durand was charged with establishing the border between Afghanistan and Pakistan. The 1,510-mile border was drawn through a mountainous region regarded by the West as no man's land, of which 800 miles were surveyed. Because the mountains are largely uninhabitable, and much of the range impassable, it was deemed a natural border. However, it cut straight through several Pashtun border tribes and through nomad routes. Afghanistan has never recognized it, and the border is in fact highly porous. The Durand Line is regarded by most Afghans as yet another imposition by the British.

The Iron Emir died in 1901 and his son Habibullah inherited the throne, and his father's best traits. He was one of Afghanistan's most liberal leaders, who attempted to introduce modern medicine. He was assassinated on a hunting trip in 1919. However, the same year, Afghanistan did manage to wrest some control of its foreign affairs back from Britain when Habibullah's third son Amanullah became emir (and later king). Taking after his father, he attempted to modernize Afghanistan: opening co-educational schools and encouraging Western dress in Kabul. He married the daughter of Mahmud Tarzi, a liberal politician who published Afghanistan's first newspaper, the political and current affairs

journal *Seraj al Akhbar*, in 1911. Tarzi was forced into exile by conservative factions, but in Paris he forged strong links between the
urban liberals of Afghanistan and France. Amanullah was much
influenced by his father-in-law, and he and his wife Queen Soraya
Tarzi visited Europe, and he returned with many ideas about how
to change his country. So unpopular were these modern ideas that
some Kabul newspapers reported that they were returning with a
machine designed to make soap out of corpses.

Tarzi recommended his son-in-law use the British–Russian
rivalry to accept aid payments from both sides, and Russia began
payments immediately, also supplying thirteen aeroplanes, pilots,
mechanics, transport specialists and telegraph operators. Between 1925 and 1926, Russia laid telephone lines between Herat,
Kabul, Kandahar and Mazar-i-Sharif. By 1928, it was possible to
fly from Moscow to Kabul via Tashkent.

Amanullah's reforms were too much for the conservatives and
he was overthrown in early 1929, although he was allowed to
abdicate and he and his wife moved to Switzerland. He was
succeeded after a tussle by Mohammad Nadir Khan (1883–1933),
formerly a general in the Afghan army. He was also a modern-
izer, but a much stealthier one than Amanullah, and he placated
the religious leaders. His lasting achievement is the road network he began to put in place, including the Great North Road
through the Hindu Kush. In June 1933 the Afghan ambassador,
and father of the future Afghan prime minister Mohammad
Daoud, was visiting Berlin when he was assassinated by student
Sayyid Kemal, who accused him of being pro-British. In September, schoolteacher Mohammad Azim entered the British
Embassy in Kabul and killed three people, one English, one
Indian, one Afghan. Then, on 8 November, Nadir Shah (as he
had styled himself) attended a high-school ceremony and was
assassinated by fifteen-year-old Hazara schoolboy Abdul Khaliq.

Khaliq was executed after 'Security officers tortured Khaliq by cutting his tongue and gouging his eyes and soldiers killed him with bayonets while his family and friends were forced to watch.'[7]

Nadir Shah was succeeded by his son Mohammad Zahir Shah (1914–2007), who was the last king of Afghanistan. Urbane, charming, fluent in French after finishing his education at the University of Montpellier, Zahir Shah was determined to modernize Afghanistan. In 1934, Afghanistan joined the League of Nations and received formal recognition from the United States. He applied for financial aid and expert advice from the US and the Soviet Union. His lasting legacy is the Helmand dam project, which he had built to try and revitalize the Helmand Valley.

The Helmand River Valley Project

The Helmand River Valley Authority was established on 4 December 1952. Helmand province lies in the south central part of Afghanistan, bordering Pakistan to the south. It is Afghanistan's largest and longest province, and its biggest producer of opium. In the north are the fearsome mountains of Baghran, and to the south Dasht-e-Margo or the Desert of Death. The Helmand River is Afghanistan's longest and rises in the Hindu Kush around fifty miles west of Kabul, running for 710 miles until it disperses into Iran's Sistan Basin. It is responsible for draining 40 per cent of the country; a river of immense power, which Zahir Shah was determined to harness through a series of dams so that the water could be controlled for irrigation and hydro-electricity.

Zahir Shah and the Afghan government engaged American firm Morrison Knudsen, which had built the Hoover Dam.

Work began in 1946 and finished on 4 December 1952. In a bloodless coup in September the following year, Mohammad Daoud, Zahir Shah's first cousin and brother-in-law, became prime minister, and was in office for a decade. Like Zahir Shah, he was progressive and in favour of women's rights. His aggressive policies towards Pakistan led to the latter closing the border in 1961, making Afghanistan more dependent on the Soviet Union for supplies such as petroleum. Since the end of the Second World War, the USSR had been in northern Afghanistan looking for oil and minerals, and attempting to win over the locals. The Afghans had, however, seen the steppes round-ups of the 1930s, and so were suspicious about Russia's presence on their doorstep. So, faced with the huge American project going on in the south, Russia paid to pave Kabul in 1953 as a visible symbol of her good intentions.

The Arghandab Dam and the Kajaki Dam were finished by 1953. The scale of the project is immense: the Kajaki Dam alone is thirty-two kilometres long. The restored irrigation canals were such a success that there was not enough labour to harvest the crops, and from 1954 onwards the government resettled farm labourers in new villages just outside Lashkar Gah. In the first phase, Daoud placed diverse tribes together in an attempt at peaceful coexistence, but they were soon fighting, and after that the villages were separated by ethnicity.

What they hadn't realized was that the effective irrigation of the Helmand Valley was also dramatically raising the salt content of the land, and soon its productivity fell. In his work *A Short Walk in the Hindu Kush*, the British travel author Eric Newby recounts speaking with an old man in the town of Geresk in Helmand: 'It is all salt below the American Dam. They did not trouble to find out and now the people will eat *hamak* [salt] for ever and ever.'[8]

In 1955, Russia lent Afghanistan $100 million for development; in 1956, the US built Kandahar airport and developed Ariana Afghan Airlines. Aware that the aid being offered was becoming increasingly territorial, Daoud began getting the Russians to pay for projects in the south and the Americans for projects in the north, subverting their notions of involvement with a particular area of the country. He was also encouraging Afghans to become more liberal, and 1960s Kabul was particularly Westernized, with the wearing of veils being a matter of personal choice, and some women even wearing miniskirts, although perhaps not quite as many as the Internet now implies. It had a strong student culture, and many of those studying there finished postgraduate degrees in America, where the left-wing movement was gathering huge momentum.

When Zahir Shah was out of the country for medical reasons, Daoud took the opportunity to seize power on 17 July 1973. (Zahir Shah is now remembered as Afghan leader for the 1964 constitution, which promoted universal suffrage and women's rights.) Daoud did not, however, call himself king, but instead declared a republic and appointed himself president. He was having ongoing problems with the Pashtun people who straddled the border. They baulked at having had the Durand Line forced upon them and were agitating for independence. In the north, Daoud was aware that the Russians were becoming more influential with the Afghan people, particularly the young, as left-wing ideas spread throughout the 1960s and 70s. In 1977 Daoud went to Moscow and met with Leonid Brezhnev, voicing his displeasure at Russia's presence in northern Afghanistan, to which the Russian leader replied that Afghanistan would be better off inside the fold of the USSR, to secure the safety of Central Asia. He also warned Daoud that there were too many North Atlantic Treaty Organisation (NATO) experts in northern

Afghanistan, who Russia regarded with suspicion. Daoud
responded derisively, and left. Returning to Kabul, he made
arrangements to lessen Afghan ties with Russia, and to increase
them with Iran, Saudi Arabia and the West. A year later, the
Afghan army and police force were being trained by Egypt rather
than Russia, infuriating Brezhnev.

In April 1978, at a socialist ideologue's funeral, up to 3,000
people came to hear speeches given by the leaders of the People's
Democratic Party of Afghanistan, including one by Nur Mohammad Taraki, a former journalist turned politician. Daoud ordered
their arrests, but Taraki escaped to the USSR. Then, on 28 April,
a *coup d'état* began at military barracks near Kabul airport, and
gathered force over the next few days. In the end, Daoud and
twenty-eight members of his family, including grandchildren,
were killed by the Communists and dumped into two mass
graves on the edge of Kabul. Their remains were discovered in
2008.

After the Saur Revolution, Afghanistan was governed by Nur
Mohammad Taraki and his Khalq faction of the PDPA; the
Parchams were the opposing faction within the same party, and
it did not take long for them to come to grief. In September 1979,
Hafizullah Amin overthrew Taraki and had him executed. The
PDPA then changed the Afghan flag to a green copy of the
USSR one, and banned usury. For the peasant farmers who
existed on the *salaam* credit system to get their crops planted
every year, this was a disaster. Agricultural production fell, and
the party seized upon land ownership as the real issue. To that
end, they would put a stop to feudalism and redistribute Afghanistan's farmland so that everyone had a share. This was as
unworkable as it sounds, and led to a further fall in food production as Afghans began to squabble over who had the best plot.
This food shortage, coupled with the bizarre political and social

repression implemented by the PDPA, whilst at the same time proclaiming women's rights, led the Soviet Union to decide that the time was ripe for an invasion.

The Russians Are Coming: Soviet Afghanistan, 1979–1989

Brezhnev deployed the 40th Army on Christmas Eve 1979, and on arriving in Kabul they killed Hafizullah Amin and installed Soviet loyalist Babrak Karmal as president. The Islamic Conference, an alliance of the Muslim nations of the world, condemned the action, and demanded 'the immediate, urgent and unconditional withdrawal of Soviet troops'.[9] The UN protested the intervention. In excess of 5 million Afghans fled to Pakistan and Iran, and Afghan rebels received copious amounts of aid, in Pakistan and China, to train them to fight the Soviets. This aid came from the US via the CIA's Operation Cyclone, and also from the Gulf States and wealthy individuals, such as Osama bin Laden, who left university in 1979 to fund a training camp for mujahideen in Pakistan. Mujahideen is the plural of mujahid, or fighter. When the Afghan rebels first assumed this group label, it meant 'to struggle with a noble aim'. The warping of Islamic terminology is a specific feature of the Afghan conflicts and in part reflects the fluid and increasingly violent nature of what it means to exist in modern Afghanistan.

The mujahideen, at this point, were hailed as heroes. President Ronald Reagan dedicated the space shuttle *Columbia* 'to the people of Afghanistan', calling their struggles 'the highest aspiration of mankind'.[10] The mujahideen mainly fought a guerilla war from the countryside, and the majority of the nation remained outside Soviet control, but they dominated the cities and the road network, doling out relentless punishment via airstrikes to villages suspected of harbouring the rebel fighters. Weapons and armaments flooded in from the West, particularly America, to support the rebel efforts.

The Russians also bombed the irrigation canals and the road network. The farmers of Helmand and other agricultural provinces could no longer get their produce to market and a period of severe economic decline set in. Russia rapidly robbed the subsistence farmers of the ability to provide for their families. The melons, peaches, pomegranates and apricots for which Afghanistan was famous, rotted on trucks stuck on broken roads or at checkpoints. The pistachios and dates couldn't be sold by those growers, who then couldn't buy enough grain to feed large families that often numbered fifteen or more in one household. So those who were already growing opium poppies increased their planting, because opium latex can be stored indefinitely and was a source of much-needed hard cash.

However, there was one aspect to Afghan farming that the Russians were unfamiliar with. In the highlands, where the opium poppy is the predominant crop, along with enough subsistence farming to get by, irrigation, far from the Helmand infrastructure, is done by *karezes*. These are tunnels running just beneath the surface of the earth and following the natural lines of the land, with channels cut to the sides to irrigate the fields. From the surface they look like large molehills, as the farmers climb inside and excavate silt or rocks that have entered the channels. Otherwise, they are hidden from view. They are maintained by the communities through the system of *hashar*, where if a field benefits from irrigation, the farmer spends a few days each year clearing silt and rubbish from the tunnels. *Karezes* are of particular use in the cultivation of opium poppies in difficult terrain, and escaped the destruction that was inflicted on the larger and more visible American-built canals.

For the Afghans who remained in their country during the Soviet occupation, life was desperate, particularly for the rural communities. On the ground, Soviet troops shot livestock and destroyed machinery. Life wasn't much better in the cities, and in 1987 a concerted effort by the Russians saw Kandahar reduced from over 200,000 inhabitants to under 25,000, with much of the city bulldozed. There is no accurate figure on the number of landmines laid in agricultural land and by roadsides, but the Red Cross puts the figure at somewhere around 15 million, and predicts that the country will never be free of them. To date, tens of thousands of Afghans have been killed or maimed. It is perhaps not surprising that when Afghan Communist sympathisers were exposed, they were executed by stoning, or that there was so much widespread support for the mujahideen.

In the same way that the Afghan tribesmen had picked off Elphinstone's army in the winter of 1841, the mujahideen picked off the troops of the Soviet army, despite being faced with tanks and artillery that far outmatched their own firepower. As early as 1983, and certainly by 1985 under the aegis of Mikhail Gorbachev, the Russians knew they had lost and were looking for a way out. They began offloading the responsibility of fighting the mujahideen to the Afghan army, and those backing the mujahideen such as the US, Saudi Arabia and Pakistan saw their chance, upping their levels of aid to the rebel fighters. The Western powers favoured the forces led by the charismatic Ahmad Shah Massoud, an ethnic Tajik Sunni Muslim nicknamed the Lion of Panjshir for his military prowess in fighting the Russians. In 1988, aware that Russia was fading, Osama bin Laden founded al-Qaeda.

Over the following three years, the Russians began a slow retreat from Afghanistan. Sadly, but true to form, things would not run smoothly. Russia was leaving a Communist puppet

government in place, in the face of overwhelming hatred from
the Afghan tribes. Only the massive artillery Russia supplied
them with allowed them to maintain control of the urban
centres of the country. Massoud, backed by Western powers, had
the stronghold in the north, and a loyal following.

When the Soviet Union began to fall apart in 1992, aid for the
PDPA government slowed to a trickle and the army could not
continue effectively without food or fuel. That year, all parties
came to a power-sharing agreement, the Peshawar Accord. The
only mujahid not to agree to it was Gulbuddin Hekmatyar, the
notorious Butcher of Kabul, who wanted to rule alone. Hekmatyar, an extremist by any measure, was funded by the Pakistani
Secret Service, the ISI, and is a highly divisive character in
Afghanistan's recent history. His rivalry with Massoud is one of
the defining relationships of the end of Soviet-era Afghanistan.

With the withdrawal of Russia from Afghanistan and the
threat of Communism no longer immediate, the US interest in
the situation waned. In rural Afghanistan the Communist governor of Helmand province announced that he would recognize as
police any group of ten or more men who were willing to fight
the mujahideen, a policy that created hundreds of miniature
police militias that were virtually indistinguishable from rebel
militias. For the beleaguered residents of Helmand, it was impossible to tell the difference.

Requests such as this from the waning Communist governments encouraged the rise of the Afghan warlord. In a country
prone to tribalism and banditry, and now with the worst standard of living anywhere outside of the poorest African nations,
recognition for a private army was exactly what many of
Afghanistan's opportunistic thugs and gangsters needed to
found their own small empires. At the same time, during the
1980s, Pakistan had been undergoing a surge in heroin use and

addiction, providing an outlet for Afghanistan's new emergency cash crop. Heroin refineries were flung up along remote stretches of the border between the two countries, providing a cheap, easily accessible supply. Some members of Pakistan's ISI (Inter-Services Intelligence Agency) participated in the trade, along with the Afghan traffickers, and the result was a rise from an estimated 5,000 Pakistani heroin addicts in 1980 to over 1 million in 1985.[11] Thus, in the early 1990s, more farmers were giving over more land to poppies, and the warlords extorted them for a share of the crop, or control of the crop itself. Many of the farmers, on their knees financially, had no choice, and were soon paying more than one militia. The militias' reputation for corruption and vice also outraged many, but their propensity for violence kept people in line. Afghanistan, used to existing in chaos, was drowning in it. Into the breach came what seemed like the solution: a group of young Pashtun scholars, *talibs*, and their strict, one-eyed mullah, Mohammed Omar.

'There is no god but God; Muhammad is the messenger of God.'[12]

It was not just the mujahideen who were trained in Pakistan. The Soviets left many orphans, and many families sent their children over the border to Pakistan to get them out of harm's way. Thousands of boys entered the madrasas of the northern Pakistan refugee camps. Many of these strict religious schools were funded by the Saudi Arabian royal family, a legacy of King Faisal's dream to spread his version of Islam – known as Wahhabism – throughout the Islamic world. Wahhabism emerged in the eighteenth century as a reductive, literal version of Islam similar to the Protestant Puritanism of the seventeenth century. Its overall world view was nihilistic, and life in the madrasas was little more than bed, board and a rote learning of the Qur'an. In traditional Afghan society, women are responsible for discipline within the home, and the role of fathers is to be indulgent, or at least indifferent, in the face of childish misdemeanours. The absence of women in the madrasas, and, for many of the orphaned boys, in their lives at all, meant that they grew up devoid of female contact, understanding only the Wahhabi religious viewpoint. Their sparse emotional lives, coupled with this youthful, all-male society, led to a kind of passionate fundamentalism that took even the conservative Afghans by surprise on 12 October 1994.

Spin Boldak, meaning 'white desert', is an enormous truckstop on the Durand Line in Kandahar province. Ostensibly it's a legitimate location for goods exchange, as well as a rest stop for truckers routinely driving non-stop for up to twenty-four hours. In reality, it is one of the largest smuggling hubs in Afghanistan. Radio equipment and narcotics are the two main commodities. After the Soviets had torn up the telephone lines, they were left lying on the sides of the roads, and the local people harvested them to sell for the wiring (Afghanistan remains more reliant on radios than fixed-line telephones).

The truck-driving community of Afghanistan is predominantly Pashtun, and they were sick of being robbed and extorted by the warlords, so it is little surprise that the predominantly Pashtun Taliban began in Spin Boldak, taking it over rapidly with minimal resistance. They moved on rapidly to Kandahar, which proved more difficult, but still fell with few losses to the Taliban.

Almost immediately they began to implement their view of Sharia law, which banned education and jobs for women, and imposed the head-to-toe covering, the burkha. One quarter of public-sector jobs had previously been in the hands of women, which meant that the civil service verged on instant collapse. The Taliban smashed every television set they came across and forbade all sports. All men capable of doing so were to grow long beards. Once established as the controlling force in Kandahar in 1996, they conducted a series of calculated massacres of the Hazara people, burned thousands of homes, many thousands of acres of farmland, and destroyed livestock. They did, however, succeed in suppressing the warlords, often simply by murdering them, although it was claimed that it was done in the name of Islam and Afghanistan. The irony is that many of these young men had never spent time in Afghanistan, having lived all their lives as refugees in Pakistan.

Unlike the Soviets, who never truly controlled the country outside the cities, by 1997 the Taliban controlled 85–90 per cent of Afghanistan, and Mullah Omar had been installed as the emir.[13] The same year, the Pashtani Tjarati bank – the Taliban central bank – imposed an at-source tax on 10 per cent of farmers' profits, and opium merchants had to pay 2.5 per cent on all transactions. The ban on the education of women created a huge pool of free labour that sustained the boom in opium production. Opium poppies were brought down from the mountains, and the farmers of Helmand and Nangarhar provinces in particular were encouraged to give their land over to the opium poppy, in exchange for the reasonable 10 per cent tax or *zakat*. This tax also bought them and their farms protection. For many farmers, having witnessed the chaos of the preceding government's collapse and the horrors of the Soviet years, this seemed like a relatively small price to pay. As one small farmer, Wali Jan, said, 'The Taliban have brought us security so we can grow the poppy in peace. I need the poppy crop to support my fourteen family members.'[14] Wali Jan was earning $1,300 per year from forty-five kilograms of raw opium gum, which was enough to

lift him out of absolute poverty. These farmers were not neces-
sarily in favour of the Taliban's draconian interpretation of the
Qur'an, but many experienced stability and a new prosperity.
This was at odds with the way the world wanted to see life in
Afghanistan under the Taliban. As Kofi Annan of the United
Nations said, 'In a country of 20 million people, fifty thousand
armed men are holding the whole population hostage.'[15] The
Taliban's unique world view was further reinforced by the appointment of their own anti-narcotics chief, Abdul Rashid, who was
in charge of rooting out hashish because it was consumed by
Afghans and Muslims. 'Opium is permissible because it is consumed by *kafirs* [unbelievers] in the West and not by Muslims
or Afghans.'[16]

In the north of Afghanistan, Ahmad Shah Massoud established
the moderate Northern Alliance in protest against the Taliban's
occupation. The Northern Alliance became the de facto government of the country since no other viable option was available.

Afghanistan began to break all records for opium production,
year upon year. The only year it was checked was 2000–1, when
Mullah Omar put in place a ban and decreed that farmers
plough up their fields, declaring the poppy 'un-Islamic'. He
relented for the 2002 season, however, and it is widely suspected
that the ban was not in fact a matter of spiritual conscience, but
to ensure they did not flood the market. In north-east Badakh-
shan, home to Marco Polo's poppies and Massoud, poppy
cultivation remained static. After that, poppy production in the
country continued to climb steeply again, until in 2006–7 it was
estimated that Afghanistan was supplying over 90 per cent of
the world's heroin, cultivated on land whose area was more than
that of all the land used for coca cultivation in Latin America.
Various well-meaning outside influences have tried to decrease
the amount of opium poppy being grown through alternative

means, such as the British offers of compensation to poppy farmers in the late 1990s, which just meant that the farmers planted more in order to receive more compensation.

However, by late 2007, after year-on-year rises in total production, it had become clear that there was a divide in Afghanistan, and in more ways that one. In the north, despite the problems and the poverty, opium production had remained low-level and static, or had diminished. The UN attributed this to 'leadership, incentives and security [which] have led farmers to turn their back on opium'.[17] With the collapse of the Soviet Union into fifteen countries in 1991, the Russian threat to Afghanistan was instantly reduced, and borders opened up, presenting opportunity for the drugs traffickers of Afghanistan to send their product north. Russia had been relatively untroubled by a domestic heroin problem, but in the eighteen months after the collapse of the USSR they saw a ninefold increase in heroin addicts. New HIV infection rates doubled every year from 1995 to 2001, along with hepatitis and drug-resistant tuberculosis, coinciding with the Taliban's output, and now 1.3 million of the population are estimated to be heroin addicts.[18] Afghanistan is taking its revenge on Russia.

In south-west Afghanistan, despite relatively higher levels of income, opium cultivation rose to unprecedented levels. The Durand Line runs through the most densely planted series of poppy fields in the world, and in 2007, 70 per cent of the poppies in Afghanistan were grown along the border, and more than half of the whole poppy crop came from Helmand.

United States Invasion of Afghanistan

The US and British invasion of Afghanistan on 7 October 2001, in retaliation for the 9/11 attacks and the suspected harbouring of Osama bin Laden by the Taliban, came hard on the heels of the Taliban's complete ban on opium farming during the previous two seasons. The Western forces succeeded in defeating the Taliban, and in doing so they not only marched into a war, but into a crisis situation where people could not feed their children or seek medical care because they had made no money for two seasons. Many of them were deeply in debt to the Taliban drug traders, and desperate. Sandeep Chawla, head of research at the United Nations Office on Drugs and Crime (UNODC), said 'in drug control terms it was an unprecedented success, but in humanitarian terms it was a major disaster'.[19] In addition, the shortage led to heroin stocks being adulterated to keep up supply, and the accompanying drop in purity resulted in high numbers of deaths in Iran and Estonia.

In late 2001, at a conference in Bonn, the United Kingdom was charged with overseeing Afghanistan's counter-narcotics efforts. From 2001 onwards, there was a boom in poppy production. Eradication attempts by NATO soldiers led not only to ill feeling between Afghan farmers and the invaders, but only worsened living conditions and were unsuccessful in the long term as poppy production only increased overall. The Taliban regime had improved the roads and the NATO intervention led to improved infrastructure. Many of the Taliban and al-Qaeda were never captured because they couldn't be identified, and simply carried on in the opium trade. Afghanistan is also now the world's largest supplier of cannabis.[20]

The futility of this situation is obvious in the reports from the UNODC: 'In 2007, Afghanistan cultivated 193,000 hectares of opium poppies, an increase of 17 per cent over last year ... Afghanistan's opium production has thus reached a frighteningly new level, twice the amount produced just two years ago.'[21] The eradication attempt stood at 19,047 hectares in total. Eradication attempts have continued since, and, alarmed by the jump in poppy cultivation, the US devised a spraying eradication programme for the spring harvest of 2008, such as Agent Orange (chemical) or Agent Green (biological). These agents had been used both in the Vietnam War, and to eradicate coca fields in Colombia in 2000. Both had caused severe health problems, particularly in children, and they never went ahead in Afghanistan.

There have been attempts to provide Alternative Livelihood programmes, such as Food Zone, which operated in Helmand from 2008 to 2012, encouraging the use of greenhouses to grow year-round crops that will sustain families, as well as wheat, saffron, black cumin and licorice, although its limited success may be to do with the concept of applying 'milestones and key performance indicators' to Afghan villagers.[22] The failure of the programmes is apparent in the 2014 UNODC report showing at least 224,000 hectares under poppy cultivation, an increase of 7 per cent on the previous year, with eradication going down by 63 per cent. The farm-gate prices and export quality of this heroin are also going down, the heroin falling to 52 per cent pure in 2014.[23] This is leading dealers to adulterate their heroin before it reaches the end user, so that there is enough of a hit to keep them coming back. Fentanyl, a synthetic opioid first produced in 1959 by Paul Janssen in Beerse, Belgium, is an extremely powerful drug estimated to be up to fifty times stronger than heroin, and is currently the most dangerous adulterant commonly used by dealers.

Even since then, genetically modified poppies and investment in irrigation and farming techniques, as well as changes in climate, have seen farmers able to grow more per year. The seeds are believed to originate in China, although the farmers buy them locally so are unsure of the origin. This has resulted, in

2016, in a 43 per cent rise in opium tonnage from 2015, from less land. The figures are stunning.[24]

Meanwhile, NATO forces were still fighting insurgents. In 2014, Western forces withdrew, almost, although have kept a presence in Helmand. Camp Bastion was a British army airbase located just north-west of Lashkar Gar, and the largest of its kind, able to hold 32,000 personnel, with a full-tented and solid field hospital.

Between 2006 and 2014, it gained an 'international reputation as the world's leading field hospital. It was this province that saw some of the fiercest fighting of the invasion.'[25] Camp Bastion was an ambitious project in the middle of a major deployment, and also marked a modification in combat medicine since the Gulf War, which still used MASH. The many developments in field medicine made in the Gulf War contributed to making Camp Bastion what it was, but the last MASH team – the 212th – was retired in 2006, and now casualties in the field depend on fully equipped Humvees containing forward surgical teams, the FSTs.

The medical personnel involved in both the Gulf conflicts and Afghanistan have since made notable contributions to civilian trauma care, particularly in the treatment of patients involved in car accidents, and also burns and gunshot wounds. At the hospital, 75 per cent of all cases were blast wounds from improvised explosive devices (IEDs), leading to advances not only in amputation, but in before and aftercare. Levels of post-traumatic stress disorder involved with these injuries are significantly reduced with sufficient pain medication and treatment within one hour, known as the Golden Hour. To this end, medics in the field used fentanyl lollipops in cases of severe injury. The reduction of pain is almost instantaneous, and unlike intravenous opioids, if the user passes out or becomes slack-jawed, the stick causes it to fall out. Anecdotally, British and US medics differ in that the US medics will tape the stick to the casualty's thumb, so that it is not lost or dropped, and so it will definitely fall from the mouth to prevent a potential overdose.

Camp Bastion also made strides forward in the treatment of children with severe trauma. Eighty-five children in total were admitted. The average age was eight. Fifty-three had battle-related injuries, around half of which were caused by IEDs. The others were mainly burns sustained in the home and car accidents.[26] Civilians also brought in their children for smaller injuries not requiring admission. A Camp Bastion surgeon, interviewed for this book, said that the children of Helmand have a high threshold for pain medication, and for opiates in particular. It seems no one in Afghanistan escapes the poppy.

The distasteful truth of the situation, in the two prime poppy-growing centres of the world, is that Western interference and demand has created an industry that refuses to be crushed. And there is no sign of peace in Afghanistan. The *talibs*, who believe they are inheriting a second golden age – now made of dust and catastrophe – have a complicated and uneasy relationship with poppy farming, but want the money to fund their wars. Now their rivals ISIS – the Islamic State of Iraq and Syria, also known as the Islamic State of Iraq and the Levant (ISIL), or Daesh in Arabic – tax the farmers on their captured territories with amoral relentlessness. Both factions are products of this interference, and both know the importance of the illegal industry under their control. The UN's attempts to eradicate Afghanistan's poppies have had the opposite effect: in times of war, food poverty and instability, opium production only increases. People may smuggle and deal in heroin to get rich; people farm the poppy to survive.

ISIS are a group of Sunni Muslims who follow the fundamentalist

teachings of the Saudi Arabian tradition of Wahhabism. Wahhabism emerged on the Arabian peninsula in the eighteenth
century, founded by Muhammad ibn Abd al-Wahhab, an ultra-
conservative religious leader who wanted to return to the glory
days of the old, austere caliphates, when the Muslim Empire
stretched as far as Spain. Many in the upper echelons of the
organization are former officers from Saddam Hussein's Iraqi
army. They emerged as a coherent organization in 2014 and began
to seize towns near major supply routes, a lesson they had learned
from the Taliban, and pressed forwards to consolidate their holdings on the Iraqi–Syrian border. ISIS is one of the richest terror
groups in history. After its first year alone, the dozen oil fields it
had captured were estimated to be bringing in more than
$1 million per day.[27] It also deals in weapons that it has stolen
from Iraqi and Syrian military compounds. Lastly, it deals in
drugs. This also is an inheritance from the Taliban. In 2008, the
then head of the Drugs Enforcement Agency (DEA) compared
the Taliban's close ties with the opium farmers and smugglers to
the Farc's involvement in the Nicaraguan cocaine business. And
it seems that ISIS is keen to copy the Farc's success. Much of the
cocaine that arrives in Europe comes across the Atlantic on what
is known as Highway 10, running along the 10th parallel. Over
the last ten years, Mali and Niger have been destabilized by
infighting, allowing the local branches of al-Qaeda to smuggle
cocaine more easily through these countries. Now, Boko Haram,
the African Islamist group, has taken over the ancient trading
routes through these countries, combining drug smuggling with
rape and kidnap as it seeks to control the flow of drugs and
money by any means necessary. To the east, Afghan drug lords
have their own equivalent of Highway 10, known as the Southern
Route. With land routes to the north becoming more difficult,
particularly as European borders close, the best way out is by sea.

North Africa and Egypt have traditionally been gateways to Europe for both cocaine and heroin, particularly Afghan heroin, after it was trekked across Saudi Arabia by camel. During the Egyptian heroin crisis of the late 1920s, things became so bad that the Camel Corps installed an X-ray machine to check if camels were being used to smuggle opium in metal containers that had been pushed down their throats. Now, ISIS actively refines opium into heroin before it is moved, and then drives it out. One side effect of ISIS refining more heroin inside the borders of Afghanistan has been a nationwide boom in the number of heroin addicts. Those in rural areas, with their higher tolerance for opiates, are particularly affected. In 2015, the UNODC estimated that there were 3 million addicts, making up 12 per cent of the population: the highest rate of addiction in the world. The heroin that does go for export moves through Iran and Pakistan, down to the Makran Coast of Balochistan. Then it is loaded onto small, seagoing dhows and motored across to Somalia, destined eventually for Uganda and Kenya. The Combined Maritime Forces (CMF), consisting of thirty-one nations who patrol the area, cannot arrest or detain the sailors, so the drugs are dumped at sea and the smugglers released. The chances of being caught are negligible, and CMF powers mean that there is no risk of imprisonment. Hezbollah and al-Shabaab also take their share of the profits from this route. Entebbe airport in Uganda has become a major heroin hub, where human mules desperate for money swallow up to a hundred heroin parcels before making the journey to the airport. Some fly with the drugs inside them; others wait for them to pass through their systems, before washing them and handing them over to a smuggler further up the chain who stockpiles them. The superintendent of Uganda's anti-narcotics department, Tinka Zaragaba, knows that they are fighting a losing battle, only discovering twenty kilos last year: 'It can be put in the breasts of women, it can be put in their private parts in the form of pads . . . [there are] very many ways of concealment.'[28]

In 2015, a 1,032-kg shipment of heroin was discovered in a dhow off Mombasa, East Africa's largest ever haul. The figures had been rising steadily since 2010, indicating that was the time the Middle Eastern groups began to dominate and encourage the Southern Route. There were also large shipments of acetic anhydride, used to refine heroin, going from East Africa towards the Golden Triangle and Crescent. Whilst it is a widely used chemical reagent, a sudden rise in supply along the route indicated to the CMF a distinct rise in heroin traffic. The CMF and other authorities turned their attention to the waters off East Africa, which has led to the Arab groups looking for somewhere else to land their cargoes. Hence why more and more heroin is also coming into South Africa since 2015, as the Southern Route utilizes as much of Africa's vast and porous coastline as possible, often called the Smack Track. The local cities are seeing the typical rise in drug use along any trafficking route. HIV infections from intravenous use are rising, and low-grade heroin and marijuana mixtures, known as *nyaope* or *whoonga*, are causing dramatic social problems around Johannesburg and Durban. All of this is caused by the trade in Afghan heroin.

ISIS, like the Taliban before it, needs to control its territory to keep the revenue from these three sources coming in. It plies its fighters endlessly with amphetamines, and in 2017 more than 11 million pills were seized at the Syrian border, destined for ISIS fighters.[29]

ISIS also bears more than a passing resemblance to the Mughal king Babur's idea of how to rule, remaining endlessly mobile over a vast amount of land, resources and peoples. Unlike the Mughals, though, it uses instability and terror to keep the people in check and the money coming in. The ISIS claims to be willing to pay any price for a pure Muslim faith for countries such as Afghanistan are belied by its exploitation of the same people, keeping them in such fear that crops and taxes are handed over willingly. The escalating drug problem also plays into the jihadists' hands, with a pliable and ever-rising number of addicts. As the ISIS structure comes to mimic those of Mexico in terms of sophisticated military organization, control of social media, and fraternization with other gangs in the same territory, its power is unlikely to be undermined. It will only be by breaking its hold on oil and opium that its stranglehold can be broken.

In a meeting with a young Afghan from Nangarhar province, I asked him what he thought of ISIS. He shrugged with typical Afghan understatement. 'Nothing much. My uncle is Taliban, so they leave us alone. Bad for women though.' Nangarhar, close to the Durand Line, is both a centre for farming opium and a conduit for passing it out to Pakistan.

'What do your family do there?' I asked.

He guessed that I already knew the answer as he replied, 'Oh, they're farmers.'

'And do they grow poppies?'

'Sure. Who doesn't?' came the deliberately guileless response.

Most Afghans resent the ISIS occupation, just as they loathed the British and Russian ones, but it is a situation they have become used to over two centuries of invaders. As always, they will continue to farm opium as long as it is more profitable than something else.

Chapter Ten

HEROIN CHIC, HIV
AND GENERATION OXY

'I owe it my perfect hours.'[1] Jean Cocteau

Jean Cocteau was born in 1889 and became addicted to opium in London in 1904, after a twenty-day bout of neuralgia. 'It was a Sunday afternoon, wet and cheerless; and a duller spectacle of this earth of ours has not to show than a rainy Sunday in London,' he recalled in his memoir of addiction, when a bored and tired druggist dispensed him some opium gum on Oxford Street, only yards from where Thomas De Quincey first purchased his laudanum over a century before.

Cocteau, an extraordinary Parisian socialite, quickly fell into 'the abyss of divine enjoyment'.[2] He maintained his habit for twenty-five years, after which he decided to become sober, and in 1929, during his most wretched hours, his most remembered works were written. Louche, attractive and absurdly charismatic, Cocteau was a poster boy for addiction, and recovery. His experiences encompassed a new understanding of what it meant to be an addict, and the accompanying sense of isolation, and salvation: 'Everything one does in life, even love, occurs in an express train racing toward death. To smoke opium is to get out of the

330

train while it is still moving. It is to concern oneself with something other than life or death.'[3]

Jean Cocteau's experience of opium, which he ate, smoked and drank, as laudanum, encapsulates the upper-middle-class European model of addiction. He remained in control of his life and faculties, yet he yearned to be free.

During the time Cocteau was writing, the world was undergoing a shift in how opium, principally heroin, was marketed. The period between the wars was a particularly difficult time in drug legislature, and also in terms of illicit global supply routes, which had been significantly disrupted by the First World War. Still painfully aware of their commitment to the Hague Convention, European countries were realizing not only the extent of their legitimate medicinal opiate needs, both in wartime and peace, but also the scale of their internal narcotics problems. Whiffens, one of the major British opiate exporters, had its licence revoked in 1923 after a smuggling scandal. La Société Roessler et Compagnie in Mulhouse, France took over as chief producer in western Europe, and in 1928 produced 4.35 tons of heroin, enough to satisfy the medical needs of the world population more than three times over.[4] French pharmaceutical companies completed meticulous export papers for 346 kilos of morphine to the United States, 440 kilos to Germany and sixty-two kilos to Jakarta, all of which were countries where morphine was now illegal. Yet those countries showed no evidence of morphine's arrival, and the French firms refused to supply the names and details of the importers to the governments of the countries receiving the drugs.[5] At the same time, Switzerland showed exports to France, which went unrecorded on import papers, and Germany and Finland supplied Estonia.

British and Dutch pharmaceutical companies in particular were finding ways to subvert their Hague Convention agreements to supply drug racketeers by importing poppy straw as raw material and processing it through an ever-widening net of company names. Also, in 1928, Estonia made a desperate plea to the League of Nations, asking that governments take over the factories producing heroin and cocaine 'on an enormous scale'.[6] Finland, outside of the League and where tuberculosis was rife, refused to give up heroin-based cough medications throughout the 1930s, such as the charmingly named Pulmo, and they continued to import vast quantities of morphine and heroin to be made into pills for a small army facing up to Stalin, which hit a peak in the Winter War of 1939–40.

Yet even as the modern commercialization of heroin spread, Cocteau's eloquent writing on opium influenced another generation of users, where all drugs, including heroin, were part of the creative, fashionable experience. Cocteau was writing in a new era of psychoactive drugs, but as an established member of the Parisian bourgeoisie, he favoured the old methods of smoking, eating or drinking opiates. He abhorred morphinists, and routinely took his opium in the morning, afternoon and evening. Yet, in the end, he knew he needed to stop, and recorded his experience as *Opium: Diary of a Cure*. Cocteau, writing in the late 1920s, along with the works of De Quincey, established drug addiction as a noble artistic undertaking for two generations of the twentieth century.

Like De Quincey, Cocteau marks the divide between addiction as a noble, mind-altering pursuit and the realities of the street trade. Coupled with the continuing American clampdown on delivery of pharmaceutical diamorphine, the Second World War disrupted the supply of heroin to the US, and official addiction figures fell to the lowest levels on record. A heroin epidemic in the young poor black community of Chicago in the late 1940s indicated that international suppliers were finding a new route into the USA, selling daily hits for pocket money in order to secure a fresh market. The problems amongst the 'Chicago Negro youth' between 1949 and 1953 were closely recorded, and demonstrated the failure of the police and judiciary to get to grips with the epidemic as it happened, with a lag of up to two years in terms of investigations and arrests, leading analysts to conclude that 'failure to respond effectively during the early stages of disease spread may be a characteristic feature of heroin epidemics, and should be considered in the design of addiction control programs'.[7]

In western Europe, the children born at the end of the Second World War were exposed to a host of new intoxicants in the form of psychoactives such as LSD. In the United States, marijuana had become a staple recreational narcotic in the 1950s and 60s, rapidly overtaken by barbiturates such as Quaaludes, benzodiazepines, and heroin smoking in the 1960s and 70s.

Jean Cocteau's articulate experience of addiction was co-opted by the American beat poets, who used all of the drugs available to expand their minds and empty their pockets. They were preoccupied by notions of personal and sexual freedom, and the ills of what they saw as a repressive, capitalist society. The ancient story of the poor writer assumed a new nobility when coupled to an existential hunger that ate up any experience narcotics had to offer.

William Burroughs, along with Jack Kerouac and Allen Ginsberg, was one of the defining figures of the Beat Generation. Burroughs was born in 1914 and was a committed drug user. He became a heroin addict in his late twenties after he was turned down for the navy during the Second World War, and he became a dealer in 1950s New York, writing later that 'Junk is not, like alcohol or weed, a means to increased enjoyment of life. Junk is not a kick. It is a way of life.'[8] His novels *Junkie* (1953) and *Naked Lunch* (1959) are testament to the debasement heroin addiction can bring, and were banned in the United States not for their narcotic-related content but for violations of sodomy laws, namely paedophilia. Widely lauded as an artistic genius, Burroughs also shot his common-law wife, Joan Vollmer, in the head during a delirious game of William Tell. They had one son, William Jr., who died aged thirty-three, soon after he was found in a ditch, suffering acute symptoms of liver failure owing to chronic drug and alcohol abuse.

Burroughs' depiction of his experiences of opiate addiction is particularly powerful, and his account of using morphine will be familiar to any user. He writes that it 'hits the backs of the legs first, then the back of the neck, a spreading wave of relaxation slackening the muscles away from the bones so that you seem to float without outlines, like lying in warm salt water.'[9] Burroughs, despite his gentlemanly exterior, had, like Kerouac and Ginsberg, spent time in a mental institution by the time he was thirty, although Kerouac's drug of choice was alcohol, while Ginsberg opted for LSD and cannabis. But like Cocteau and Thomas De Quincey, Burroughs was committed to opiates.

And like De Quincey, Burroughs, unlike those around him, lived a long life and died aged eighty-three. His legacy to a new creative generation was coupled with his staunchly traditional American upbringing and Harvard education, things that many of those who so slavishly read his works could not hope to experience.

In later editions of *Naked Lunch*, Burroughs wrote that the only successful cure for heroin addiction that he had come across was apomorphine, stating that it 'is qualitatively different from other methods of cure. I have tried them all. Short reduction, slow reduction, cortisone, antihistamines, tranquilizers, sleeping cures, Tolserol, reserpine. None of these cures lasted beyond the first opportunity to relapse.'[10]

Apomorphine occurs naturally in blue lotus flowers and white water lilies of the species *Nymphaea*. The Mayans of Central America used *Nymphaea* in rituals, as a hallucinogenic and aphrodisiac, as also indicated in ancient Egyptian tomb artwork. Apomorphine can also be synthesized from morphine and sulphuric acid, and was produced as early as 1845 by the German chemist A. E. Arppe. It was used originally to treat aggressive behaviour in farmyard animals and by 1884 it had been used in trials for the treatment of Parkinson's disease, trials that recommenced only as late as 1951, with considerable success.[11] It became part of the treatment programmes for alcohol in London in 1931 under radical addiction doctor John Yerbury Dent, who also used it to treat drug addiction. It was later restricted as a dangerous drug in its own right, with actions too similar to morphine to be of significant use when weighed against the side effects, which can include convulsions, but are mainly associated with violent vomiting. Owing to the vomiting, many medical professionals have labelled apomorphine a form of aversion therapy, in which the patient comes to connect the vomiting with the heroin or morphine habit. However, the average heroin addict is accustomed to vomiting and purging to the point where this is unlikely. Apomorphine is used now for veterinary purposes when dogs swallow poisons. Professor Andrew Lees of London's National Hospital for Neurology and Neurosurgery, and the world's leading Parkinson's specialist, remains convinced of apomorphine as an effective treatment for Parkinson's, and says that it should also be trialled again for heroin addiction, 'but we are up against punitive and draconian legislation. The heroic era of neuropharmacological research has now vanished.'[12]

Lees points to Burroughs as one of the successful examples of

the apomorphine cure, and Burroughs himself remained convinced of its efficacy, writing that before he took apomorphine
at the hands of Dr John Dent, 'I had no claims to call myself a
writer and my creativity was limited to filling a hypodermic. The
entire body of work on which my present reputation is based was
produced after the apomorphine treatment, and would never
have been produced if I had not taken the cure and stayed off
junk.'[3] Apomorphine kept Burroughs clean for two creatively
productive years before subsequent relapse, but his belief in apomorphine for breaking down the metabolic actions of addiction
didn't waver, and he became a sage to other artists struggling
under the burden of their own habits.

In 1974, *Rolling Stone* magazine recorded a conversation
between the British musician David Bowie and William Burroughs. Whilst it is hard to have much sympathy for Burroughs,
one can only feel for him agreeing to a grim simulation of a
Jamaican meal 'prepared by a Jamaican in the Bowie entourage',
with Bowie dressed in 'a three tone NASA jumpsuit' and whose
most memorable contribution to the exchange was 'I change my
mind a lot. I usually don't agree with what I say very much. I'm
an awful liar'. Bowie was then in the grip of an overwhelming
cocaine addiction, and eighteen months later had to change his
life entirely in order to recover, moving to Berlin and living in a
cheap apartment above a Turkish cafe where he ate all his meals:
'I had approached the brink of drug-induced calamity one too
many times, and it was essential to take some kind of positive
action.'[4]

Their interview, however, highlights the divides in popular
culture, something of which the sixty-year-old Burroughs had
only scant knowledge and from which the twenty-seven-year-
old Bowie had fashioned an existence. As Burroughs remarked,
wonderingly, 'The escalating rate of change. The media are really

responsible for most of this. Which produces an incalculable effect.'[15]

For many, management of their habit had become the new reality. Bowie, like Burroughs, would not be clean for decades, but they both went on to enjoy long and productive lives. For others, it was not so easy, and in 1964, despite the United States having allegedly reduced its legal morphine consumption to negligible levels, the market for heroin on both coasts was booming, particularly in New York City. Intravenous heroin use was becoming the norm amongst users, but the series of wars and particularly Korea, with its advanced blood-banking facilities in the MASH tents, had revealed that transfusions weren't simply a matter of giving the blood from one to another. Hepatitis was rife in the donations.

Intravenous heroin use emerged simultaneously in Alexandria, Egypt and Indiana, USA, as a widespread problem in 1925. There is still no evidence why this happened in both places at the same time, although Indiana has acted historically as a conduit to the south for contraband coming into Chicago. Egypt went from negligible heroin use in the First World War to a full-blown intravenous heroin epidemic by 1925. In 1926 one Armenian chemist sold 600 kg of heroin, quite legally as there were still no restrictions. By 1929, almost one in four Egyptian males aged between twenty and forty were addicted to heroin, and only an outbreak of subtertian malaria, from needle-sharing, seemed to slow it down.[16] From Indiana intravenous heroin use spread across the United States as the quickest mode of consumption. By the 1960s, to be 'on the spike' was nothing remarkable.

In 1964, America announced that it had a medical solution to the problem of heroin addiction: methadone, a treatment pioneered by doctors Vincent Dole, Mary Jeanne Kreek and Marie Nyswander at the Rockefeller University in New York. Although it had been synthesized in the winter of 1937–8 by Gustav Ehrhart and Max Bockmuhl for Hoechst AG near Frankfurt, the Second World War had put development on hold and it only went into experimental use in the late 1940s, when methadone required the backing of private funding to achieve mainstream recognition. Administered in a controlled environment, methadone maintenance treatment (MMT) 'eliminates the drug craving which drives many detoxified addicts to resume heroin addiction'.[17] Methadone produced neither 'euphoria nor other distortion of behaviour', and 'frees the heroin addict from the exigencies of the street life', but it also robbed them of the will to get out of bed and take a shower.[18] Addiction doctors treating inpatients in rehabilitation units knew that they were battling a gargantuan problem, and that management might be the best they could hope for, because 'Almost without exception, these units merely separate the addict from heroin for a brief period.'[19]

For many, MMT was 'a system of chemical parole', and there remains substantial evidence that treatment programmes do not dispense adequate doses to keep patients from the discomfort associated with heroin withdrawal.[20] Hence, many in MMT continue to use street heroin or other drugs outside of their programme. MMT also robbed the user of the routine that surrounded their habit: a supervised dose administered by or in front of a physician in clinical surroundings bore little resemblance to the score many users were accustomed to. For Burroughs, methadone was 'completely satisfying to the addict, an excellent painkiller, and at least as addicting as morphine'.[21] Owing to the 1971 initiation of the War on Drugs, there was a disruption in the supply of street heroin to the East Coast of America at the same time as there was a surge in the number of methadone patient places, with New York City Council making 40,000 available by 1973, of which 34,000 were taken up.[22] This is in contrast to Dole's original 1969 clinic, which had places for only 1,000 carefully screened addicts. For health services, MMT had the distinct advantage over the early twentieth century Public Health Service clinic programmes because it was an outpatient service, making it significantly more cost-effective.

Outpatient care had the disadvantage of not removing the addict from their street surroundings, and in a changing market, where the quality of street heroin was dropping as it was cut further and further to make up for reduced supply, addicts began to turn to pharmaceutically produced methadone for a reliable high, and the market on the street for methadone began in earnest. To enrol in a treatment programme had significant advantages too, not least the 100-mg daily maintenance dose: those in a programme were issued with a methadone identity card, to be presented in clinic. However, these cards were extremely useful for those also scoring on the street, as they could be shown to any arresting officer as proof of the need to carry methadone. So within two years of the beginning of the War on Drugs, street demand in New York City had moved towards methadone liquid. MMT remained controversial, because, unlike in China, the USA had refused to maintain addicts when it passed the Harrison Act, and 'According to the Bureau of Narcotics, any doctor who uses methadone maintenance as treatment for heroin addicts violates federal law'.[23] Challenges to Harrison, demanding that addicts be maintained, had been rebuffed definitively by *Webb* v. *United States* in 1919. The cases of Linder (1925) and Boyd (1926), occurring less than seven years later – when doctors had been entrapped by federal agents for prescribing more than one morphine dose – allowed the Supreme Court to fudge the issue by declaring that if a doctor acted 'for the purpose of curing disease or relieving suffering', then an acquittal was in order.[24]

These fudges allowed MMT to become part of the official governmental rehabilitation of addicts in the early 1970s. Private clinics used other drugs, such as apomorphine, and also ibogaine, throughout the 1960s and 70s, when those who could afford it sought cures in comfortable surroundings. Ibogaine remains controversial. Derived from iboga root bark or the plant *Tabernanthe iboga,* ibogaine is a psychedelic that some claim breaks the metabolic chain of addiction in as little as forty-eight hours. The promotion of ibogaine as a cure for addiction was mainly the work of one man, Howard Lotsof, who as a nineteen-year-old heroin addict in 1962, took ibogaine and claimed to be cured instantly. His life's work was to bring ibogaine to the attention of governments and major pharmaceutical companies, in which he had a measure of success. Various offshore ibogaine treatment centres still exist around the world, and in most Hague Convention nations, it is either unregulated or illegal. Lotsof died in 2010, still a committed proponent of both ibogaine and methadone, and ibogaine remains a persistent presence on the fringe of addiction treatment. Trials in the 1990s proved that it is effective in mitigating the early effects of withdrawal, but like most heroin cures, ibogaine's success depends largely upon the commitment of the patient, as Keith Richards said of his attempt with apomorphine in 1971: 'I once took that apomorphine cure that Burroughs swears by. Dr Dent was dead but his assistant whom he trained, this lovely old dear call Smitty, who's like a mother hen, still runs the clinic . . . But it's a pretty medieval cure. You just vomit all the time. In 72 hours, if you can get through it, you're clean. But that's never the problem. The problem is when you go back to your social circle – who are all drug pushers and junkies. In five minutes you can be on the stuff again.'[25]

By the time Richards was taking the apomorphine cure, drugs, and particularly heroin, had become associated with a new generation of musicians. Jimi Hendrix and Janis Joplin died in 1970, both aged twenty-seven. The official cause of Hendrix's death was a barbiturate overdose, but he was a regular user of both heroin and hashish. Joplin was a heroin addict, whose use escalated alarmingly when she was stressed or unhappy. Bob Dylan claimed, perhaps untruthfully, to have been both a heroin addict and a prostitute, in interviews in the 1960s. Of his heroin addiction, he told the BBC that 'I kicked a heroin habit in New York City [when he was involved with the Beat movement] . . . I got very, very strung out for a while, I mean really, very strung out . . . I had about a $25-a-day habit and I kicked it'.[26] This may or may not be true, but the drug culture that arose from the Beat movement encouraged experimentation and breaking the shackles of society's expectations. Even popular journalism changed for good with the arrival of the American drug-taking titan Hunter S. Thompson, who used heroin to counteract the vast quantity of cocaine he used daily, as well as the mescaline he also enjoyed. He seemed to live in a state of perpetually intoxicated chaos, and when he committed suicide aged sixty-seven, in 2005, had his ashes fired from a cannon at his funeral. Yet he appeared to have few regrets. *Where the Buffalo Roam*, a film of 1980 based on Thompson's own autobiographical stories, attributed to him the line, 'I hate to advocate drugs, alcohol, violence, or insanity to anyone, but they've always worked for me.'

In the last half of the twentieth century there was a sea change in the way society, particularly American society, viewed and used recreational drugs. Thompson's life was so extreme it approached parody, but the interview recorded between Burroughs and Bowie had highlighted a moment of wider change in narcotic culture. For Burroughs, 'junk' was an essential part of his lived experience, which eventually fuelled and was inextricably linked to his creativity, true of the other beats with their intoxicants of choice. For David Bowie, it was a personal pitfall that had ultimately threatened calamity. For Keith Richards, it was part of a lifestyle. In the following decades, many musicians wrote about the experience of heroin, ranging from Lou Reed with his 'Perfect Day', Pink Floyd and the dreamily expansive 'Comfortably Numb', The La's with the deceptively cheerful 'There She Goes', to Iggy Pop's looming withdrawal symptoms in 'Lust for Life'. For many, the greatest song written about the experience of heroin addiction and its attendant mental and physical torments was the 1994 release of 'Hurt' by American band Nine Inch Nails. In the same year, Kurt Cobain of the grunge band Nirvana was found dead of a self-inflicted gunshot after failing to overcome his heroin addiction, which he used to temper stomach pain (possibly itself the result of his heroin use), and depression.

The death of Kurt Cobain brought the realities accompanying chronic heroin dependence into the open for a new generation, and also reinforced the connection between opiates and the temporary relief from fear and anxiety.

From John Leigh in the 1780s, to Sertürner's work in 1804, chemists and pharmacists had worked diligently upon isolating the active compounds present in opium latex, aware that these drugs had an effect on the human nervous system, one that had the dual action of allaying pain and anxiety, but they did not fully understand why. The boom in recreational drug use of all kinds across the Western world in the 1960s made official bodies keener than ever to discover the mechanisms of opiates and their synthetic counterparts, opioids, but it wasn't until 1973 that a rebellious graduate student finally arrived at the answer.

Candace Pert was born in 1946 in Manhattan. She was due to enter Johns Hopkins School of Medicine in Baltimore as a graduate researcher in pharmacology in 1970 when she broke her back in a horse-riding accident. The subsequent effect morphine had upon both her brain and her body inspired a lifelong career in researching the connections between the two. Working under Solomon Snyder, she neglected her authorized work on insulin receptors to focus upon the effects of opioids on the brain, and in 1973 ordered the materials she would need to conduct her own experiments, including morphine and brain tissue. (Receptors are proteins in the brain to which molecules or short peptides are designed to bind specifically, comparable to the way a key fits into a lock, effectively blocking out pain and discomfort.) The morphine was labelled with a radioactive atom that made it traceable when it bound itself to the brain matter. Preferring to work when the laboratory was empty, Pert brought her five-year-old son Evan with her on a Friday night so that she could conduct her experiment in peace. When she returned to work on Monday morning, the radioactive atom pathway had identified the first known opioid receptor in the human brain.

Two years later, in 1975, a pair of researchers in Scotland, Hans W. Kosterlitz and John Hughes, identified encephalin, the first of the endorphin family to be discovered and one of the peptides which act in the brain as painkillers, manufactured by the central nervous system and the pituitary gland. Physical exercise, breast-feeding, voluntary sexual intercourse and laughter all produce endorphins in humans.

In 1978, as a result of these findings, Snyder, Kosterlitz and Hughes shared the Albert Lasker Award for Basic Medical Research, which frequently precedes the award of the Nobel Prize. Pert, however, was excluded, owing to her status as a graduate student and, many felt, including Pert herself, her gender. She wrote a sharp protest letter to *Science* magazine in January 1979, stating that 'I played a key role in initiating this research and following it up'. Snyder credited Pert in his acceptance speech: 'I am honored that the Lasker Foundation has chosen this year to recognize the field of opiate receptor and opiate-like peptide research ... Among the many people who contributed to this area, my own special thanks go to Candace Pert who, as a graduate student, identified the opiate receptors in my laboratory.'[27] In an ongoing campaign, Pert refused to stand aside and let a senior associate take the credit for her work, scotching one of the most promising careers of the century, in terms of research into analgesics. An embittered Pert went on to have a groundbreaking career in peptide research, and after her death in 2013 in Potomac, Maryland from the complications of heart failure aged sixty-seven, Snyder remembered her in a tribute in the *New York Times* as 'one of the most creative, innovative graduate students I have ever mentored'.[28]

And Behold, A Pale Horse: HIV

One of the peptide therapies Candace Pert hoped to develop was Peptide T, designed to block the action of Human Immunodeficiency Virus. She was unsuccessful, largely due to the mutable nature of HIV itself. It is an extraordinarily adaptable disease, with a virus body one-sixtieth the size of the human red blood cell. The rapid spread amongst intravenous drug users in the early 1980s was cause for alarm, although this new disease appeared to primarily manifest in the sexually active members of the gay community of the coastal continental United States.

The 1925 outbreak of malaria had deterred many in the Middle East from injecting heroin, but the same had not been true in America, and the country that had happily supplied so many mail-order syringe kits for a century was inevitably going to suffer. HIV-1, the primary manifestation of the disease that leads to AIDS, emerged in the 1920s in the Belgian Congo, but did not begin to spread widely in the USA until 1981. The mysterious death of a fifteen-year-old boy, Robert R[ayford], in St Louis in 1969 is one of the few indicators that AIDS was present in the USA before the epidemic that began in 1981. Rayford had never travelled, and those treating him speculated that he had been involved in sex work. The first confirmed case in Europe came in 1976, when Norwegian sailor and truck driver Arne Vidar Røed, known as Arvid Noe, his wife and eight-year-old daughter, died in quick succession after being diagnosed the previous year.

HIV is a particularly cunning virus that can lie dormant when untreated for more than a decade before it emerges as a crippling immune condition that renders the host helpless in the face of bacterial infections, skin cancers and respiratory ailments. Its sudden dominance in the coastal United States homosexual male community, at a time when gay pride had asserted itself as a social and political force, was interpreted by many as a form of divine justice. That it also infected the intravenous drug-using population only reinforced this belief. Since the Second World War, America had also undergone a long and undignified debacle involving blood transfusions from and within the armed forces, where hepatitis B and C were rife, transmitting the disease within the ranks and to civilians. The hypodermic needle was rapidly becoming tainted with the association of sickness rather than cure.

When AIDS emerged as an issue amongst the prostitutes of the San Francisco Tenderloin district in 1985, the mainstream media seized upon the issue. It was no longer simply a homosexual problem, it had passed into the straight male population via the disease vector of sexual intercourse and needle-sharing.

Silvana Strangis was one of the first reported San Francisco prostitutes to exhibit the symptoms of AIDS, most likely contracted from her pimp, Tony, who was a fellow heroin addict as well as her sexual partner, and in the advanced stages of the disease. At the time, more than 98 per cent of the San Francisco AIDS cases were homosexual men, and it had been easy to dismiss the disease as a gay problem, but 'Suddenly there were children with AIDS who wanted to go to school, labourers with AIDS who wanted to work, and researchers who wanted funding, and there was a threat to the nation's public health that could no longer be ignored.'[29]

This public-health issue formed the bedrock of a new White House campaign against drugs. Drawing deeply upon America's well of sentimentalism, Ronald and Nancy Reagan founded the Just Say No campaign, targeting 'this cancer of drugs' upon American soil. The Christian message of the Reagan campaign against drugs is clear, coupling an 'unyielding and inflexible' attitude to drug use with the steaming righteousness accompanying such phrases as 'We Americans have never been morally neutral against any form of tyranny.'[30] The sudden coincidence between the Just Say No campaign and the spread of HIV to the heterosexual male population in 1985–6 is remarkable, representing the governmental response to the spread of the disease to what was perceived as the mainstream population.

The sense of immunity from illness that had come with the widespread usage of penicillin had lasted a scant five decades before a new sexually transmitted, blood-borne virus arrived to haunt the West, and HIV/AIDS comprised 'a disease that from its first days was as much a social as a medical problem'.[31] The inability to acclimatise to a new cultural reality regarding alternative sexuality and drug use left the Reagans calling upon the nobility of the Second World War dead as a reason not to use drugs in their White House address of 1986.

In the USA in 1990, 10 per cent of intravenous drug users who volunteered for testing returned a positive result for HIV.[32] Yet, five years after the Reagan campaign, there was still little practical advice for people living and sleeping with an IV heroin user or sex worker. 'Just Say No' wasn't quite as simple and effective as it first appeared. Randy Shilts, the determined and eloquent journalist who wrote the definitive text on the early years of the epidemic in San Francisco, *And The Band Played On*, died aged forty-two from AIDS complications. 'It is a tale that bears telling', he wrote, 'so that it will never happen again, to any people, anywhere.'[33]

The stigma of HIV became irretrievably entangled with American stigmas against homosexuality and also drug addicts. The rapidity of the spread of HIV amongst the high-risk homosexual populations of San Francisco and New York, who were now increasingly mobile in a new era of cheap air travel, was genuinely terrifying, yet the prejudice against this relatively small subset of the American population grew out of all proportion. A huge gulf remains even in Shilts's measured writing, specifically between the homosexual and intravenous drug-using communities, each of whom blamed the other for spreading HIV. Heroin use was suddenly associated not with smoking or snorting, but the process and ritual of injecting, tainting the user and further separating them from society. The studies which were conducted into HIV also focussed on the racial background of those carrying HIV, with black and Hispanic drug users and prostitutes targeted as not more vulnerable, but more ignorant to the reality of HIV infection. The association of Latin and black Americans with danger to society re-emerged with a vengeance less than a century after Harrison, despite the evidence for the fastest vector of infection being the white, male homosexual population. Extensive studies by the National Center for Health Statistics upon the pregnant Latina population commenced, highlighting religious superstition and lack of safe-sex practice. The enemy was not so much a mysterious and parasitic disease as a type of person.

As the AIDS epidemic came to pass, the methadone programmes gained popularity: a safe oral daily dosage, administered in a supervised environment, seemed the perfect way to stop Americans turning to the hypodermic. Heroin had become inextricably linked to a soiled street life of prostitution, hustle, and the instant gratification of a $10 high.

Throughout the 1960s and 70s, the peak of street heroin usage, a series of utopian initiatives to combat global opium farming had been introduced. The Royal Project in Thailand, initiated by King Bhumibol in 1969, was and remains one of the world's most successful opium-poppy replacement projects. In the northern highlands of Thailand, which had been taken over by the opium trade from Burma, the hill tribe people were struggling to survive. On the Thailand–Burma border, the elephants used for the logging trade were routinely drugged with opium to render them docile. The Royal Project, which aimed to replace opium cultivation with market gardening, has offered rehabilitation for humans and animals alike, but has also created a series of model villages more suited to tourist visits than to the needs of the communities who had previously farmed opium to survive. The divide between those engaged in heroin use, and those who grew opium for a living, is widening constantly.

The Royal Project succeeds because of the sheer amount of money involved, and because of the late King Bhumibol's philanthropic commitment. Similar projects have been initiated in Afghanistan, namely the growing of almonds by Californian farmers as a replacement for the opium poppy, but Afghanistan is simply too dangerous, and the irrigation infrastructure too irregular, for such projects to work. Crop replacement remains the ideal solution to opium farming in some of the world's poorest places, but it requires huge amounts of money and a support network. As the farmers of Afghanistan have realized repeatedly, growing melons is foolhardy if there are no roads on which to take them to market, or the market has been bombed out of existence.

Crop-replacement initiatives are, in the main, vanity projects for philanthropists. The displaced Akha people, now numbering some 80,000 in Chiang Mai and Bangkok, would profit from such projects more than the imported workers who farm them currently. In 2007, the Thai government passed a law curbing the people's access to fertile farmland, claiming it instead for the queen under the Community Forest Act, curtailing the traditional Akha way of life still further. Many of the young non-literate Akha women entered the Thai sex trade, unable to survive otherwise. The mountain existence they had been raised to, one of monthly ancestor and spirit veneration, slash and burn agriculture, and opium smoking or eating, was replaced with sex work, cheap heroin, AIDS and social ostracization. The parallel existence of the Royal Project and the systematic theft of the Akha way of life typifies the hypocrisy of current opium farming replacement schemes. The Akha people are now left to beg on the streets of Chiang Mai and Bangkok, sell their bodies, or commit to remaining in their homeland in 'simple lives of unremitting tedium, enlivened by two things: addiction to opiates and being used as a tourist attraction'.[34]

A Return to the Fragrant Harbour

Hong Kong, the opium-trading centre created on a barren out-crop in the Pearl River Delta, has gone from strength to strength. While Afghanistan probably still claims the title in terms of endemic corruption, Hong Kong takes the crown in terms of revenue, and quasi-legitimate infrastructure. The founding of the Hongkong and Shanghai Banking Corporation (HSBC) in 1865 made it possible to channel credit and liquid funds from the opium trade into other shipping and mercantile businesses. No longer confined to Hong Kong Island, British, American and Australian companies took over Kowloon, and 235 more tiny islands in the delta, creating a sprawling mass of high-rises and a financial industry unrivalled anywhere in the world.

Hong Kong's population increased dramatically when Mao Tse-tung created the People's Republic of China in 1949, as hundreds of thousands of Chinese decided to avail themselves of Hong Kong's privileges of extraterritoriality, and the opportunities for free trade available there – or, as the English translation of a Chinese history of the area states, 'the familiarity of the entire region to achieve economic gains by illegal means'.[35] The economic hierarchy of Hong Kong lends itself to organized crime in a unique way: the series of laws and bylaws brought in under British rule coupled with institutionalized corruption in the police force and judicial system meant that, from the 1930s onwards, Hong Kong became not only a settlement built on the opium trade, but the focus of global heroin trafficking. Largely, this is due to the borderless nature of Greater China, making Hong Kong the financial funnel of a country that takes up approximately 3,657,765 square miles of territory and has a conservative population estimate of 1.5 billion. It is a vast territory, embracing extreme climates: Kashgar, in north-west China, is lucky to see four inches of rainfall a year, while Canton can have as much as thirteen. As with the Pashtuns of Afghanistan and the Was and Akhas of Burma, many different peoples straddle official borders, all of whom conduct business between themselves and outlying tribes. This tribal business structure was echoed in the early Triad societies of Hong Kong, which was taken over in the early twentieth century by one of the Green Gangs. The Green Gangs assimilated with the criminal *chiu chau* gangs of Hong Kong and the original secret societies of the seventeenth century to form one solid mass of incestuous corruption three centuries later, pushing drugs and cash through the Pearl River Delta on an unprecedented scale.

In 1963, embattled by the Marseilles heroin trade and looking for a global answer, Interpol sent out a memo from its Paris headquarters: 'Since 1958 the General Secretariat's attention has been drawn – more especially by the authorities in Hong Kong – to the arrival of a certain number of Chinese in Europe. Supplied with passports, and claiming to be representatives for genuine or non-existent clothing manufacturers in the Far East, they make numerous journeys in all European countries . . . their real purpose is to establish contact and relationships with certain suspicious characters in an attempt to set up a system of drug traffic and distribution, aimed ultimately at the USA.'[36]

Traditional Triad business on the mainland stretched to people trafficking, and kidnap and protection rackets, but Hong Kong offered the potential to create a global heroin network. The Green Gangs, who specialized in the three original Triad mainstays, gave way to a new generation who saw the revenue potential in narcotics and learned that only savage violence would protect their interests, resulting in splinter groups such as the Thin Blade Gang.

The level of Hong Kong heroin traffic was reflected in customs seizures, which escalated from eighty-four kilos between 1947 and 1951 to 2,337 kilos in 1977 alone. Seizure rates are typically taken to be around 10 per cent of the real amount of any given illicit commodity passing through a customs centre, rendering Hong Kong the largest heroin hub in the world outside of Rotterdam. By the mid-1970s, the US Drug Enforcement Agency had listed heroin as fifteenth in comparative sales listings for the top 500 American corporations, only just below Shell Oil, and above Goodyear Tyres, Xerox, and the Campbell Soup Company.[37]

As the heroin business supplanted Hong Kong's traditional opium trading, the established commercial systems were co-opted into the modern world. Compradors became 'controllers', who travelled on the planes from Chep Lap Kok airport with the drug mules who carted kilos of heroin No.4 in suitcases or internally; in the early 1970s, the sex and drugs trades united as Chinese women leaving Hong Kong for Amsterdam had their vaginas packed with heroin to the point where it was difficult for them to sit through the flight. This made it considerably easier for them to be identified as persons of interest by the Dutch authorities. Once the mules reached their ultimate destination in Vancouver or the coast of the United States, they were abandoned with their passport and some money, deemed payment enough for services rendered. Should they be caught, the controller would visit the family and deliver compensation in cash.

The criminal grip on urban commerce and politics that began in the nineteenth century, implemented by Du Yuesheng in Shanghai in the 1930s and cemented by his move to Hong Kong in 1951, meant that not only British Hong Kong but also Chinese Hong Kong was always teetering on the brink of legitimacy. Added to this was the fact that most of the ethnic Chinese who had arrived in Hong Kong spoke or adopted the dialect of the *chiu chau* people, which is notoriously difficult and exclusive, making commercial transactions opaque at best, and an impartial and increasingly independent Hong Kong took in not only the economic migrants but an organized-crime hierarchy that established itself with rapacious efficacy. Throughout the twentieth century, disillusioned soldiers, sailors and fugitives from the law gathered and entered the heroin trade in Hong Kong. They later followed natural routes of emigration through the massive port cities of Europe, such as Naples, Marseilles, Amsterdam and Rotterdam, and then New York, San Francisco and Vancouver in the US and Canada. Italy, France, Holland, America and Canada all possess largely uncontrolled and porous borders that allow for the movement of people and narcotics. The alleged activities of the Ma brothers, *chiu chau* speakers from Canton, illustrate the almost mainstream aspect of Hong Kong organized crime. The brothers arrived in Hong Kong in the 1960s and, in 1969, established the *Oriental Daily News*, a popular tabloid newspaper with a current daily readership of over 3 million people. Ma Yik Shing, also known as 'White Powder Ma', was charged by the Hong Kong government in the summer of 1977 with conspiracy to traffic in morphine and opium. The brothers fled to Taiwan and Ma Sik Yu died in 1992, still a fugitive. The Hong Kong government's main witness, Ng Sik Ho, popularly known as 'Limpy' owing to a leg injury, died in 1991, his testimony and evidence perishing with him. The true whereabouts of Ma Yik Shing are unknown, although, since the death of Limpy Ho, his British lawyers have made repeated requests for him to be permitted to return to Hong Kong at the end of his life. These requests have been met with continued refusal and the promise of immediate arrest should Ma Yik Shing return to the island. Taiwan will not tolerate any discussion about extradition, but maintains that it is strenuous in its efforts to combat organized crime, and will collaborate with Chinese police to that end. The *Oriental Daily News* remains the most popular newspaper in Hong Kong.

Drugs, along with vice and racketeering, were the mainstays of the colony's organized criminal network. Corruption in the Royal Hong Kong Police Force was a major problem, with many officers supplementing their relatively low wages through bribery and blackmail, known as 'tea money'. Arrest warrants for those suspected of smuggling were often issued after the subject had left the harbour area. In 1973, the Chief Superintendent of the RHKPF, Peter Fitzroy Godber, was found to have amassed millions of dollars in various bank accounts. He was tipped off, and fled to Britain, but was later extradited and stood trial, serving four years in prison. The Godber incident led to the creation of the Independent Commission Against Corruption in 1974, which has been called 'one of the best parting gifts from the colonial government'.[38] The ICAC made huge inroads in cleaning up police corruption, and just in the nick of time.

A sharp rise in the numbers of resident heroin addicts to around 45,000 in the early 1980s resulted in a renewed attempt by the government and law enforcement agencies to get a hold on the trade. It was concentrated inside the 9.25-acre site of the old Chinese fort, which had become a slum known as the Walled City, where drugs, prostitution and gambling went on in plain sight with little attempt to control the Triad gangs who operated there. With around 20,000 residents packed into the crumbling, labyrinthine, centuries-old site, the police had been faced with an impossible task in controlling the Walled City since at least the 1950s. A police report from 1955 gives an insight into the character of the neighbourhood at that time, where there were 648 buildings, some as high as 14 storeys, and 120 huts, between them housing 120 narcotics divans, 20 brothels, 5 gambling houses, 9 dentists, 94 shops (many of them specializing in dog meat) and 4 schools. The same year, police seized over 17,000 packets of heroin and morphine powder alone within the Walled City, but they were fighting a losing battle.[39] With only a few entrances and exits, and a warren of passageways within, 'swarming with mendicants suffering from all sorts of diseases', suspects could be lost to sight within a moment. The Triads were also quick to react to any attempt to bring in new legislation. Owing to the long history of opium use in Hong Kong, it was not illegal to be an addict, only to possess narcotics. Inside the Walled City, the gangs set up impromptu 'clinics' where users could come for their hit, and then go back to the streets empty-handed. As IV heroin use took over from the heroin pipe the older Chinese had favoured, these clinics were a fast and efficient way to do business.

The Godber scandal and creation of the ICAC heralded the beginning of the end for the Walled City and its endemic heroin trade (it was finally demolished in 1994, and replaced with a municipal park). Wider changes to the law meant that ships found carrying narcotics in Hong Kong waters, which was still the primary method of smuggling it in, meant that the vessels' owners were now liable. Between 1976 and 1978, in a push to disrupt police corruption, the Triads and the heroin trade, the ICAC managed to shut down the notorious Yau Ma Tei fruit market in West Kowloon, which had been a centre for narcotics import and the Hong Kong heroin trade. The resulting arrests of eighty-seven local officers left the police station there virtually unmanned.

The continued success of the ICAC has seen a vast improvement in Hong Kong's law enforcement structure, but the late 1970s and early 1980s saw a huge rise in both seizures and the trade itself. As the CIA shored up the Golden Triangle of Burma, Thailand and Laos, the boom in production and advances in refinement meant that Hong Kong became an international centre for the production of high-quality heroin. New technology such as mobile phones and pagers also gave the criminal gangs the edge over law enforcement agencies, which were slower to adopt them. Despite two bumper years for heroin seizures in 1983 and 1984, including a record haul of 298 kilos found in a fishing net off Ping Chau, the 1980s cemented Hong Kong's position as one of the world's key locations for the refinement and movement of heroin.[40]

Up in the hills of the Triangle, extended families laboured to produce the opium latex that then made its way to Hong Kong, from where it fanned out across the world. Each small family group, averaging five workers, could produce up to fifteen kilos of latex from a good harvest, although more usually nine or ten, which would still produce over a kilo of morphine.

The production of heroin is not a magical process, but an industrial one. It can be done in a bathtub, as demonstrated by a defiant group of Polish university students in 1976 (leading to the invention of *Kampot*, a cheap and unreliable version of home-cooked heroin still popular in Poland), but the easiest and most common method is to stack clean oil drums onto bricks or blocks thirty or forty centimetres above the ground and to build a wood fire beneath them.[41] Into each drum, 115 litres of water are poured and then ten to fifteen kilos of opium latex are added. The resulting mixture is sieved for impurities before slaked lime or calcium hydroxide is added, which binds to the morphine solution and makes it rise to the top. When it is almost cool, it is scooped out and put into different cooking pots for reheating or 'cooking'. Ammonium chloride is added as the morphine heats, creating a telltale strong smell of urine, making it risky to have a heroin kitchen in the stacked apartments of New York City and Hong Kong, but irrelevant in the vast expanses of Turkey, Afghanistan and the Mexican highlands.

The pH levels of the solution are monitored until it precipitates, or crashes, to the bottom of the drum, from where it is poured through muslin filters then spread out on baking trays to dry. This morphine base is then ready to be processed into smoking or IV heroin. The process can be scaled up or down, and some of the most basic heroin kitchens only possess a wok, a measuring cup, a plastic funnel, coffee filter papers, litmus paper and a steel pan. Industrial kitchens feature bottled-gas ovens, food mixers and fan extractors, still all ordinary items featured in homes around the world.

To cook heroin from morphine base takes between four and six hours. The simplest form is 'black tar' heroin, popular in Mexico and some parts of West Africa. This is the quickest and cheapest way to produce a heroin that can be sticky like tar, but also hard, or rock-like.

To produce the brown or white forms of heroin, the dried morphine base is crushed in a food mixer, then put into a pan to which acetic anhydride is added. Acetic anhydride has been a common compound used in chemical processes for years, and since it has been used to modify starch for food purposes, bulk imports of it into the USA are either ignored or passed without question. It is easily available in large quantities and when added to morphine base, after two hours of continuous heating at eighty-five degrees Celsius, will produce impure heroin. The skill of the heroin cook comes into play at this point, when No.3 or No.4 are created. Sodium carbonate is added for stability, until the mixture stops fizzing, and the heroin is now only up to two-thirds of the weight of the morphine, which was only one-tenth of the weight of the opium latex. To create smoking heroin is simple: the

base is mixed with hydrochloric acid, another industrial compound found easily across the globe. Each kilo is stirred slowly
with the acid until heroin hydrochloride is formed, after which
various adulterants can be added, such as caffeine, quinine or
strychnine. This is heroin No.3, the brown-coloured pieces of
which are ground up and packaged for sale. It is most easily consumed by snorting or smoking, but can be mixed with lemon juice
or vinegar and filtered through cotton wool for intravenous use.

To create the coveted heroin No.4, chloroform is added to the
mixture and left to stand, which binds to the impurities in the
solution and creates a heavy red grease at the bottom of the pan.
The pourable solution is drained off, and purified repeatedly
with activated charcoal, until it is colourless. Again, sodium carbonate is added until the powder becomes very white, after
which it is dried, mopped with filter paper and then ground into
powder and pressed into 700 gram or 350 gram bricks of 85–95
per cent purity, which is easily soluble for IV use.[42]

Cooking highly refined heroin using basic kitchen equipment
in trying surroundings is what the best of the Cantonese heroin
cooks specialize in, and they are transported around the world
for their work. Just like Mecca during the *hajj*, spring in Chiang
Mai is a market for bulk heroin and a recruitment fair for the
best chefs.

Throughout the 1970s, various members of the Thai government set fire to, or otherwise destroyed, seized shipments of
heroin in the public eye, to convince the West that they were on
the side of narcotics enforcement. Yet each successive military
enforcer was holding back a portion of the seized drugs for personal gain. Their main traffic is with the Netherlands, and neither
Thailand nor the Netherlands have conspiracy laws, so possession
is the only possible charge – there is no 'intent to supply' indict-
ment.

The world's second-largest Triad, the 14K gang, operated with impunity throughout northern Europe during the 1970s, culminating in the obvious and flamboyant murder of Kay Wong, a Chinese restaurant owner from Essex who was kicked to death in London's Soho during a game of mah-jong over a botched heroin delivery in Amsterdam. The body of the errant dealer was found decomposing in the sand dunes of The Hague's Scheveningen two weeks later, with eight bullets in his chest and hundreds of guilders stuffed into his suit pockets, done to prove that the killing had been one of honour, not just another tiresome mugging. Despite fleeing to the north of England and Wales, the killers of Kay Wong were found guilty of manslaughter in London's Old Bailey in November of 1976 and served terms of five to fourteen years.

The 1970s marked a period of intense global turf war for the Triads, who were establishing themselves in Western cities and using the narcotics trade to gain a foothold. The trial of Shing May Wong – no relation to Kay Wong – is a prime example of the relationship between East and West at the time. Shing May Wong was educated mainly in Britain and latterly at the exclusive private school Roedean, then went on to own a beauty salon. After her bullion-dealer father was kicked to death in a Triad honour killing in Singapore, she ascribed her entry to organized crime as an act of revenge, in order to find his murderers. In reality, she was importing and distributing vast quantities of heroin through Heathrow airport with her Chinese Muslim lover, Li Jafaar Ma (also known as Li Mah). In a short time they were earning £9,000 a day, supplying between 250 and 900 addicts at any one time. The accounts were kept carefully, in red double-entry books, in an unoccupied flat in North London, along with kilos of heroin. When the police arrested Li Mah, he took them to the flat, which contained an estimated £700,000

in heroin and two automatic weapons.[43] Shing May Wong tes-
tified that she was a married mother of three, and that she had
trafficked drugs only in order to penetrate the Overlord gang
which ran London's narcotics business, and which she believed
had murdered her father. She had, according to her testimony,
only engaged with Li Jafaar Ma to this end. Judge Michael
Argyle was not convinced. When sentencing her to fourteen
years in prison (later commuted to twelve on appeal), Argyle
told her: 'When your tiny shadow fell upon Gerrard Street,
metaphorically the whole street was darkened and you and your
confederates walked through the shadow of the valley of death.'
Addressing them both, he said, 'When you drove to the West
End of London it was to become spreaders of crime, disease and
corruption, even death.'[44] Shing May Wong was divorced *in
absentia* by the husband she had married in 1966, in Penang's
High Court in March 1980, on the grounds of desertion.

The 1980s saw the Triads dominate global heroin trafficking,
although the numbers of addicts in Hong Kong itself fell. The
Chinese youth were turning instead to cannabis and barbiturates
to relax from high-pressure urban lifestyles. The Triads were
increasingly cleaning up their business, separating the money and
drugs on almost all levels, so that cash and heroin rarely changed
hands in a straightforward trade. Money-laundering became
highly complex, and highly rewarding, allowing the proceeds to be
filtered into restaurants, wholesaling, and other legitimate businesses. Such transactions are hard to pin down, but the DEA in
the United States began to make concerted efforts to identify how
the profits from the narcotics trade were moving around the world,
and who was moving them. A series of investigations culminated
in 1999 with the introduction of the Foreign Narcotics Kingpin
Designation Act. Kingpin works to halt the movement of money
in and out of the drugs trade by seizing the assets of any person

or entity thought to be involved in it. Now seventeen years old, Kingpin is under review: many of those it has designated to be kingpins are dotted around the globe and disappear from sight with the majority of their funds intact, and legitimate, low-paid American employees face losing their jobs in companies and corporations moving the money. The Act has been more successful in South America, owing to banking practices there.

Meanwhile, Hong Kong has returned to Chinese control. The global narcotics trade remains, unsurprisingly, a cornerstone of many of its banking transactions, cloaked as it is by long-established privileges and traditions. This laundering does not only support the lifestyles of the world's kingpins, it also has the ability to fund terrorism. Offshore banks have been linked to facilitating the use of heroin profits to fund terrorism in Afghanistan, and more specifically, the 2008 Islamist terrorist attacks in Mumbai that left 164 people dead and 308 wounded. Dawood Ibrahim, the world's biggest heroin kingpin and, as a drug lord, second only to the late King of Cocaine Pablo Escobar, enabled the terrorists to operate through his network in Mumbai, where he was born the son of a policeman in 1955. The UK Treasury department's Consolidated List of Financial Sanctions Targets listed him in 2003 and, as of November 2017, his entry contains twenty-one aliases (his wife has two), fourteen known passports, multiple addresses across the world and hundreds of millions in suspect assets in the UK alone.[45] His total wealth is estimated by *Forbes* magazine at $6.7 billion and international authorities have a bounty on his capture in the region of $25 million. His main business is heroin trafficking, but he is also heavily involved in weapons and counterfeiting, and is believed by the Indian government to be involved in the flooding of the Indian economy with fake currency, causing economic crisis in 2016. He is believed to move between Pakistan and Dubai, but his true

whereabouts are unknown. His holdings in the Indian construction industry, as well as Bollywood, are legitimate and growing
rapidly, despite the fact that Ibrahim fled India in 1984, impli-
cated in a murder. Ibrahim's D-company organized crime outfit
operates in at least sixteen countries, and his money moves
constantly through the global banking network of tax havens. In
2017, it was reported that he was in a state of depression, as his
only son, aged thirty-one, had chosen to pursue a life of religion,
rather than take up the reins of the family business.

In 2012, the US government handed HSBC a landmark fine
of $1.9 billion for money laundering, the biggest fine for the
crime in history.[46]

Women on Drugs

'Heroin is a very particular drug. It gets inside your head, it
gets under your skin . . . it becomes you'

The role of women in the War on Drugs remains controversial,
much as it was during the Gin Craze in 1740s London. In the case
of Shing May Wong, women, whilst more likely to first be injected
with heroin by a male sexual partner, are still viewed as harbingers
of doom in terms of drug use, forever casting the 'tiny shadow'.

Women, and specifically young women, became the target of
both the narcotic and the counter-narcotic public-relations campaigns of the 1980s and 90s. Increasingly, marketing and image
were becoming important to the heroin trade. Just as the original
morphinists had struggled with sores, blisters and ulcers owing
to infected needles and repeated injection sites, the adulteration
of No.4 heroin with everything from baking to talcum powder
meant that a new generation of opiate users were suffering the
side effects of their habits, never mind the possibility of con-

tracting HIV, hepatitis, or sepsis. The perception of female use of intoxicants was heavily influenced, as it had been during the Gin Craze, by the mainstream media, using alarmist language and shocking images to create sensational stories that remained in the public consciousness. Heroin users in England and Scotland suffered particularly badly with an infected batch of the drug in the mid-1990s, when *Clostridium novyi*, a bug found in soil and faeces, was also found in heroin scores. The infection caused instant sepsis and more than thirty intravenous users died in a matter of days, yet little news of these deaths made it into the papers. Instead, the death of Essex schoolgirl Leah Betts (1977–95), from taking a single MDMA or Ecstasy tablet, was the focus of the media reports in the same week. Her image, yoked to a life-support machine after taking the tablet and drinking seven litres of water in ninety minutes, causing her brain to swell fatally, was front-page news for months, linked inextricably to the plague of narcotics thought to be spreading across Britain. In reality, a young generation in Britain was experiencing a new kind of high through the combination of music and chemical stimulants. As with any youth movement, traditional elements of the media were shocked and outraged, and further stigma became attached to drug use, with heroin representing the apex of a terrifying pyramid. Ecstasy and cannabis were referred to as gateway drugs with increasing frequency, as if once the decision to use drugs was taken, the path to ultimate destruction through intravenous heroin use was inescapable.

The idea of female youth corrupted by the influence of narcotics reached a peak five years later in 2000, with the death in Exmouth, Devon of Rachel Whitear. Whitear had begun taking drugs aged fourteen, and by 1999 was using heroin, for which she sought help. She had overdosed on frequent occasions, likely due to her lack of experience with the drug. Born in Devon, the family had moved to Herefordshire during her childhood, but she had made the move back to Devon as soon as she was independent. As she distanced herself from her family, she grew closer to her boyfriend Luke Fitzgerald, a fellow drug user, with whom she had begun a turbulent relationship in 1997. After a series of family arguments and a failed attempt to study at Bath University, Rachel made the commitment to cease using heroin and to find a safe space for herself in 2000, away from Luke Fitzgerald. She agreed to meet him on the beach at Exmouth, to say goodbye, on Wednesday 10 May. 'She told me she wanted to start a new life for herself. I left her sitting on the beach at about 9.30 p.m. and went straight home. I have not seen Rachel since that time.'[47] The *Telegraph* pursued the story relentlessly over the following seven years. Rachel Whitear's body was found on the floor of her apartment in Exmouth. She was crouched on her knees with a capped syringe in her hand. Whilst the cap of the syringe contained traces of diamorphine, the syringe itself tested negative for controlled substances, indicating that a used cap had been placed on a new syringe. Rachel's body was heavily discoloured and she had been bleeding from her mouth. The efforts of the judiciary were minimal, and there was no immediate post-mortem, likely owing to Rachel's status as a junkie. The coroner, Richard van Oppen, eventually returned an open verdict, unsure of the exact circumstances that had led to her death.

Whitear's family believe there were other people in the room when their daughter died, people who know precisely what happened and who staged her body to make it look like she had overdosed. In an attempt to prevent others suffering the fate of their daughter, her parents allowed the images of her body to be used in a drugs awareness video for teenagers. Little dignity is afforded to any of us in death, and to Rachel Whitear less than most. The use of her image, not as an advisory for other vulnerable young people, but as a scare tactic implying that it could happen to anyone, neglects the evidence that she may not have died of a heroin overdose at all. The exact circumstances of her death remain a mystery, and the small injuries on her body, as well as the blood coming from her mouth, point to final hours that held more than that one last high. Her parents have fought consistently for her to be remembered as a person, regardless of the media's insistence on referring to her as a 'bloated' corpse.[48] Yet Rachel was disinterred in 2004 so that a post-mortem could be carried out, and found to be still wearing the blue and white striped dress and cardigan she died in. The results of the post-mortem were inconclusive.

The dehumanization of Rachel Whitear, even nearly twenty years on from her death, is symptomatic of the treatment of women who do not conform to the rules of society. It also discounts the textbook induction of a young woman into a heroin habit by a controlling male partner. Luke Fitzgerald has since been called to testify about what happened the day Rachel died. Now clean of heroin for some years, the inconsistencies in his story may not be criminal, but they are reprehensible, as evidenced by his own words: 'I was not happy with her, she was not happy with me. The question did I love Rachel – I did not really know what love was.'[49] It is partly answers such as these, when coupled to the statistics regarding female IV heroin use, that lead government researchers to conclude that 'Gender inequalities remain a driver of ill health.'[50]

Smack Attack

Where opiates and opioids are available, people will consume them. The difficulties with the increase in worldwide heroin production have come largely since the 1960s, when heroin networks widened, and it became easier and cheaper to obtain. In 1956, Britain had only fifty-four registered heroin users. After first becoming a problem in Liverpool in the early 1970s, heroin addiction spread rapidly to Manchester and then Glasgow and Edinburgh throughout the 1980s, becoming an epidemic in the 1990s. These four cities were suddenly flooded with high-quality smokeable heroin, although most users began injecting quickly. Unemployment and poor living standards made the temporary but warm oblivion of heroin seem an inviting choice. The Muirhouse Estate in Edinburgh was famous as the setting for the film *Trainspotting*, based on Irvine Welsh's novel, published in 1993, about four friends who use heroin together, living chaotic and ultimately tragic lives, before attempting to seek redemption. *Trainspotting* appeared in 1996, when heroin was devastating those cities. HIV was rife, along with hepatitis, and for long-term users, diabetes was associated with their general lifestyles. The people who became addicts then and who survived are in poor health now, particularly in Muirhouse. Many remain addicted, living in social housing, and still unemployed. Even those who have succeeded in getting clean are often little better off.[51]

A scant five years after the beginning of Britain's heroin troubles, Portugal found itself in the same situation. After the revolution of 1974 overthrew the authoritarian government, people became consumers, at the same time as the heroin trafficking route across Portugal and to Brazil became much more attractive for smugglers, just as the former USSR would experience less than two decades later. Heroin was an epidemic. By 2001, Portugal, previously the warehouse of Europe and a mighty naval presence across the world, had become one of the most drug-ridden and poorest countries in the West. The drug-using population of perhaps 50,000–60,000 drug addicts were living mainly in the Lisbon area, so the problem there seemed over-whelming, much like in Edinburgh. Faced with the need to take drastic action, the country initiated what was effectively a sur-vival drive: it legalized all drugs in July 2001. The legalization of heroin, coupled with needle exchange and a bare-bones yet sup-portive healthcare system, yielded fast and unexpected results: not only did illicit drug use fall, so did rates of overdose and chronic drug-related illnesses, and HIV infection fell by 95 per cent. Health-workers handed out packs of clean needles and talked with users from mobile dispensaries. Support for those wanting to adopt MMT is widely available and supported by local pharmacies, who dispense either methadone or buprenor-phine, a semi-synthetic opioid dropped on or under the tongue, which has the advantage of not suppressing the respiratory system in the same way as morphine. Checking in regularly with the treatment programme is also strongly encouraged.

Portugal's thirteen-point plan for decriminalization is clear and thorough, and number one is to reinforce international cooperation, before decriminalization at number two. Anyone caught with less than a ten-day supply for personal use does not face prosecution. Dealers are still imprisoned if intent to supply is proven. Written by João Goulão, a doctor specializing in addiction, it is the most impressive piece of drug legislation in recent history, after the UN's 1988 Convention Against Illicit Trafficking in Narcotic Drugs, which outside decriminalization shares the same ethos, and concentrates on cooperation and also the monitoring of precursors used to make finished narcotic products. Although many are in favour of the Portuguese model, it has reaped such rewards for reasons that may not work in other countries. Different users around the world purchase and consume their highs in vastly different ways, and Portugal's heroin users were mainly collected in one place, stigmatized, often homeless, and a visible problem. In more scattered populations of users, it would be hard to get the same effect. Spain and Italy both decriminalized the possession of small amounts of narcotics before Portugal, but have seen rising heroin use, and cannabis is almost endemic. But there is no denying Portugal's achievements, and its determination to keep addicts connected to the treatment system.

Portugal's remarkable success in abandoning any attempt on a war on the users of drugs since 2001 is material evidence of the fact that there is no need for one. It is all the more remarkable for being implemented at almost the same moment as people began to buy their drugs on a new free market: the Internet.

In 1971–2, students at Stanford and MIT used ARPANET, or the less-catchy Advanced Research Projects Agency Network, to conduct a marijuana deal, the first known electronic exchange (although some argue that the first true financial transaction was on 11 August 1994 for a copy of Sting's *Ten Summoner's Tales*). Just as the original mail-order catalogues provided a way to have your fix delivered to your door, the Internet soon not only delivered, it peer-reviewed. Deals conducted online or on the street were suddenly subject to scrutiny, with ratings correlating to 'Rush, Legs and Count' or quality, longevity and weight per glassine packet, with such gems as 'Fire as fuck, small bags though,' for the Mad Dog brand of heroin available in New Brunswick, New Jersey.[52] Packets are stamped with everything from guns to skulls and Louis Vuitton logos.

Internet-based peer-reviewing systems work remarkably well in the illegal narcotics business. The forums are free to access, and consumers are quick to complain if their scores are substandard. Adulteration (the addition of other drugs) and dilution (the addition of inert substances to bulk out the product) are not as common as might be expected in an illegal enterprise. While the quality of heroin itself is variable, owing to point of origin, testing of 228 heroin samples in the UK between 1995 and 1996 revealed that nearly half the samples had not been adulterated at all.[53] Another study, ten years later in New York, found that where heroin was cut, it was over 60 per cent pure, with the most frequent other additions including 'acetaminophen, caffeine, malitol, diazepam, methaqualone, or phenobarbital'.[54] Urban myths involving the cutting of street heroin with ground glass, or caustic soda, are simply myths, but the Internet offers a not inconsiderable element of consumer protection in a fraught market, particularly with the cutting of heroin scores, with fentanyl becoming more prevalent in recent years.

What is widely referred to as the darknet is not hard to find, or to buy from. The main business of the darknet is the sale of narcotics and pharmaceuticals, followed closely by child pornography. Of these, cannabis and then pharmaceuticals take up the lion's share, with heroin only around 5–6 per cent. The preferred currency is bitcoin, which emerged in 2008 as a new and anonymous way of facilitating online purchases. Few people truly know who created bitcoin, although the most common name given is Satoshi Nakamoto. This is an alias, and many sources point to Nick Szabo or Hal Finney, American cryptographers. Finney was the first person to receive a payment via bitcoin, and died in 2014. Szabo denies involvement. The adept and varied use of English colloquialisms – earning or 'mining' bitcoins requires the miner to find a number called the 'nonce', for example – indicates that the originator of bitcoin is not Japanese, may be more than one person, and is probably not American. Recently, Craig Steven Wright, a forty-seven-year-old Australian computer scientist, claimed to be the originator. Collectively, the founders of bitcoin are worth billions of dollars.

Bitcoins are a source of endless speculation, but they are only a credit system, based upon the same lines as opium, tea and bullion in the eighteenth and nineteenth centuries. The bitcoin system is the work of a solitary or collective genius, as is the narcotic infrastructure of the Internet. One of the biggest drug networks was known as the Silk Road, part of the hidden or Tor services of the Internet, where users browse anonymously. The original Silk Road was shut down in 2013, and in the criminal charges against its founder Ross William Ulbricht from Austin, Texas, the FBI stated that from 'February 6, 2011 to July 23, 2013 there were approximately 1,229,465 transactions completed on the site'.[55] The resulting bitcoin commission Ulbricht earned could have been up to $80 million in a single year, mainly from the sale of narcotics. In February 2015 he was given a life sentence without the possibility of parole. Whether Ulbricht was ultimately responsible for the Silk Road remains unknown. His alias, 'Dread Pirate Roberts', is a reference to *The Princess Bride*, a novel of 1973 and a cult film of 1987. Likewise, the Silk Road's replacement, Hansa, was a nod towards the original Hanseatic League, and shut down in July 2017. Its main competitor was Alphabay, the darknet's version of eBay, which facilitated the sale of illegal arms, drugs and extreme pornography, also shut down in the same month.

The USA has spearheaded the prosecution of narcotics retailers on the darknet, in the continued campaign by the FBI, DEA and CIA to police an industry they have no hope of controlling and can only fuel by attempting to do so. On Alphabay alone there were more than a quarter of a million listings at the time it was shut down, as the warning went out across popular mainstream web forums such as Reddit: 'Time to clean your house and make it tidy for law enforcement.'

Reddit itself is increasingly involved in the wider narcotics experience. The web forum site, where people gather to chat online, has various forums dedicated to narcotics, including opioids and heroin. First-time users ask questions, and people celebrate their purchases – 'Approximately 0.3g of some lovely #4 H (not fentanyl), approximately 0.1 of some absolutely top shelf shard and two 2mg clonazepam :)' is not an untypical post. 'Shard' is crystal methamphetamine and clonazepam is a benzodiazepine that is sometimes, ill-advisedly, mixed with heroin. There are also many long-term users looking for advice on how to quit, and friends and families seeking help. It is a strictly peer-monitored site and no selling or sourcing is allowed. The opioid and heroin forums are, in the main, positive and supportive, particularly for people wanting to change their lives.

Addictions are even made into apps now, in which you can see how many minutes, hours, days or months you've stayed clean, speak to other addicts in a forum, or try to find help. Some even geolocate your phone if you're 'cold-copping' from a dealer you don't know, in case something bad happens. In all the forums there are stories of hustling, violence, misery, loneliness, frustration, but also great kindness and human camaraderie, from the local warnings about fentanyl-spiked heroin, to a lady whose partner has been prescribed opiates for back pain, and doesn't know if he should eat before or after his medication. Her first post was, 'A question about high fat meals, please?'

Generation Oxy

'Change is coming, it has to'

As the use of the Internet to buy and sell narcotics became popular in the 1990s, the pharmaceutical industry was producing better and more sophisticated synthetic opioids. In 1996, Purdue Pharma, founded in New York and with a long history of producing pain medication, brought out a new drug that was quickly adopted across the worldwide medical industry for chronic pain: OxyContin. It had already developed MS Contin twelve years before, a slow-release version of morphine. Purdue prided itself on the slow-release system of its drugs, which release over a twelve-hour period providing measured pain relief, and marketed them aggressively to doctors and prestigious medical journals. They also funded non-profit pain-management organizations and research groups with the sole aim of promoting opioids, namely OxyContin, as an all-round pain-management method. But opiate addicts can achieve a high by snorting or injecting Oxy, as it became known. By presenting themselves to different doctors, or 'doctor-shopping', they could obtain large amounts of pills to either sell on or use. When the medical profession began to report that they were under pressure from obvious shoppers – coupled with a negative report from an addiction monitoring body sponsored by Purdue themselves, Researched Abuse, Diversion and Addiction-Related Surveillance (RADARS) – widespread concern surfaced. RADARS found that OxyContin and hydrocodone were by far the most abused prescription opioids. However, they were followed, in order, by other oxycodones, methadone, morphine, hydromorphone, fentanyl and then buprenorphine. The report's findings included that the OxyContin abuse was most prevalent with recreational drug users and street addicts; no surprise, given the appearance of morphine and buprenorphine on the list, raising multiple questions about how legal supplies were being diverted. But that wasn't the whole story, and other studies found heroin addicts who had started out with an OxyContin prescription and later turned to heroin, an echo of the naive morphinated patients of the nineteenth century. 'But they don't think of them as drugs, they think of them as medication, and this is the problem,' relates Cat Marnell, former New York beauty editor and drug blogger.[56] There were rumours of gross overselling by Purdue, coupled with inappropriate prescriptions from doctors: from 1991 to 2011, opioid prescriptions dispensed by US pharmacies went from 76 million to 219 million. Purdue was fined over $600 million in 2007 and was put under serious pressure by the Connecticut Attorney General Richard Blumenthal to reformulate the drug. As as result, in 2010 Purdue released a gel form of OxyContin that could not be crushed and powdered, much to the disappointment of its millions of American fans. This sudden cut-off came just as massive amounts of heroin began to move from Mexico into the US, as well as coinciding with very high Afghan production. Suddenly, heroin was everywhere, and seizures by the DEA found it was high-purity, and cheap, so in lieu of the previous OxyContin pill, users turned to it. A study by the Centers for Disease Control and Prevention (CDC) found that not only had use increased in the typical user, white males aged eighteen to twenty-five, it had more than doubled in women and other non-typical user groups, such as those in the top wage bracket.[56] America was suddenly under siege from the Middle East and Mexico. It became rapidly worse. The CDC found doctors in certain states, such as West Virginia, all of the Southern states and particularly Florida, had prescribed large amounts of opioid painkillers to their patients.[58] In Florida, a huge number of pill mills sprung up, selling opioids without prescriptions. The pill presses are made in China, and the synthetic opiates can also be ordered on the Internet, with instructions for how to make the pills. They arrive in the mail, and are virtually risk-free; and fentanyl, or its analogues such as another street drug China White, are so powerful that they can be packed as a sachet of silica gel inside a box of urine test strips. The Chinese are making up for the addiction once thrust upon them.

The people who are cutting the fentanyl with other drugs, including heroin, often misjudge the dosage, because a fatal dose is so small. There is also a new demand for another Paul Janssen creation, a synthetic opioid analogue far more powerful than fentanyl, known as carfentanil, whose brand name was Wildnil: an elephant anaesthetic. It has been found by the narcotics police in New Hampshire, where overdoses and deaths from synthetic opioids are becoming unmanageable for the state services. In 2015, every two out of three drug deaths was due to fentanyl. In two weeks in March, the police department of Manchester, New Hampshire were called out to sixty-four overdoses, which were either fentanyl or carfentanil.[59] Police and paramedics are carrying naloxone, known as Narcan, on their standard issue equipment. Naloxone, when injected – or sprayed into the nose of someone who has overdosed – blocks the opiate receptors, but it must be administered quickly. New Hampshire has a high rate of opioid prescriptions, coupled with the second-lowest substance and addiction assistance spending in the country, so perhaps it's hardly surprising they are only second behind West Virginia in terms of opioid deaths. Fentanyl, the painkiller that had proved its worth to countless cancer and spinal-surgery patients, as well as on the battlefields of the Middle East, has become a popular recreational high among the rural poor of America.

Owing to deaths in or around libraries, which are seen as a safe place to inject, librarians in San Francisco, Denver and Philadelphia are now trained to administer naloxone. But the numbers are still rising, and in 2016 there were 20,000 American deaths from fentanyl alone, exceeding heroin for the first time, including the musician and long-term opiate user Prince Rogers Nelson in the spring of 2016.

America's drug epidemic has been born not only out of

Mexico, the Middle East or China, but its own pharmaceutical industry and poor healthcare support. Two decades of rampant over-prescription of opioid medications in the US, reaching a high of 255,207,954 in 2012, and equating to 81.3 prescriptions for every 100 people, directly preceded the start of the current American heroin epidemic which commenced the following year.[60] Some counties, such as Walker County, Alabama, saw rates as high as 335.1 opioid prescriptions per 100 persons.[61] By 2014, Walker County had also seen a vast spike in incarceration for drug-related offences, and had the highest rate of drug over-dose deaths in the state.[62] From 2012 to 2016, US physicians cut the prescription rate for opioids to just under 215 million nation-wide, but deaths from illegally obtained opioids continue to rise, and by the end of 2016 total opioid overdose deaths were five times higher than in 1999.[63] For many, such as the State's Attorney for Lake County, Illinois, Michael Nerheim, 'The source of this crisis is not on street corners; it's in boardrooms'.[64] Some of the biggest names in the business are currently defending their actions in opiod scandals, and in the year leading up to September 2017, more than thirty US cities, states and counties either filed law suits, or began the process of filing them, against manu-facturers and distributors of opiod medication.[65]

Atul Gawande, the renowned American surgeon and public-health specialist, has stated that 'We are running out of ways to emphasize how dire the opioid crisis has become,' and placed the blame at the door of doctors and pharmaceutical companies in an article in April 2017. America's current opioid crisis is more complicated than the short soundbites put out by public com-mentators and politicians might indicate, and it will not be resolved quickly, if at all. The appetite for bigger, better, faster and stronger, to the point where there is now an active trade in opioid that will sedate elephants, indicates a deeper malaise in the American psyche, as does the inability to take any sort of effective action. Yet dissent is rising, with high-profile experts such as Gawande in the vanguard. As he says, 'We cannot sit idly by. We surgeons turn out to be suppliers of the excess prescription opiates fueling addiction and death by overdose. We have to change that. And we now know how we can.'[66]

Change will not be as simple as that. Gawande's statement is only the repetition of a fact that has been evident for over a century. Doctors will always seek to doctor, and the pharmaceutical companies and banks with their gigantic profits are unlikely to abandon their revenue without a fight. Organized crime has responded in step with the threats to their business. The Mexican cartels are working, no longer in competition, but in collaboration with each other to supply the rapacious demands of the continental United States for cheap heroin. Where previously they would have staged street battles over turf, they have adopted the franchise model to profit from a seemingly bottomless market. No amount of empty talk about 'The Wall' will deter them. The Italian-Americans of the East Coast, although no longer in their heyday, are now working to protect their territories in Italy with West African street gangs of such brutality it shocks even the hardened Neapolitan police. The Triads continue to make their way quietly, but surely, in the heroin kitchen and the laboratory. As the Middle East destabilizes, heroin and the funding it brings will become ever more important to whichever group comes next to destroy everything in its path. The drugs are getting more powerful, and the criminals are too. On both sides of the line.

It seems like the obvious answer, but it is unlikely in the extreme that the poppy fields of Afghanistan, the Shan states of Burma or the Sinaloa mountains will be brought under any significant governmental, let alone international control. The world is finding its medical-grade opiates through legally grown poppies in Australia and Tasmania, some of the world's best, as well as India, Turkey, France, Spain, Britain and Hungary. The main production is poppy straw, produced from mashing the whole plant, which is less time-consuming than the traditional scarifying method. Figures regarding production and quality vary as wildly as the estimates for Afghanistan, but it appears things are changing for the better, and we may soon have enough high-quality pain relief for people all around the world. This is not the will of people who would control one resource after another, pretending that it isn't about money and ever-greater power, or for the welfare and safety of their people. No one seeking to control the world's poppy fields is in it for the greater good, whichever side of the political or economic fence they are on. But one thing is for sure, under capitalism or communism, the opium poppy will thrive. It will be there when we most need it. It always has been.

Ultimately, we must never forget that this is a battle fought only with ourselves. From those Neolithic settlements at the edge of Swiss lakes, to Brooklyn street corners and end-of-life care in quiet, anonymous hospitals across the world, the poppy has held humanity's hand and will continue to do so. *Papaver somniferum* remains one of the greatest global commodities there is, and we must seek to mitigate the harm it can do while retaining our faith in the marvels it can achieve. This will be our endless opium war.

AFTERWORD

At dusk on a still and dry day, farmers of the opium poppy walk from the narrow mud alleyways and secluded sun-baked compounds of their villages to their fields, or they climb in cheap rubber boots to jungle terraces, armed with a machete and sweat. They begin work. Three months earlier, the same farmers, and often their wives and children, were in the fields and terraces, planting. They share-crop, which gives them enough labour without impacting profit, or introducing outsiders, idlers or welchers. These bonds stretch through generations and are webbed with intermarriage, fraternity and tribal hierarchy. Planting is hard, hurried work, and the subsequent months of constant weeding, particularly as the seedlings establish themselves, is intensive. Large extended families who are already short of food knit tighter, and work as a unit.

They have waited out the tense days when the poppies have announced their presence, through their brightly coloured petals, to anyone in the vicinity, and now it is time for the harvest. These skilled workers slice each green seed capsule three to four times with a small, sharp knife. The slashes exude a white substance, poppy milk. The men, women and children work carefully and methodically, to keep their clothing and bodies from brushing the capsules, thus sealing them back up with a smear of latex like a sticking plaster and stopping them producing their tears; many favour walking backwards while working, to prevent this happening. Often, they will tie a coloured thread around the neck of the most productive poppies. Those capsules will be harvested when their opium gum is exhausted, and their seeds saved for next season's crop. An acre of poppies is a decent harvest for a family group, and usually the fields are also planted with maize, which protects the vulnerable young plants, both from the climate and from prying eyes, and which along with the poppy stalk is a reliable food for the hardy livestock of the village. They work as quickly as caution will allow; not only will dark soon be upon them, but spending too long among the clacking and rustling stems stirs up the fumes of the gathering milk. In more than one sense, poppy-harvesting is heady work.

Overnight, the milk gathers in rapidly darkening teardrops in the capsule and by morning has solidified into a latex ready for harvesting. In the dawn light they scrape the gum from the capsule with a crescent-shaped spatula, often shiny with generations of use, and lay it out to dry in open wooden boxes. Over the next three to five still days, the process is repeated. When the gum has dried a little, it may be boiled to allow capsule scrapings or bits of stalk to come to the top, before being strained through cheesecloth or sieves. Then it is ready to be packed into marked bags or moulded into balls which are stamped with the farmers' own identifying marks. The opium is now ready to depart on the first step towards its final destination.

From that compound or jungle gate, in some of the poorest countries in the world, heroin will fan across the globe in a constantly churning cycle of cash and consumption.

Four years after beginning to write this book, the reality I live in is altered immeasurably. Last week, my husband watched me watching two men and a woman order a drink at a small bar in the south of France. With gaunt, lantern-jawed faces, stilted, mannered language, and hands that raked their itchy skin, they placed their glasses down with elaborate care as they passed the time. 'That's heroin,' he said. 'I think.'

'Yes,' I replied, and thought of those Afghan compounds and farm gates, as the woman in the group took a naked baby from a pushchair containing not bedding but only a plastic liner, and sat him on her lap, touching his spine with the absent, gentle care of petting a cat, half stroke and half scratch. They sat and talked, full of conversation and communal affection for the fractious child. A smartly dressed man came to sit with them and ordered a drink: the local doctor. He lit a cigarette before asking them how their days had been.

'It's everywhere, isn't it,' my husband remarked, to no one in particular, looking out into the sunny street.

'Yes,' I said again.

As we sat and watched, the very ordinariness of it all made me remember the reasons I so badly wanted to write this book: that addictions of all kinds surround us, making us neither good nor bad, nor less human. They make us who we are. Our petty daily tallies, the small triumphs in the face of finality, are measured out in teaspoons for the billionaire and the street addict alike.

Our reality is that humanity is yoked to opiates for the foreseeable future, whether we are casualties of war, surgery, chronic illness or pain; whether we are facing up to a compromised life or death itself. The mode of delivery may differ, but in every form, from a patch to a pill or an intravenous driver, we are all seeking the key that fits the lock in our bodies, minds and hearts. And this won't end, nor should it. To struggle, to endure and to survive is all we can do, and it is as noble an endeavour as any. The natural world has offered humanity a compound that has evolved to ease our worst fears, and soothe horrendous physical torment. This single fact pulls social, economic, scientific and humanitarian factors into a churning morass of bliss, horror, luxury, depredation, good and evil. The gross crimes concerning opiates committed by gangsters, and by governments in the name of commercial freedom or human rights over the last two centuries, reveal the utter hypocrisy of those who purport to rule their kingdoms. Just as addicts seek to absent themselves from reality and physicians seek to doctor, businesses seek to profit and governments attempt to control. Within all of these parameters, economies are built, both legal and illegal, petty and international. And whether they be sidewalk dope dealers or pharmaceutical giants, merchants know no country, just as the search for even a glimpse of paradise is constant and without end.

ACKNOWLEDGEMENTS

The writing of this book has been a long process, the final form of which inevitably changed as the opioid crisis in America exploded. Huge thanks go to my editor, Georgina Morley, for her patience, encouragement and wisdom. Thanks also to David Milner, Laura Carr and everyone at Pan Macmillan for their great efforts on this book's behalf. As ever, thanks to my agent Kirsty McLachlan, and all the team at David Godwin. Andy Johnston and Lucy Fisher have very kindly given me more professional and expert advice than they needed to, and certainly more of their time. The London, Wellcome and British Libraries have been, again, havens of knowledge and warmth, both human and physical. The London Library remains precious for its dedication to protect its community of writers, and their often precious hours.

Thanks to the team of friends who are always looking out for and taking care of me: Fiona Kirkpatrick, Rory Maxwell, David Child and Clementine Fletcher.

I must also thank Benno Grotz, finest of all neighbours, for his endless kindnesses great and small, and his Bavarian food. Richard Courtney and Kaye Michie have been wonderful cheerleaders and staunch allies. And many thanks to my oldest friend, Max Johnstone, soldier and trekker, because if at half past two on a Friday afternoon my phone rings, I know who it is.

Thank you to my mother, Irene, and my sister, Sally, who have been invaluable sounding boards, and their faith in me and the manuscript has seen me through some very long Lincolnshire days and nights.

Last and first, all my love and thanks to Richard, Mr Inglis, who has supported me through the writing of this book as he always does; with humour, stoicism and stern advice. Without him, it could not have been written.

NOTES

Introduction

1. Khan Bacha, poppy farmer, Nangarhar province, Afghanistan, as reported by Associated Press, 14 November 2013.

Chapter One: The Ancient World

1. Mark Merlin, *On the Trail of the Ancient Opium Poppy* (Fairleigh Dickinson University Press, 1984), pp.53–4.
2. A. M. Niggorski, 'Polypus and the Poppy: two unusual Rhyta from the Mycenean Cemetery at Mochlos' in P. Betancourt, V. Karageorgis, R. Laffineur and W. Niemer (eds.), *Meletemata: Studies in Aegean Archaeology Presented to Malcolm H. Wiener as He Enters His 65th Year* (Université de Liège, 1999), pp.537–42.
3. Carl Trocki, *Opium, Empire and the Global Political Economy* (Routledge, 2012), p.16.
4. Niggorski, pp.537–42; Daniel, Zohary, *Domestication Of Plants In The Old World: The Origin and Spread of Cultivated Plants in West Asia, Europe, and the Nile Valley* (Oxford University Press, 2001), p.109.
5. Merlin, p.28.
6. Susan McCarter, *Neolithic* (Routledge, new edn, 2007), p.xii.
7. Andrew Moore, Gordon Hillman and Anthony Legge, *Village*

on the Euphrates: From Foraging to Farming at Abu Hureyra (Oxford University Press, 2000).

8. Juliet Clutton-Brock, 'Origins of the dog: domestication and early history' in James Serpell (ed.), *The domestic dog: its evolution, behaviour and interactions with people* (Cambridge University Press, 1995), p.11.

9. Ofer Bar-Yosef, Avi Gopher, Eitan Tchernov and Mordechai Kislev, 'Netiv Hagdud: An Early Neolithic Village Site in the Jordan Valley', *Journal of Field Archaeology*, Vol. 18, No. 4 (Winter, 1991), pp.420–1.

10. Disciplinary Committee Inquiry of the Greyhound Board of Great Britain, 13/10/2015, p.1.

11. Jordi Juan-Tresserras and María Josefa Villalba, 'Consumo de la adormidera (*Papaver somniferum L.*), en el Neolítico Peninsular: el enterramiento M28 del complejo minero de Can Tintorer', *Il Congrés del Neolític a la Península lherica SAGVNTVM-PLAV*, Extra-2 (1999), pp.397–404.

12. Robert Kunzig and Jennifer Tzar, 'La Marmotta', *Discover*, November 2002.

13. Ibid.

14. Ferran Antolín and Ramon Buxó, 'Chasing the traces of diffusion of agriculture during the Early Neolithic in the Western Mediterranean Coast', *Congrés Internacional Xarxes al Neolític – Neolithic Networks Rubricatum. Revista del Museu de Gavà*, 5 (2012), p.96.

15. Nicholas Postgate, *Bronze Age Bureaucracy: Writing and the Practice of Government in Assyria* (Cambridge University Press, 2013), p.112.

16. Mark Golitko and Lawrence H. Keeley, 'Beating back ploughshares into swords: warfare in the Linearbandkeramik', *Antiquity*, 81 (2007), pp.332–42.

17. Jan Harding and Frances Healy, *A Neolithic and Bronze Age Landscape in Northamptonshire: The Raunds Area Project* (English Heritage, 2008), p.36.

18. Mark Robinson, 'Macroscopic Plant Remains from The

Wilsford Shaft, Wiltshire', *Ancient Monuments Laboratory Report*, 55/88, pp.1–11.

19. Jane McIntosh, *Handbook of Life in Prehistoric Europe* (Oxford University Press USA, 2009), p.107, and for details of the bodies, Gerald Brenan, *South From Granada* (Penguin, 2008), p.189.

20. Trocki, p.16.

21. R. Campbell Thompson, *Assyrian Medical Texts From The Originals In The British Museum* (Oxford University Press, 1923), p.112.

22. Charles E. Terry and Mildred Pellens, *The opium problem, For the Committee on Drug Addictions in collaboration with the Bureau of social hygiene, inc.* (New York, Bureau of Social Hygiene, 1928).

23. Dr Erica Reiner, Assyriologist and philologist, Oriental Department, University of Chicago, quoted in Abraham D. Krikorian, 'Were the Opium Poppy and Opium Known in the Ancient near East?', *Journal of the History of Biology*, Vol. 8, No. 1 (Spring, 1975), p.102.

24. Elena Marinova and Soultana-Maria Valamoti, 'Crop Diversity and Choice in Prehistoric Southeastern Europe: Cultural and Environmental Factors Shaping the Archaebotanical Record of Northern Greece and Bulgaria' in Alexandre Chevalier, Elena Marinova and Leonor Pena-Chocarro (eds.), *Plants and People: Choices and Diversity through Time* (Oxbow, 2014), p.72.

25. Merlin, p.184.

26. S. Marinatos, 'The Volcanic Destruction of Minoan Crete', *Antiquity* (1939), 13, pp.425–39.

27. Joan Aruz, Sarah B. Graff and Yelena Rakic, *Cultures in Contact: From Mesopotamia to the Mediterranean in the Second Millennium BC* (Metropolitan Museum of Art, 2013), pp.40–1.

28. Mari tablet ARMT 21.432, 4–12, quoted in A. Bernard Knapp, 'Spice, Drugs, Grain and Grog: Organic Goods in East Mediterranean Bronze Age Trade' in *Bronze Age Trade in the Mediterranean, Studies in Mediterranean Archaeology*, 90 (P. Astroms Forlag, 1991).

29. Helen Askitopoulou, Ioanna A. Ramoutsaki and Eleni

Konsolaki, 'Archaeological Evidence On The Use Of Opium In The Minoan World', *International Congress Series*, Volume 1242 (December 2002), p.3.

30. P. G. Kritikos and S. P. Papadaki, 'UNODC – Bulletin On Narcotics – 1967 Issue 3 – 003', *Unodc.org*. N.p., 2015. Web. 6 June 2015.

31. C. Pedro Behn, 'The Use of Opium in the Bronze Age in the Eastern Mediterranean', Listy filologické / Folia philologica, Roč. 109, Čís. 4 (1986), p.195.

32. V. Karageorghis, 'A Twelfth-century BC Opium Pipe from Kition', *Antiquity* (1976), p.125.

33. Kritikos and Papadaki, 'UNODC . . .'.

34. Askitopoulou, Ramoutsaki and Konsolaki, pp.23–9.

35. Ferribyboats.co.uk, 'Information On The Possible Performance Of The Ferriby Boats'. N.p., 2015. Web. 6 December 2015.

36. Hadjisavvas Sophocles, *The Phoenician Period Necropolis of Kition, Volume I*, Shelby White and Leon Levy Program for Archaeological Publications (2013), p.1.

37. Behn, p.194.

38. Silvia Ferrara, *Cypro-Minoan Inscriptions: Volume 2: The Corpus* (Oxford University Press, 2013), pp.81, 126–7.

39. Karageorghis, p.125.

40. Behn, p.195.

41. Giorgos Papantoniou, *Religion and Social Transformations in Cyprus: From the Cypriot Basileis to the Hellenistic Strategos* (Brill Academic Publishing, 2012), p.265.

42. Kathryn Eriksson, 'Cypriot ceramics in Egypt during the reign of Thutmosis III: the evidence of trade for synchronizing the Late Cypriot cultural sequence with Egypt at the beginning of the Late Bronze Age', *Proceedings of a Colloquium held in the Royal Academy of Letters, History and Antiquities, Stockholm, May 18–19, 2000*, p.63.

43. Behn, pp.193–7.

44. Ibid.

45. L. Kapoor, *Opium Poppy: Botany, Chemistry, and Pharmacology* (CRC Press, 1997), pp.2–3.
46. Cynthia Clark Northrup, *Encylopedia of World Trade From Ancient Times to the Present* (Routledge, 2015), p.292.
47. Merlin, p.213.
48. Homer, *The Odyssey*, trans. A. T. Murray (Loeb, 1995), Vol.1, p.135.
49. P. G. Kritikos and S. P. Papadaki, 'The history of the poppy and of opium and their expansion in antiquity in the eastern Mediterranean area', *Journal of the Archaeological Society of Athens*, 1967, pp.17–38.
50. Amelia Arenas and Hippocrates, 'Hippocrates' Oath', *Arion: A Journal of Humanities and the Classics*, Third Series, Vol. 17, No. 3 (Winter 2010), pp.73–4.
51. *Hippocratic Writings*, ed. G. E. R. Lloyd (Penguin, 1983), p.262.
52. Helen King, *Hippocrates' Woman: Reading the Female Body in Ancient Greece* (Routledge, 1998), pp.118–19.
53. http://classics.mit.edu/Aristotle/sleep.html, Part 3.
54. John Scarborough, 'Theophrastus on Herbals and Herbal Remedies', *Journal of the History of Biology*, Vol. 11, No. 2 (Autumn, 1978), pp.370–1.
55. Trudy Ring (ed.), *International Directory of Historic Places, Vol.3: Southern Europe* (Dearborn Fitzroy, 1995), p.374. Opium and hemlock mixture: *Valerius Maximus. II 6. 8*, and Gabriel Welter, 'Aristeides, Lawgiver of Keos', *Archaeological Journal*, 1953–4, Vol. III, pp.158–9, as quoted in Kritikos and Papadaki, 'The history of the poppy . . .', pp.17–38.
56. Flavia Frisone, 'Norms and Change in Greek Funerary Rituals', *Construction of Consensus* (Macmillan, 2011), pp.179–99.
57. Zohara Yaniv and Nativ Dudai (eds.), *Medicinal and Aromatic Plants of the Middle East* (Springer, 2014), p.308.
58. Wilhemina Jeemster Jashemski, *The Natural History of Pompeii* (Cambridge University Press, 2002), p.139.
59. John Scarborough, 'Theophrastus on Herbals and Herbal

Remedies', *Journal of the History of Biology*, Vol. 11, No. 2
(Autumn, 1978), p.372.

60. Pliny the Elder, *Natural History*, trans. Philemon Holland
(1601); Edward Hamilton, *The Flora Homeopathica*, Vol. 1 (H.
Balliere, 1852), p.293.

61. J. Scarborough and V. Nutton, 'The Preface of Dioscorides' De
Materia Medica: Introduction, Translation and Commentary',
*Transactions and Studies of the College of Physicians of
Philadelphia*, Vol.4, No.3 (1982), p.195.

62. Dioscorides, *De materia medica*, Book IV, 64, quoted in Roy
Porter and Mikulas Teich, *Drugs and Narcotics in History*
(Cambridge University Press, 1995), p.13.

63. John Scarborough, 'The Opium Poppy in Roman and
Hellenistic Medicine', in Roy Porter and Mikulas Teich, *Drugs
and Narcotics in History* (Cambridge University Press, 1995),
p.16.

64. Dioscorides, quoted in Mojtaba Heydari, Mohammad Hashem
Hashempur and Arman Zargaran, 'Medicinal Aspects Of
Opium As Described In Avicenna's Canon Of Medicine', *Acta
Medico-Historica Adriatica 11 (1)* (2013), p.103.

65. Nicander of Colophon (2nd century BC), quoted in Roy Porter
and Mikulas Teich, *Drugs and Narcotics in History* (Cambridge
University Press, 1995), p.16.

66. Galen, *Anatomical Procedures*, IX; 10:10 (Oxford University
Press for the Wellcome Historical Medical Museum, 1956),
pp.226–36.

67. Maud W. Gleason, 'Shock and Awe: the performance
dimension of Galen's anatomy demonstrations', in Christopher
Gill, Tim Whitmarsh, John Wilkins, *Galen and the World of
Knowledge* (Cambridge University Press, 2009), p.103.

68. Julius Rocca, 'Galen and the Uses of Trepanation', in Robert
Arnott, Stanley Finger, Chris Smith (eds.), *Trepanation* (Taylor
& Francis, 2005), p.259.

69. Gleason, pp.103–4.

70. Galen XIV, 4, quoted in Thomas W. Africa, 'The Opium

Addiction of Marcus Aurelius', *Journal of the History of Ideas*, 22 (1961), p.99.

71. Ibid.

72. V. Nutton, 'The Drug Trade in Antiquity', *Journal of the Royal Society of Medicine*, Vol. 78 (1985), pp.138–45.

73. Svetlana Hautala, 'The Circulation of Pharmaceutical Recipes in Antiquity as a Kind of Folklore', PhD dissertation, University of Siena, p.1.

74. Nutton, p.145.

75. Quoted in Tom Holland, *In the Shadow of the Sword: The Battle for Global Empire and the End of the Ancient World* (Abacus, 2013), p.194.

Chapter Two:
The Islamic Golden Age to the Renaissance

1. Robert Clarke and Mark Merlin, *Cannabis: Evolution and Ethnobotany* (University of California Press, 2013), p.243.

2. Ilza Veith, *Huang Ti Nei Ching Su Wen; The Yellow Emperor's Classic of Internal Medicine* (University of California Press, 1966), p.3.

3. Herodotus, *The Histories, Book 8: Urania* (Simon & Schuster, 2015), p.99.

4. R. Walz, quoted in Daniel Potts, 'Bactrian Camels and Bactrian-Dromedary Hybrids', *Silk Road Foundation Newsletter*, Vol. 3, No.1: www.silkroadfoundation.org.

5. David Christian, 'Silk Roads or Steppe Roads? The Silk Roads in World History', *Journal of World History*, Vol. 11, No. 1 (Spring, 2000), p.5.

6. Burton Watson, *Records of the Grand Historian of China* (Columbia University Press, 1961), p.123.

7. Subhakanta Behera, 'India's Encounter with the Silk Road', *Economic and Political Weekly*, Vol. 37, No. 51 (21–7 December 2002), p.5078.

8. Watson, p.33.
9. Seneca the Younger, *Declamations Vol. I*; Pliny the Elder quoted in Valerie Hansen, *The Silk Road: A New History* (Oxford University Press, 2012), p.20.
10. Eugene Hugh Byrne, 'Medicine in the Roman Army', *The Classical Journal*, Vol. 5, No. 6 (April 1910), p.271.
11. Pliny the Elder, *Natural History*, Vol.6 (Henry G. Bohn, 1855), p.18.
12. Yulia Ustinova, 'New Latin and Greek Rock-Inscriptions from Uzbekistan', *Hephaistos: New Approaches in Classical Archaeology and Related Fields*, 18/2000, pp.169–79.
13. Lionel Casson, *The Periplus Maris Erythraei: Text With Introduction, Translation, and Commentary* (Princeton University Press, 1989), p.49.
14. Lionel Casson, 'Rome's Trade with the East: The Sea Voyage to Africa and India', *Transactions of the American Philological Association* (1974–), Vol. 110 (1980), p.32.
15. R. N. Frye, *The Cambridge History of Iran, Vol.4: The Period from the Arab Invasion to the Saljugs* (Cambridge University Press, 1975), p.396.
16. Firdausi, *Shanameh*, quoted in Cyril Elgood, *A Medical History of Persia and the Eastern Caliphate* (Cambridge University Press, 2010), p.298.
17. http://www.iranicaonline.org/articles/haoma-ii.
18. Example of botanical argument for *haoma* ingredients: George Erdosy (ed.), *The Indo-Aryans of Ancient South Asia: Language, Material Culture and Ethnicity*, Vol.1 (Walter de Gruyter, 1995), pp.385–9; Mark Merlin, 'Archaeological Evidence for the Tradition of Psychoactive Plant Use in the Old World', *Economic Botany* 57(3), 2003, p.302.
19. *Chronicon ad Annum Christi 1234 Pertinens: 1.237*, quoted in Tom Holland, *In the Shadow of the Sword* (Abacus, 2013), p.3.
20. L. D. Kapoor, *Opium Poppy: Botany, Chemistry and Pharmacology* (Haworth, 1995), p.7.
21. Qur'an, 5:90.

22. J. Edkins, *Opium: Historical Note, or The Opium Poppy in China* (American Presbyterian Mission Press, 1899), p.6.

23. Selma Tibi, *The Medicinal Use of Opium in Ninth-Century Baghdad* (Brill, 2006), p.29.

24. Islamic Medical Association of North America Ethics Committee, 2005, *Publication 2*, p.2.

25. Du Huan, Jinxing Ji, cited by X. Liu, *The Silk Road in World History* (Oxford, 2010), p.101.

26. Saeed Changizi Ashtiyani, Mohsen Shamsi, Ali Cyrus and Seyed Mohammad Tabatabayei, 'Rhazes, a Genius Physician in the Diagnosis and Treatment of Nocturnal Enuresis in Medical History', *Iranian Red Crescent Medical Journal*, August 2013, 15(8), pp.633–8.

27. Paul Barash et al., *Clinical Anaesthesia* (7th edn., Lippincott, 2013), p.5.

28. Cyril Elgood, *A Medical History of Persia and the Eastern Caliphate* (Cambridge University Press, 2010), p.298.

29. Tyler M. Muffly, Anthony P. Tizzano, and Mark D. Walters, 'The history and evolution of sutures in pelvic surgery', *Journal of the Royal Society of Medicine*, March 2011, 104 (3), pp.107–12.

30. Elgood, p.299.

31. Yassar Mustafa, 'Avicenna the Anaesthetist', AAGBI History of Anaesthesia Prize Submission (March, 2014), pp.1–16.

32. Elgood, p.299.

33. Kapoor, p.3.

34. Avicenna, quoted in Mojtaba Heydari, Mohammad Hashem Hashempur and Arman Zargaran, 'Medicinal Aspects Of Opium As Described In Avicenna's Canon Of Medicine', *Acta Medico-Historica Adriatica* 11 (1) (2013), p.109.

35. Avicenna, *Canon of Medicine* (London, 1930), p.717.

36. Lenn Evan Goodman, *Avicenna* (Cornell University Press, 2006), pp.43–4.

37. Andrew Crislip, 'A Coptic Request for Materia Medica', *Zeitschrift für Papyrologie und Epigraphik, Bd. 157* (2006), p.165.

38. Charles Thomas, *Christianity in Roman Britain to AD 500* (University of California Press, 1981), p.197.

39. Diodorus Siculus, quoted in Jacob G. Ghazarian, *The Mediterranean legacy in early Celtic Christianity: a journey from Armenia to Ireland* (Bennett & Bloom, 2006), p.49.

40. H. J. Edwards (trans.), *Caesar: The Gallic War* (Heinemann, 1909), pp.109–11.

41. Quoted in Wilbur Fisks Crafts, *Intoxicants & opium in all lands and times* (International Reform Bureau, 1900), p.283.

42. John H. Harvey, 'Garden Plants of Moorish Spain: A Fresh Look', *Garden History*, Vol. 20, No. 1 (Spring, 1992), pp.71–82.

43. Pernille Rohde Sloth, Ulla Lund Hansen and Sabine Karg, 'Viking Age garden plants from southern Scandinavia – diversity, taphonomy and cultural aspects', *Danish Journal of Archaeology*, 1:1, pp.30–1.

44. *Corpus Hippocraticum*, quoted in Peter McDonald, *Oxford Dictionary of Medical Quotations* (Oxford University Press, 2004), p.47.

45. Piers D. Mitchell, *Medicine in the Crusades: Warfare, Wounds and the Medieval Surgeon* (Cambridge University Press, 2004), pp.12, 32.

46. Quoted in Conor Kostick, *The Social Structure of the First Crusade* (Brill, 2008), p.89.

47. M. Chibnall (trans.) and Orderic Vitalis, *The Ecclesiastical History of Orderic Vitalis* (Clarendon Press, 1968–80), Vol. V, pp.80–1.

48. Mitchell, pp.120–2.

49. William of Tyre, *Historia rerum in partibus transmarinis gestarum*, XIX, 23, *Patrologia Latina* 201, 770–1, trans. James Brundage, *The Crusades: A Documentary History* (Marquette University Press, 1962), pp.136–8.

50. Richard Swiderski, *Poison Eaters: Snakes, Opium, Arsenic, and the Lethal Show* (Universal, 2010), p.63.

51. Mitchell, pp.232–5.

52. Ibid., p.19.

53. T. S. Miller, 'The Knights of St John and the Hospitallers of the Latin west', *Speculum*, No. 53, pp.709–33.

54. Ibid.

55. Jonathan Riley-Smith, *The Knights Hospitaller in the Levant, c.1070–1309* (Palgrave Macmillan, 2012), p.72.

56. J. Prawer, *The World of the Crusades* (Weidenfeld & Nicolson, 1972), p.119.

57. Monica H. Green, *The Trotula: A Medieval Compendium of Women's Medicine* (University of Pennsylvania Press, 2001), p.103.

58. Borgognoni, quoted in Mitchell, p.200.

59. E. Campbell and J. Colton (trans.), Theodoric Borgognoni, *The Surgery of Theodoric, ca. AD 1267* (Appleton-Century-Crofts, 1955–60), Vol. 2, p.135.

60. Lluís Cifuentes, 'Vernacularization as an Intellectual and Social Bridge. The Catalan Translations of Teodorico's "Chirurgia" and of Arnau De Vilanova's "Regimen Sanitatis"', *Early Science and Medicine*, Vol. 4, No. 2 (1999), pp.127–48.

61. Luca Mocarelli, 'The guilds reappraised: Italy in the Early Modern period', delivered at the Return of the Guilds Utrecht, Utrecht University, 5–7 October 2006, p.10.

62. Henry Yule (trans.), *The Book of Ser Marco Polo* (John Murray, 1903), pp.140–142.

63. Bruce Lincoln, 'An Early Moment in the Discourse of "Terrorism": Reflections on a Tale from Marco Polo', *Comparative Studies in Society and History*, Vol. 48, No. 2 (April 2006), p.246.

64. Gabriel G. Nahas, M.D., 'Hashish In Islam 9th To 18th Century', *Bulletin of the New York Academy of Medicine, Department of Anesthesiology Columbia University College of Physicians and Surgeons*, Vol.58, No.9 (1982), pp.814–31.

65. Frances Wood, *Did Marco Polo Ever Go To China?* (Avalon, 1998).

66. Yule (trans.), pp.158–9.

67. Christiane Nockels Fabbri, 'Treating Medieval Plague: The

Wonderful Virtues of Theriac', *Early Science and Medicine*, Vol. 12, No. 3 (2007), p.257.

68. Ibid., p.260.

69. Barry Stow Architect Ltd and Associates, 'A Conservation and Management Plan For Merton Priory and Merton Abbey Mills', The Merton Priory Trust and the London Borough of Merton (August 2006), p.40.

70. Daniel Poore, David Score and Anne Dodd, *Excavations at No. 4A Merton St., Merton College, Oxford: The Evolution of a Medieval stone house and tenement and an early college property* (Oxoniensia, 2006), p.229.

71. Christine Winter, 'Prisons and Punishments in Late Medieval London', PhD dissertation, University of London Royal Holloway, University of London (2012), p.88.

72. Louis Sanford Goodman, Alfred Goodman Gilman, *Goodman & Gilman's The Pharmacologie Basis of Therapeutics* (11th edn, Macmillan, 2006), p.50.

73. Sherman M. Kuhn (ed.), *Middle English Dictionary* (University of Ann Arbor, 1980), p.238.

74. *De corporis humani fabrica libri septum*, Syndics of Cambridge University Library (MS Dd.6.29, f79r-v).

75. William D. Sharpe (trans.), *Isidore of Seville, The Medical Writings* (American Philosophical Society, 1964), 54, part 2, p.62.

76. https://www.measuringworth.com.

77. D'Arcy Power (ed.), *John of Arderne, Treatises of Fistula in ano, haemorrhoids and clysters* (Kegan Paul, 1910), p.101.

78. Katharine Park, 'The Criminal and the Saintly Body: Autopsy and Dissection in Renaissance Italy', *Renaissance Quarterly*, Vol. 47, No. 1 (Spring, 1994), pp.8–9.

79. Yule (trans.), p.xcix.

80. Falloppio quoted in Park, p.20.

81. David Jayne Hill, *A history of diplomacy in the international development of Europe*, Vol. 2 (Longman's, 1924), p.268.

Chapter Three: The Silver Triangle and the Creation of Hong Kong

1. Jin Wu, *Zheng He's Voyages of Discovery*, 600th Anniversary Lecture, UCLA Asia Institute, 12 April 2005.
2. Ibid.
3. Christopher Columbus, *The Journal of Christopher Columbus (During His First Voyage, 1492–3)* (Cambridge University Press, 2010), p.41.
4. Robert S. Wolff, 'de Gama's Blundering: Trade Encounters in Africa and Asia During the European Age of Discovery 1450–1520', *The History Teacher*, Vol.31, No.3 (May 1998), p.297.
5. Quoted in Kevin H. O'Rourke and Jeffrey G. Williamson, 'Did Vasco da Gama Matter to European Markets?', *Economic History Review*, 62, 3 (2009), p.655.
6. Ibid., p.657.
7. Gonçalo Gil Barbosa, quoted in Sanjay Subrahmanyam, *The Career and Legend of Vasco Da Gama* (Cambridge University Press, 1997), p.233.
8. Mansel Longworth Dames (trans.), *The Book Of Duarte Barbosa* Vol. 1 (Hakluyt Society, 1918), p.34.
9. Ibid., p.38.
10. Armando Cortesao (trans.), *The Suma Oriental of Tomé Pires* (Hakluyt Society, 1944), p.xxiv.
11. Ibid., p.159.
12. Ibid., p.213.
13. Bartolomé de las Casas, quoted in Peter Frankopan, *The Silk Roads* (Bloomsbury, 2015), p.209.
14. Fernão Lopes de Castanheda, quoted in Manoel Cardozo, 'The Idea of History in the Portuguese Chroniclers of the Age of Discovery', *Catholic Historical Review*, Vol. 49, No. 1 (April 1963), p.7.
15. Cortesao (trans.), p.228.
16. F. W. Mote, *Imperial China, 900–1800* (Harvard University Press, 1999), p.745.

17. A. Kobata, 'The Production and Uses of Gold and Silver in Sixteenth- and Seventeenth-Century Japan', *Economic History Review*, New Series, Vol. 18, No. 2 (1965), p.247.

18. Dennis O'Flynn and Arturo Giraldez, 'Cycles of Silver: Global Economic Unity through the mid-eighteenth century', *Journal of World History*, Vol.13, No.2 (Fall, 2002), p.406.

19. Edward Rothstein, 'A Big Map That Shrank The World', *New York Times*, 10 January 2010.

20. Patricia Ebery, *Women and the Family in Chinese History* (Routledge, 2002), p.208.

21. J. Horton Riley (ed.), *Ralph Fitch, England's Pioneer to India and Burma* (Fisher Unwin, 1899), p.100.

22. Song Gang (ed.), *Reshaping the Boundaries: The Christian Intersection of China and the West in the Modern Era* (Hong Kong University Press, 2016), p.15.

23. Frei Sebastien Manrique, *Itinerario de las Missiones Orientales*, C. E. Luard (trans.) and Fr. H. Hosten (ed.), 2 vols (Hakluyt Society, 2nd series, LIX, 1926), I, VI, pp.59–60.

24. James Brown Scott (trans.), Hugo Grotius, *The Freedom of the Seas* (Oxford University Press USA, 1916), pp.28, 7.

25. Wyndham Beawes, *Lex mercatoria rediviva: or, The merchant's directory. Being a Compleat Guide to All Men In Business* (James Williams, 1773 edn), p.813.

26. Ramusio quoted in Helen Saberi, *Tea: A Global History* (Reaktion Books, 2010), p.83.

27. Adam Olearius, *The voyages and travells of the ambassadors sent by Frederick, Duke of Holstein, to the great Duke of Muscovy and the King of Persia*, trans. John Davies (Thomas Dring and John Starkey, 1662), p.324.

28. C. R. Boxer (ed.), *South China in the sixteenth century: being the narratives of Galeote Pereira, Fr. Gaspar da Cruz, O.P. [and] Fr. Martín de Rada, O.E.S.A. (1550–1575)* (Hakluyt Society, 1953), p.287.

29. Saberi, p.87.

30. http://www.pepysdiary.com/diary/1660/09/25/.

31. Francisco de Arino, *Sucesos de Sevilla de 1592 a 1604*, quoted in Frankopan, p.218.
32. Anthony Reid, 'From betel-chewing to tobacco-smoking in Indonesia', *Journal of Asian Studies*, Vol. 44, No. 3 (May 1985), p.535.
33. Lucie Olivova, 'Tobacco Smoking In Qing China', *Asia Major*, Third Series, Vol. 18, No. 1 (2005), p.226.
34. Reid, p.533.
35. Olivova, p.226.
36. Yongming Zhou, *Anti-Drugs Crusades in Twentieth Century China: Nationalism, History and State Building* (Rowman & Littlefield, 1999), pp.12–13.
37. Yao Lu quoted in Frank Dikotter, Lars Laaman and Zhou Hun, *Narcotic Culture: A History of Drugs in China* (University of Chicago Press, 2004), p.26.
38. Quoted in E. H. Nolan, *The British Empire in India and the East* (James Vertue, 1858), p.33.
39. https://www.measuringworth.com.
40. Philip D. Curtin, *Cross-Cultural Trade in World History* (Cambridge, 1984), p.142.
41. Dikotter, Laaman and Hun, p.26.
42. Quoted in Frank Dikotter, *Narcotic Culture: A History of Drugs in China* (C. Hurst, 2004), p.34.
43. Ibid., p.33.
44. United Nations Office On Drugs And Crime, Bulletin On Narcotics, *A century of international drug control*, Vol. LIX, Nos.1 and 2 (2007), p.12.
45. Quoted in Alfred J. Andrea and James H. Overfield (eds.), *The Human Record: Sources of Global History, Volume II: Since 1500* (Cengage Learning, 2009), p.217.
46. Peter Mundy quoted in Jane Pettigrew, *The Tealover's Companion: A Guide to Teas Throughout the World* (The National Trust, 2005), p.13.
47. Austin Coates, *Macao and the British 1637–1842: Prelude to Hong Kong* (Hong Kong University Press, 2009), p.8.

48. Peter Mundy, *The Travels of Peter Mundy in Europe and Asia, 1608–1667*, ed. Sir Richard Carnac Temple (Hakluyt Society, 1919), Vol. 3, p.207.

49. Ibid.

50. Quoted in Coates, p.15.

51. Weddell quoted in Coates, p.19.

52. Peh T'i Wei, 'Why Is Hong Kong Called "Fragrant Harbour": A Synthesis', *Journal of the Royal Asiatic Society Hong Kong Branch*, Vol. 54 (2014), p.45.

53. Ibid., p.39.

54. Translation from *Research study on Hangzhou Trade in the Late Qing and Republican Eras* (Hangzhou Publishing House, 2011), p.2.

55. *Journal of the House of Commons*, 1714–1718 (House of Commons, reprinted 1803), p.665.

56. F. W. Mote, *Imperial China, 900–1800* (Harvard University Press, 1999), p.745.

57. George Bryan Souza, 'Opium and the Company: Maritime Trade and Imperial Finances on Java, 1684–1796', *Modern Asian Studies*, Vol. 43, No. 1, *Expanding Frontiers in South Asian and World History: Essays in Honour of John F. Richards* (January 2009), p.130.

Chapter Four: The Romantics Meet Modern Science

1. A. S. Beveridge (trans.), *Babur-Nama* (Oriental Books Reprint Corporation, 1970), p.52.

2. Pierre Belon, *Travels in the Levant* (Gilles Courrozet, 1554), p.183.

3. Mehrdad Kia, *Daily Life in the Ottoman Empire* (Greenwood, 2011), p.245.

4. Quoted in Roger Stevens, 'European Visitors to the Safavid Court', *Iranian Studies*, Vol. 7, No. 3/4, Studies on Isfahan:

Proceedings of the Isfahan Colloquium, Part II (Summer–Autumn, 1974), p.429.

5. Quoted in ibid., p.442.

6. Cristobal Acosta, *On the Drugs and Medicines from the East Indies*, quoted in Richard Davenport-Hines, *The Pursuit of Oblivion: A Social History of Drugs* (Hachette, 2012), p.18.

7. Lisa Balabanlilar, 'The Begims of the Mystic Feast: Turco-Mongol Tradition in the Mughal Harem', *Journal of Asian Studies*, Vol. 69, No. 1 (February 2010), p.125.

8. John Henry Grose, *A Voyage to the East Indies* (S. Hooper, 1772 edn.), p.113.

9. Lisa Balabanlilar, *Imperial Identity in the Mughal Empire* (I. B. Tauris, 2012), p.91.

10. Lisa Balabanlilar, 'The Emperor Jahangir and the Pursuit of Pleasure', *Journal of the Royal Asiatic Society*, Third Series, Vol. 19, No. 2 (April 2009), p.182.

11. William Foster (ed.), *The Embassy of Sir Thomas Roe to the Court of the Great Mogul, 1615–1619* (Hakluyt Society, 1899), p.322.

12. Balabanlilar, 'The Begims of the Mystic Feast . . .', p.143.

13. William Shakespeare, *Othello, Moor of Venice*, Act 3, Scene 3.

14. Francis Bacon, *History of Life and Death* (I. Okes, 1623), p.1.

15. Adrian Tinniswood, *His Invention So Fertile* (Jonathan Cape, 2001), p.36.

16. Thomas Spratt, quoted in N. S. R. Maluf, 'History of Blood Transfusion', *Journal of the History of Medicine and Allied Sciences*, Vol. 9, No. 1 (January 1954), p.61.

17. Thomas Sydenham, *The Works of Thomas Sydenham, M.D.* (The Sydenham Society, 1851), Vol. 1, p.143.

18. Thomas Sydenham, *The Works of Thomas Sydenham, M.D.* (The Sydenham Society, 1851), Vol. 1, p.xcix.

19. Thomas Sydenham quoted in Kenneth Dewhurst, 'A Symposium on Trigeminal Neuralgia: With Contributions by Locke, Sydenham, and other Eminent Seventeenth Century Physicians', *Journal of the History of Medicine and Allied Sciences*, Vol. 12, No. 1 (January 1957), p.32.

20. *The Works of Francis Bacon, Lord Chancellor of England*, Vol. 1 (Carey & Hart, 1844), p.203.

21. Samuel Garth, *Oratorio Laudatoria* (Impensis Abel Roper, 1697), p.3.

22. Quoted in Albert Rosenberg, 'The London Dispensary for the Sick-Poor', *Journal of the History of Medicine and Allied Sciences*, Vol. 14, No. 1 (January 1959), p.44.

23. Patrick Wallis, 'Consumption, Retailing, and Medicine in Early-Modern London', *Economic History Review*, New Series, Vol. 61, No. 1 (February 2008), p.32.

24. R. S. Morton, 'Dr Thomas ("Quicksilver") Dover, 1660–1742', *British Journal of Venereal Disease* 44 (1968), p.343.

25. Thomas Dover, *The Ancient Physician's Legacy to his Country* (H. Kent, 1742), p.106.

26. Ibid., p.14.

27. James Boswell, *Boswell's Life of Johnson: including their Tour to the Hebrides* (John Murray, 1851), p.127.

28. 'William and Mary, 1690: An Act for the Encourageing the Distilling of Brandy and Spirits from Corn and for laying severall Dutyes on Low Wines or Spirits of the first Extraction. [Chapter IX. Rot. parl. pt. 3. nu. 8.]' in *Statutes of the Realm: Volume 6, 1685–94*, ed. John Raithby (sl., 1819), pp.236–8.

29. T. Poole, *A Treatise on Strong Beer, Ale, &c.* (Debrett, 1782), p.14.

30. Patrick Dillon, *Gin: The Much-lamented Death of Madam Geneva* (Justin, Charles, 2002), pp.115–16.

31. Bernard Mandeville, *The Fable of the Bees* (J. Wood, 1772 edition), p.14.

32. Quoted in Jonathan White, 'The "Slow but Sure Poyson": The Representation of Gin and Its Drinkers, 1736–1751', *Journal of British Studies*, Vol. 42, No. 1 (January 2003), p.41.

33. Charles Davenant quoted in Dillon, p.13.

34. Ernest L. Abel, 'The Gin Epidemic: Much Ado About What?', *Alcohol Alcohol* (2001), 36 (5).

35. Proceedings of the Old Bailey, February 1734, trial of Judith Defour (t17340227–32).

36. Ibid.

37. Henry Fielding, quoted in *Crime and Punishment in England: A Sourcebook* (UCL Press, 1999), p.140.

38. Stephen Hales, *A Friendly Admonition to the Drinkers of Gin, Brandy, and Other Distilled Spirits* (B. Dod, 1751), p.19.

39. John Brownlow, *Memoranda; Or, Chronicles of the Foundling Hospital* (S. Low, 1847), p.114.

40. Reginald Hugh Nichols, Francis Aslett Wray, *The History of the Foundling Hospital* (Oxford University Press, 1935), p.39.

41. Proceedings of the Old Bailey, 5 December 1711, trial of Thomas Abram (t17111205-31).

42. Proceedings of the Old Bailey, 30 August 1727, trial of Richard Montgomery (t17270830-29).

43. Robert Burton, *The Anatomy of Melancholy* (1621), p.56.

44. Ibid., pp.395-6.

45. James Boswell, *The Life of Samuel Johnson* (H. Baldwin for C. Dilly, 1791), p.339.

46. William G. Smith, 'On Opium, Embracing its History, Chemical Analysis and Use and Abuse as a Medicine' (NYSU, 1832), pp.10-11.

47. Dr John Jones, *The Mysteries of Opium Reveal'd* (Richard Smith, 1700), pp.7-8.

48. Ibid., pp.101, 106.

49. Ibid., p.371.

50. George Young, *A Treatise on Opium: Founded Upon Practical Observations* (A. Millar, 1753), p.vi.

51. Ibid., p.59.

52. Ibid., p.6.

53. John Awsiter, *An Essay on the Effects of Opium* (G. Kearsley, 1763), p.v.

54. Ibid., pp.3-5.

55. Ibid., p.62.

56. John Leigh, *An Experimental Inquiry Into the Properties of Opium* (Elliot, 1786), p.23.

57. Ibid., p.51.

58. Ibid., pp.124–5.
59. Samuel Crumpe, *An Inquiry into the Nature and Properties of Opium* (G. G. & J. Robinson, 1793), p.5.
60. Ibid., p.207.
61. James Harvey Young, *Old English Patent Medicines in America* (Smithsonian Institute, 1956), p.22.
62. J. Hector St John de Crèvecœur, *Letters from an American Farmer and Sketches of Eighteenth-Century America, 1782* (Penguin USA, 1986), p.160.
63. Anthony Benezet, *The Mighty Destroyer Displayed* (James Crukshank, 1774), p.17.
64. Benjamin Rush, *Inquiry into the Effects of Ardent Spirits on the Human Mind and Body* (Benjamin & Thomas Kite, 1784), p.8.
65. Ibid., frontispiece.
66. David W. Robson, '"My Unhappy Son": A Narrative Of Drinking In Federalist Pennsylvania', *Pennsylvania History: A Journal of Mid-Atlantic Studies*, Vol. 52, No. 1 (January 1985), pp.22–35.
67. Thomas Trotter, *An Essay, Medical, Philosophical and Chemical, on Drunkenness, and its Effects on the Human Body* (Longman & Rees, 1804), pp.12–13, 17, 44.
68. Thomas De Quincey, *Confessions of an English Opium-Eater* (George Newness, 1822), p.348.
69. *The Poetical Works of Samuel Taylor Coleridge* (D. Appleton, 1854), p.143.
70. Samuel Taylor Coleridge, *Complete Works*, Letter 493, http://inamidst.com/coleridge/letters/letter493.
71. Richard Buckley Littlefield, *Tom Wedgwood, the first photographer* (Duckworth, 1903), p.178.
72. Ibid., p.179.
73. Robert Southey quoted in Alethea Hayter, *Opium and the Romantic Imagination* (Faber & Faber, 1968), p.196.
74. De Quincey, p.431.
75. Thomas de Quincey, *Confessions of an English Opium-Eater* (Ticknor, Reed & Fields, 1851 edition), p.111.

76. Charles Rzepka, 'De Quincey and the Malay: Dove Cottage Idolatry', *The Wordsworth Circle*, Vol. 24, No. 3 (Summer 1993), pp.180–1.

77. De Quincey, p.192.

78. Ibid., p.68.

79. Robert Morrison, *The English Opium Eater: A Biography of an English Opium Eater* (Hachette, 2009), p.226.

80. Charles Richard Sanders, *The Victorian Rembrandt: Carlyle's Portraits of His Contemporaries* (Manchester University Press, 1957), p.5.

81. Derosne quoted in John E. Lesch, 'Conceptual Change in an Empirical Science: The Discovery of the First Alkaloids', *Historical Studies in the Physical Sciences*, Vol. 11, No. 2 (1981), p.312.

82. *Annalen der Physik*, 55 (1817), pp.56–9.

Chapter Five: The China Crisis

1. Hoh-Cheung and Lorna H. Mui, 'The Commutation Act and the Tea Trade in Britain, 1784–1793', *Economic History Review*, New Series, Vol. 16, No. 2 (1963), p.234.

2. Jonas Hanway, *An Essay on Tea, Considered as Pernicious to Health* (Woodfall & Henderson, 1756), p.298.

3. Samuel Johnson, *The Literary Magazine* 2, No. 13 (1757).

4. Jonas Hanway quoted in ibid.

5. Ibid.

6. Mary Waugh, *Smuggling in Devon and Cornwall, 1700–1850* (Countryside Books, 1991), p.14.

7. Ibid., p.24.

8. Hoh-Cheung and Mui, p.237.

9. Quoted in Tom Pocock, *Battle for Empire, The Very First World War, 1756–63* (Michael O'Mara Books, 1998), p.46.

10. Thomas Babington Macaulay, *Essays, Critical and Miscellaneous* (A. Hart, 1846), p.332.

11. Horace Walpole, *The Letters of Horace Walpole, Earl of Orford*, Vol. 4 (R. Bentley, 1840), p.55.

12. Quoted in Percival Spear, *Master of Bengal: Clive of India* (Thames & Hudson, 1974), p.189.

13. William Hoey, *A Monograph on Trade and Manufactures in Northern India* (Lucknow, 1880), p.142.

14. G. H. Smith, 'Abstract of a Paper on Opium-Smoking in China', *Medico-Chirurgical Review and Journal of Practical Medicine*, Vol. 36 (1842), p.584.

15. M. S. Commissariat, *Mandelslo's Travels in Western India 1638–9* (H. Milford, 1931), pp.43–4.

16. Wellesley quoted in Richard M. Eaton, *Expanding Frontiers in South Asian and World History* (Cambridge University Press, 2013), p.83.

17. Lo-shu Fu, *A Documentary Chronicle of Sino-Western relations, Volume 1* (Association for Asian Studies by the University of Arizona Press, 1966), p.380.

18. Colonel Thomas H. Perkins quoted in Jacques M. Downs, *The Golden Ghetto: The American Commercial Community at Canton and the Shaping of American China Policy 1784–1844* (Hong Kong University Press, 2014), p.123.

19. Richard J. Grace, *Opium and Empire: The Lives and Careers of William Jardine and James Matheson* (McGill Queen's University Press, 2014), p.11.

20. Ibid., p.125.

21. Matheson quoted in Dan Waters, 'Hong Kong Hongs With Long Histories and British Connections', *Journal of the Hong Kong Branch of the Royal Asiatic Society*, Vol. 30 (1990), p.223.

22. Charles-Edouard Bouée, *China's Management Revolution* (Palgrave Macmillan, 2011), p.192.

23. William C. Hunter, *The 'Fan Kwae' at Canton before Treaty Days, 1825–1844* (Kegan Paul, Trench, 1882), p.40.

24. Quoted in R. Alexander, *The Rise and Progress of British Opium Smuggling* (Judd and Glass, 1856), p.9.

25. Grace, p.133.

26. http://sourcebooks.fordham.edu/halsall/mod/1839lin2.asp.

27. *Sessional Papers of the House of Lords, Correspondence Relating to China*, No.148 (1840), p.385.

28. Michael Partridge, *Gladstone* (Routledge, 2003), p.43.

29. Alexander, p.10.

30. Quoted in ibid., p.6.

31. Queen Victoria quoted in John Cannon and Robert Crowcroft, *The Oxford Companion to British History* (Oxford University Press, 2015), p.924.

32. Robert Fortune quoted in John M. Carroll, *Edge of Empires: Chinese Elites and British Colonials in Chinese Hong Kong* (Harvard University Press, 2005), p.39.

33. Robert Fortune, *Three Years' Wanderings in the Northern Provinces of China* (John Murray, 1847), p.13.

34. https://www.jardines.com/en/group/history.html.

35. Dafydd Emrys Evans, 'Jardine, Matheson & Co.'s First Site In Hong Kong', *Journal of the Hong Kong Branch of the Royal Asiatic Society*, Vol. 8 (1968), p.149.

36. Ibid.

37. Fortune, p.13.

38. Robert Fortune, *Three Years' Wanderings in the Northern Provinces of China: Including a Visit to the Tea, Silk and Cotton Countries* (Cambridge University Press, 2012), p.24.

39. Fortune (1847), p.28.

40. John Mark Carroll, *A Concise History of Hong Kong* (Rowman & Littlefield, 2007), p.8.

41. Steve Tsang, *A Modern History of Hong Kong* (I. B. Tauris, 2003), p.59.

42. Ibid., p.61.

43. Pottinger, quoted in Evans, p.149.

44. Simon Morgan (ed.), *The Letters of Richard Cobden: Volume III: 1854–1859* (Oxford University Press, 2012), p.287.

45. Karl Marx quoted in Travis Hanes and Frank Sanello, 'The Opium Wars: The Addiction of One Empire and the Corruption of Another', *New York Daily Tribune*, 20 September 1858.

46. King James Bible, Mark 16:15.
47. Jon Miller and Gregory Stanczak, 'Redeeming, Ruling, and Reaping: British Missionary Societies, the East India Company, and the India-to-China Opium Trade', *Journal for the Scientific Study of Religion*, Vol. 48, No. 2 (June 2009), p.336.
48. Bridgman quoted in Michael C. Lazich, 'American Missionaries and the Opium Trade in Nineteenth-Century China', *Journal of World History*, Vol. 17, No. 2 (June 2006), p.205.
49. Parker quoted in Edward P. Crapol, *Tyler: The Accidental President* (University of North Carolina, 2013), p.131.
50. https://www.unodc.org/documents/wdr/WDR_2008/ WDR2008_100years_drug_control_origins.pdf.

Chapter Six: The American Disease

1. Samuel Ward, *America* (Boston, Massachusetts, July 1895).
2. John Duffy, *From Humors to Medical Science: A History of American Medicine* (University of Illinois Press, 1993), p.32.
3. Nathaniel Chapman, *Elements of Therapeutics or Materia Medica* (H. C. Carey and I. Lea, 1825), p.162.
4. Thaddeus Betts, 'To the Public', *Connecticut Journal*, 21 April 1878.
5. Elias P. Fordham, *Personal Narrative of Travels in Virginia, Mary land, Pennsylvania, Ohio, Indiana, Kentucky; and of a Residence in the Illinois Territory: 1817–1818*, ed. Frederic A. Ogg (The Arthur H. Clark Co., 1906), p.57.
6. Edwin Morris Betts, Hazlehurst Bolton Perkins and Peter J. Hatch, *Thomas Jefferson's Flower Garden at Monticello* (University Press of Virginia, 1986), p.72.
7. Winslow's standard advertisement, taken from 1895: http:// www.herbmuseum.ca/content/mrs-winslows-soothing-syrup.
8. J. Collins Warren and Thomas Dwight (eds.), *Boston Medical and Surgical Journal*, Vol. 83 (Cupples, Upham, 1873), p.432.

9.   *Ayer's American Almanac* (Ayer, 1857), no page numbers.

10. James Grant Wilson & John Fiske (eds.), *Appleton's Cyclopaedia of American Biography* (D. Appleton, 1900), p.122.

11. Jonathan Lewy, 'The Army Disease: Drug Addiction and the Civil War', *War In History*, Vol. 21, No. 1 (January 2014), p.104.

12. John Price, 'Dominique Anel And The Small Lachrymal Syringe', http://europepmc.org/backend/ptpmcrender.fcgi?accid=PMC1033979&blobtype=pdf.

13. *Edinburgh Medical and Surgical Journal*, No. 82 (1855).

14. Robert Bartholow, *Manual of Hypodermic Medication* (Lippincott, 1869), p.25.

15. J. H. Bill, 'A New Hypodermic Syringe', *Medical Record 5* (1870), pp.45–6.

16. Charles Warrington Earle, 'The Opium Habit', *Chicago Medical Review* 29 (1880), p.493.

17. Felix von Niemeyer, *A Text-book of practical medicine*, Vol. 2 (H. K. Lewis, 1869), p.291.

18. H. Gibbons, 'Letheomania: the result of the hypodermic injection of morphia', *Pacific Medical and Surgical Journal* 12 (1870), p.481.

19. Niemeyer, p.291.

20. Bartholow, p.6.

21. H. H. Kane, *The Hypodermic Injection of Morphia* (C. L. Bermingham, 1880), p.5.

22. Louisa May Alcott, *Hospital Sketches, and Camp Fireside Stories* (Roberts Brothers, 1871 edn.), p.50.

23. Ibid., p.37.

24. James M. MacPherson, *Battle Cry of Freedom* (Penguin USA, 1990), p.485.

25. Walt Whitman, *Prose Works*, 1:32 (David McKay, 1892), p.26.

26. W. W. Keen quoted in Michael C. C. Adams, *Living Hell: Dark Side of the Civil War* (Johns Hopkins University Press, 2014), p.90.

27. H. H. Cunningham, *Doctors in Gray* (LSU Press, 1993).

28. Lewy, p.104.

29. Dan Waldorf, Martin Orlick and Craig Reinerman, *Morphine Maintenance: The Shreveport Clinic, 1919–1923* (Drug Abuse Council, 1974), p.63.

30. https://www.ncbi.nlm.nih.gov/pmc/articles/PMC1286579/pdf/amjphealth00104-0034.pdf.

31. Thomas Crothers, *Morphinism and Narcomanias* (W. B. Saunders, 1902), p.76.

32. Joseph Spillane, *Cocaine: From Medical Marvel to Modern Menace in the United States, 1884–1920* (Johns Hopkins University Press, 2000), p.75.

33. Horace B. Day, *The Opium Habit* (Harper and Brothers, 1868), p.7.

34. Holmes, quoted in Cunningham.

35. Rodman Paul, 'The Origin of the Chinese Issue in California', *Mississippi Valley Historical Review*, 25:2 (September 1938), p.182.

36. B. E. Lloyd, *The Lights and Shades of San Francisco* (A. L. Bancroft, 1870), p.245.

37. Mark Twain, *Roughing It* (Harper, 1904), p.133.

38. Lloyd, p.236.

39. Ronald Takaki, *Strangers From A Different Shore* (Little, Brown, 1998), p.84.

40. Lloyd, p.234.

41. Henry Grimm, *'The Chinese Must Go': A Farce in Four Acts* (Bancroft, 1879), p.3.

42. Andrew Urban, 'Legends of Deadwood', *Journal of American History*, Vol. 94, No. 1 (June 2007), p.224.

43. Rose Estep Fosha and Christopher Leatherman, 'The Chinese Experience in Deadwood', *Historical Archaeology*, Vol. 42, No. 3, The Archaeology of Chinese Immigrant and Chinese American Communities (2008), p.97.

44. Ibid., p.100.

45. Watson Parker, *Deadwood: The Golden Years* (Bison Books, 1981), p.145.

46. *Black Hills Residence and Business Directory*, May 1898 (Enterprise Printing Co., 1898), p.51.

47. Parker, p.145.
48. Fosha and Leatherman, p.102.
49. Jeremy Agnew, *Alcohol and Opium in the Old West* (McFarland, 2013), p.160.
50. Parker, p.146.
51. Virginia Berridge and Griffith Edwards, *Opium and the People: Opiate Use in Nineteenth Century England* (Allen Lane, 1982), p.455.
52. Alonzo Calkins, *Opium and the Opium Appetite* (Lippincott, 1871), p.163.
53. Quoted in D. T. Courtwright, 'The Female Opiate Addict in Nineteenth-Century America', *Essays in Arts and Sciences*, Vol. 10, No. 2. (1982), p.164.
54. George Miller Beard quoted in Stephen R. Kandall, *Substance and Shadow: Women and Addiction in the United States* (Harvard University Press, 1999), p.29.
55. Quoted in ibid., p.37.
56. Barry Milligan, 'Morphine-Addicted Doctors, the English Opium Eater, and Embattled Medical Authority', *Victorian Literature and Culture*, Vol. 33, No. 2 (2005), p.545.
57. Ibid., p.541.

Chapter Seven: A New Addiction, Prohibition and the Rise of the Gangster

1. M. J. D. Roberts, *Making English Morals: Voluntary Association and Moral Reform in England, 1787–1886* (Cambridge University Press, 2004), p.165.
2. John Stuart Mill, *On Liberty* (Walter Scott Publishing, 1878), p.167.
3. Letter to the Editor, *Boston Medical Surgery Journal* (October 2, 1833), pp.117–20, 435.
4. Virginia Berridge and Griffith Edwards, *Opium and the People: Opiate Use in Nineteenth Century England* (Allen Lane, 1982), p.193.

5. Society for the Study and Cure of Inebriety, *Inaugural Address, April 25th 1884*, Norman Kerr MD (H. K. Lewis, 1884), p.4.

6. Ibid.

7. 'Dalrymple Home for Inebriates', *British Journal of Psychiatry*, 29 (128) (January 1884), pp.615–16.

8. N. Kerr, 'How to deal with inebriates', *Report of the III International Congresses against the Abuse of Spiritual Beverages in Christiania* (Mallinske Boktrykkeri, 3–5 September 1890).

9. Kerr quoted in Jack S. Blocker, David M. Fahey and Ian R. Tyrrell (eds.), *Alcohol and Temperance in Modern History* (ABC CLIO, 2003), p.190.

10. http://bayer.com.

11. https://www.bayer.com/en/history.aspx.

12. H. Dreser and T. Floret, 'Pharmakoligisches ueber einige morphin-derivative', *Therapeutische Monatschefte*, 12 (1898), pp.509–12, and H. Dreser, 'Ueber die wirkung einiger Derivate des Morphins auf die Athmung', *Archiv fur Physiologie*, 72 (1898), pp.485–521.

13. Tom Carnwath and Ian Smith, *Heroin Century* (Routledge, 2002), p.34.

14. José Cantón Navarro, *History of Cuba* (Union Nacional de Juristas, 2000), p.71.

15. Alma N. Bamero, 'Opium: The Evolution of Policies, the Tolerance of the Vice, and the Proliferation of Contraband Trade in the Philippines, 1843–1908', *Social Science Diliman* (January–December 2006), 3:1–2, p.58.

16. Ibid., p.59.

17. Ibid., p.62.

18. Glenn A. May, 'Why the United States Won the Philippine-American War, 1899–1902', *Pacific Historical Review*, Vol. 52, No. 4 (November 1983), p.356.

19. http://www.msc.edu.ph/centennial/benevolent.html.

20. Bamero, p.68.

21. Hamilton Wright, 'Uncle Sam is the Worst Dope Fiend in the World', *New York Times*, 12 March 1911.

22. Hamilton Wright, 'The Opium Commission', *American Journal of International Law*, Vol. 3, No. 3 (July 1909), pp.648–73.

23. Ibid.

24. Caroline Jean Acker, *Creating the American Junkie: Addiction Research in the Classic Age of Narcotic Control* (Johns Hopkins University Press, 2002), p.13.

25. Quoted in Carnwath and Smith, p.18.

26. International Opium Convention, The Hague, 1912, *The American Journal of International Law*, Vol. 6, No. 3, Supplement: Official Documents (Jul., 1912), pp.177–92.

27. Howard Abadinsky, *Organized Crime* (Wadsworth Publishing, 2009), p.2.

28. Luis Astorga, *Drug Trafficking in Mexico: A First Assessment* (UNESCO, 1999), p.11.

29. John J. Bailey, *Organized Crime and Democratic Governability: Mexico and the U.S.–Mexican Borderlands* (University of Pittsburgh Press, 2000), p.69.

30. Ryan Gingeras, *Heroin, Organized Crime and the Makings of Modern Turkey* (Oxford University Press, 2014), p.33.

31. Ibid., p.73.

32. *LIFE*, 19 July 1943, p.86.

33. Ibid.

34. Brian G. Martin, 'The Green Gang and the Guomindang State: Du Yuesheng and the Politics of Shanghai', *Journal of Asian Studies*, Vol. 54, No. 1 (February 1995), p.67.

35. Alfred W. McCoy, *The Politics of Heroin* (Lawrence Hill Books, 2003), p.49.

36. Oriana Bandiera, 'Land Reform, the Market for Protection, and the Origins of the Sicilian Mafia: Theory and Evidence', *Journal of Law, Economics, & Organization*, Vol. 19, No. 1 (April 2003), p.227.

37. Arcangelo Dimico, 'Origins of the Sicilian Mafia: The Market

for Lemons', paper delivered at Gothenburg University, 23 June 2014 (University of Gothenberg, appendix, table 3).

38. McCoy, p.29.
39. Ibid.
40. Carnwath and Smith, p.60.

Chapter Eight: From the Somme to Saigon

1. Merritt Crawford quoted in Ellen Hampton, 'How World War I Revolutionized Medicine', *The Atlantic*, 24 February 2017.
2. Lea Doughty and Susan Heydon, 'Medicine Supply During the First World War: Overcoming Shortages in New Zealand', *Health and History*, Vol. 17, No. 2, Special Issue: World War I (2015), p.37.
3. Henry Cushing, *From a Surgeon's Journal* (Little, Brown, 1936), p.16.
4. Ibid., p.33.
5. Doughty and Heydon, p.42.
6. Cushing, pp.45–6.
7. 'Rise in Opium', *The Register*, 27 April 1915, p.4.
8. H. D. Dakin, 'Biochemistry and War Problems', *British Medical Journal* (23 June 1917), p.833.
9. Richard van Emden, *The Soldier's War* (Bloomsbury, 2008), p.260.
10. *Tar Heel Junior Historian*, NC Museum of History, Spring 1993: https://www.ncpedia.org/wwi-medicine-battlefield.
11. Ikramul Haq, 'Pak-Afghan Drug Trade in Historical Perspective', *Asian Survey*, Vol. 36, No. 10 (University of California Press, 1996), p.954.
12. Cushing, p.281.
13. Jeffrey C. Larrabee, 'A Tale Of Two Trucks: American Casualty Evacuation In World War I', *Icon*, Vol. 14 (2008), p.130.
14. Axel Helmstädter and Svem Siebenand, 'Drug shortages in World War I: How German Pharmacy Survived the Years of Crisis', *Pharmaceutical Historian* 45 (2015), p.18.

15. Cushing, p.501.

16. Emden, p.205.

17. Bernard L. Rice, *Indiana Magazine of History*, Vol. 93, No. 4 (December 1997), p.316.

18. Ibid., p.318.

19. http://history.amedd.army.mil/booksdocs/wwii/medicalsupply/chapter2.htm.

20. League of Nations, *Analysis of the International Trade in Morphine, Diacetylmorphine and Cocaine, for the years 1925–1930* (League of Nations Publications, 1930), p.29.

21. Quoted in Nicolas Rasmussen, 'Medical Science and the Military: The Allies' Use of Amphetamine during World War II', *Journal of Interdisciplinary History*, Vol. 42, No. 2 (Autumn 2011), p.207.

22. John Nicholl, Tony Rennell, *Medic: Saving Lives* (Penguin, 2010), p.120.

23. S. Suter, *Health Psychophysiology* (Taylor & Francis, 1986), p.97.

24. Emma Newlands, *Civilians Into Soldiers: War, the Body and British Army Recruits, 1939–45* (Oxford University Press, 2014), p.160.

25. A. A. Berle Jr on behalf of the US Secretary of State, quoted in George W. Grayson, *Mexico: Narco-Violence or Failed State* (Transaction, 2010), p.54.

26. Interview with Edward Heath of the DEA, *PBS Frontline*, 2000.

27. Quoted in George W. Grayson, p.24.

28. Bernard L. Rice, 'Recollections of a World War II Combat Medic', *Indiana Magazine of History*, Volume 3, Issue 4, 1997, p.343.

29. Patricia Posner, *The Pharmacist of Auschwitz* (Crux, 2017), Chapter 8 of preview edition.

30. Telford Taylor statement transcribed from United States Holocaust Museum recording.

31. Rice, pp.334–5.

32. Otto F. Apel MD and Pat Apel, *MASH: An Army Surgeon in Korea* (University Press of Kentucky, 1998), p.1.

33. John. M. Jennings, 'The Forgotten Plague: Opium and Narcotic in Korea Under Japanese Rule, 1910–1945', *Modern Asian Studies*, Vol. 29, No. 4 (October 1995), p.795.

34. Ibid., p.799.

35. Pierre Arnaud Chouvy, *Opium: Uncovering the Politics of the Poppy* (I. B. Tauris, 2009), p.69.

36. Major Booker King, MD, FACS and Colonel Ismail Jatoi, MD, PhD, FACS, 'The Mobile Army Surgical Hospital (MASH): A Military and Surgical Legacy', *Journal of the National Medical Association* (May 2005), p.649.

37. Ibid., p.652.

38. Albert E. Cowdrey, *The Medic's War* (Center of Military History, United States Army, 1987), p.275.

39. Ibid., p.250.

40. Paul M. Edwards, *The Korean War* (Greenwood Publishing Group, 2006), pp.106–7.

41. Richard Nixon, War on Drugs speech, 18 June 1971.

42. King and Jatoi, p.653.

43. https://www.marxists.org/history/usa/workers/black-panthers/1970/dope.htm.

44. Mark Jacobson, *American Gangster: And Other Tales of New York* (Atlantic, 2007), p.18.

45. Philip Caputo, *A Rumour of a War* (Pimlico, 1999), p.4.

Chapter Nine: Afghanistan

1. Lillias Hamilton, *A Vizier's Daughter* (John Murray, 1900), p.5.

2. Louis Dupree, *Afghanistan* (Princeton University Press, 1973), p.14.

3. Corruption Perceptions Index, 2016: https://www.transparency.org.

4. Quoted in Dupree, p.419.

5. Hamilton, p.6.

6. Ibid., p.3.

7. Emadi Hafizullah, *Customs and Culture of Afghanistan* (Greenwood Publishing, 2005), p.35.

8. Eric Newby, *A Short Walk in the Hindu Kush* (Pan Macmillan, 2008 edn.), p.72.

9. Sixth Emergency Special Session, Provisional Verbatim Record of the Third Meeting, Document, General Assembly, United Nations, 11 January 1980.

10. Footage of Ronald Reagan dedicating the *Columbia* featured in documentary *Bitter Lake* (BBC, 2015).

11. The *Shahada*, or testimony of belief, quoted in Frederick Mathewson Denny, *An Introduction to Islam* (Routledge, 2015), p.409.

12. Pierre Arnaud Chouvy, *Opium: Uncovering the Politics of the Poppy* (I.B. Tauris, 2009), p.48.

13. Ahmed Rashid, *Taliban: Militant Islam, Oil and Fundamentalism in Central Asia* (Yale University Press), p.117.

14. Nora Boustany, 'Busy are the peacemakers', *Washington Post*, 10 January 1998.

15. Abdul Rashid as interviewed by Ahmed Rashid, quoted in Ahmed Rashid, *Taliban: Militant Islam, Oil and Fundamentalism in Central Asia* (Yale University Press), p.118.

16. http://www.unodc.org/pdf/research/AFG07_ExSum_web.pdf.

17. Mark Galeotti, *Narcotics and Nationalism: Russian Drug Policies and Futures* (New York University Center for Global Affairs, 2016), p.2.

18. Martin Jelsma, *Learning Lessons from the Taliban Opium Ban* (Transnational Institute, 2005), https://www.tni.org/en/archives/act/1594.

19. *The Afghanistan Cannabis Survey*, UNODC, 2009, p.7.

20. *Afghan Opium Poppy Survey 2007 Executive Summary* (UNODC, 2007), p.1.

21. Ministry of Counter-Narcotics, Islamic Republic of Afghanistan, *Food Zone Report*, http://mcn.gov.af/en/page/5138/5141.

22. *Afghan Opium Poppy Survey 2007 Executive Summary* (UNODC, 2014), p.6.

23. Ibid., p.4.

24. David Vassallo, 'A short history of Camp Bastion Hospital: the two hospitals and unit deployments', *British Medical Journal*, 28 February 2015, p.355.

25. G. S. Arul, et al., 'Paediatric admissions to the British military hospital at Camp Bastion, Afghanistan', *Annals of the Royal College of Surgeons* (January 2012), pp.52–7.

26. Gregor Aisch, 'How Isis Works', *New York Times*, 24 September 2014.

27. Alexandra Fisher, 'Africa's Heroin Highway to the West', *Daily Beast*, 11 May 2016.

28. Hiba Khan, 'Isis and al-Qaeda', *Independent on Sunday*, 16 April 2017.

Chapter Ten: Heroin Chic, HIV and Generation Oxy

1. Jean Cocteau, *Diary of an Addict* (Longman, Green, 1932), p.11.

2. Thomas De Quincey, *Confessions of an English Opium-Eater* (George Newness, 1822), p.81.

3. Cocteau quoted in John Baxter, *The Golden Moments of Paris* (Museyon, 2014), p.135.

4. Tom Carnwath and Ian Smith, *Heroin Century* (Routledge, 2002), p.19.

5. Alan A. Block, 'European Drug Traffic and Traffickers between the Wars: The Policy of Suppression and Its Consequences', *Journal of Social History*, Vol. 23, No. 2 (Winter 1989), pp.319–20.

6. Ibid., p.317.

7. Patrick H. Hughes, Noel W. Barker, Gail A. Crawford and Jerome H. Jaffe, 'The Natural History of a Heroin Epidemic', https://www.ncbi.nlm.nih.gov/pmc/articles/PMC1530426/pdf/amjph00729-0095.pdf.

8. William S. Burroughs, *Junky* (Penguin, 2003), p.128.

9. Barry Miles, *Call Me Burroughs: A Life* (Twelve, 2015), p.55.

10. William S. Burroughs, *Naked Lunch: The Restored Text* (Penguin, 2015), p.17.

11. Pille Taba, Andrew Lees and Gerald Stern, 'Erich Harnack (1852–1915), and a Short History of Apomorphine', *European Neurology*, 2013 (69), p.323.

12. Lees quoted by Robert McCrum, *Observer*, 14 October 2014.

13. William S. Burroughs, *Rub Out the Words: The Letters of William S. Burroughs 1959–1974* (to the editor of the *New Statesman*, 4 March 1966) (Penguin, 2012), p.168.

14. Bowie quoted by Frank Mastropolo, *Ultimate Classic Rock*, 11 January 2016.

15. Craig Copetas, *Rolling Stone*, 28 February 1974.

16. Carnwath and Smith, p.55.

17. Paul Gerwitz, 'Methadone Maintenance for Heroin Addicts', *Yale Law School Legal Repository*, 1 January 1969, p.1175.

18. Michael Agar, 'Going Through the Changes: Methadone in New York City', *Human Organization*, Vol. 36, No. 3 (Fall 1977), p.291.

19. Gerwitz, p.1179.

20. Cary Bennett, 'Methadone Maintenance Treatment: Disciplining the "Addict"', *Health and History*, Vol. 13, No. 2, Special Feature: Health and Disability (2011), p.131.

21. Burroughs, *Naked Lunch*, p.18.

22. Agar, p.291.

23. Gerwitz, p.1195.

24. Ibid., p.1200.

25. http://www.timeisonourside.com/chron1971.html.

26. Rebecca Jones, *Today*, BBC Radio 4, 23 May 2011.

27. http://www.sciencemag.org/careers/2013/09/complex-social-process.

28. http://www.nytimes.com/2013/09/20/science/candace-pert-67-explorer-of-the-brain-dies.html.

29. Randy Shilts, *And the Band Played On* (St Martin's Press, 1987), p.xxi.

30. Ronald Reagan, *Public Papers of the Presidents of the United States: Ronald Reagan, 1986* (Office of the Federal Register, 1986), p.1182.

31. William W. Darrow. 'Randy M. Shilts 1952–1994', *Journal of Sex Research*, Vol. 31, No. 3 (1994), p.249.

32. Ronald O. Valdiserri, T. Stephen Jones, Gary R. West, Carl H. Campbell, Jr. and P. Imani Thompson, 'Where Injecting Drug Users Receive HIV Counseling and Testing', *Public Health Reports* (1974–), Vol. 108, No. 3 (May–June 1993), p.295.

33. Shilts, p.xxiii.

34. *The Age*, 27 October 1992, p.127.

35. Sonny Shiu Hing Lo, *The Politics of Cross-border Crime in Greater China: Case Studies of Mainland China, Hong Kong and Macao* (Routledge, 2009), p.187.

36. Fenton Bresler, *The Trail of the Triads: An Investigation into International Crime* (Weidenfeld & Nicolson, 1980), p.1.

37. Ibid., p.2.

38. Steven Tsang, *A Modern History of Hong Kong* (I.B. Tauris, 2004) p.276.

39. Greg Girard, *City of Darkness: Life In Kowloon's Walled City* (Watermark, 1993).

40. Carol Jones and Jon Vagg, *Criminal Justice in Hong Kong* (Routledge, 2007), p.357.

41. European Monitoring Centre for Drugs and Drug Addiction, *Drug Policy Profile: Poland* (2014), p.5.

42. https://www.ncjrs.gov/pdffiles1/Digitization/141189NCJRS.pdf.

43. Philip Matthews, 'Chronicle of Malaysia, 11 January 1977', in *Chronicle of Malaysia: Fifty Years of Headline News, 1963–2013* (Editions Didier Millet, 2013), p.128.

44. James Morton, *The Mammoth Book of Gangs* (Constable & Robinson, 2012), p.187.

45. http://hmt-sanctions.s3.amazonaws.com/sanctionsconlist.pdf, p.181.

46. U.S. Vulnerabilities to Money Laundering, Drugs, and Terrorist Financing: HSBC Case History, 17 July 2012, hearing transcript:

https://www.hsgac.senate.gov/download/report-us-vulnerabilities-to-money-laundering-drugs-and-terrorist-financing-hsbc-case-history.

47. Daniel Foggo, *Telegraph*, 27 April 2003: http://www.telegraph.co.uk/news/uknews/1428462/Rachel-did-not-die-from-a-heroin-overdose.html.

48. Jason Bennetto, *Independent*, 12 November 2003: http://www.independent.co.uk/news/uk/this-britain/what-did-happen-to-rachel-77919.html.

49. Foggo: http://www.telegraph.co.uk/news/uknews/1428462/Rachel-did-not-die-from-a-heroin-overdose.html.

50. Kevin M. De Cock, *Reflections on 30 Years of AIDS*: https://www.ncbi.nlm.nih.gov/pmc/articles/PMC3358222/.

51. Max Daly, *Vice*, 18 January 2017, 'This Is What Happened to the "Trainspotting" Generation of Heroin Users'.

52. http://dequinceyjynxie.blogspot.fr/2015/07/mad-dog-new-brunswick-nj.html.

53. Ross Coomber, *Perceptions of Illicit Drugs and Drug Users: Myth-Understandings and Policy Consequences*, PhD thesis, 1999, University of Greenwich, p.27.

54. Ann Higgins, 'Cut The Shit', *VICE*, 1 December 2005.

55. *United States* v. *Ross William Ulbricht* (United States Court of Appeals, Second Circuit, Southern District of New York, 27 September 2014).

56. Cat Marnell, *New York Times*, 27 January 2017: https://www.nytimes.com/2017/01/27/style/cat-marnell-addiction-memoir-how-to-murder-your-life.html.

57. https://www.cdc.gov/mmwr/volumes/65/ss/ss6506a1.htm.

58. https://www.cdc.gov/drugoverdose/data/prescribing.html.

59. Casey Leins, 'New Hampshire: Ground Zero for Opioids', *US States and World Report*, 28 June 2017.

60. Centers for Disease Control and Prevention, U.S. Prescribing Rate Maps: https://www.cdc.gov/drugoverdose/maps/rxrate-maps.html.

61. Centers for Disease Control and Prevention, U.S. County

Prescribing Rates, 2012: https://www.cdc.gov/drugoverdose/
maps/rxcounty2012.html.

62. Amy Yukanin, 'Poor, Rural and Addicted', www.al.com, 24
    August 2017.

63. Centers for Disease Control and Prevention, U.S. Prescribing
    Rate Maps: https://www.cdc.gov/drugoverdose/maps/rxrate-
    maps.html, and Centers for Disease Control and Prevention,
    Drug Overdose Death Data: https://www.cdc.gov/
    drugoverdose/data/statedeaths.html

64. Michael Nerheim quoted by James Fuller, 'Suburban Counties
    Sue Drug Makers Over Overdose Deaths', *Daily Herald*, 21
    December 2017.

65. David Crow, 'US Seeks Fix For Its Opioid Addiction',
    Financial Times, 11 September 2017.

66. Atul Gawande, *Annals of Surgery*, Vol. 265, Issue 4 (April 2017),
    p.693.

INDEX